A Clinical Guide to Surface Palpation

THE ART AND SCIENCE OF THE PERFECT TOUCH

SECOND EDITION

Michael Masaracchio, PT, DPT, PhD, OCS, FAAOMPT
Long Island University

Chana Frommer, PT, DPT, OCS, SCS, RISPT, CCI
Long Island University

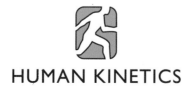

HUMAN KINETICS

Library of Congress Cataloging-in-Publication Data

Names: Masaracchio, Michael, 1976- author. | Frommer, Chana, author.
Title: A clinical guide to surface palpation : the art and science of the
  perfect touch / Michael Masaracchio, Chana Frommer.
Other titles: Clinical guide to musculoskeletal palpation
Description: Second edition. | Champaign, IL : Human Kinetics, [2022] |
  Preceded by Clinical guide to musculoskeletal palpation / Michael
  Masaracchio, Chana Frommer. [2014] | Includes bibliographical references
  and index.
Identifiers: LCCN 2021006350 (print) | LCCN 2021006351 (ebook) | ISBN
  9781492596684 (paperback) | ISBN 9781492596691 (epub) | ISBN
  9781492596707 (pdf)
Subjects: MESH: Palpation--methods | Musculoskeletal Pain--etiology |
  Musculoskeletal System--anatomy & histology | Musculoskeletal
  System--injuries | Touch | Case Reports
Classification: LCC QM100 (print) | LCC QM100 (ebook) | NLM WB 275 | DDC
  612.7--dc23
LC record available at https://lccn.loc.gov/2021006350
LC ebook record available at https://lccn.loc.gov/2021006351

ISBN: 978-1-4925-9668-4 (print)

Acquisitions Editor: Jolynn Gower; **Developmental and Managing Editor:** Amanda S. Ewing; **Copyeditor:** Annette Pierce; **Proofreader:** Pamela S. Johnson; **Indexer:** Andrea J. Hepner; **Permissions Manager:** Dalene Reeder; **Graphic Designer:** Julie L. Denzer; **Cover Designer:** Keri Evans; **Cover Design Specialist:** Susan Rothermel Allen; **Photograph (cover):** © Human Kinetics; **Photographs (interior):** © Human Kinetics; photos on pages 55 and 107 courtesy of Chana Frommer; **Photo Production Specialist:** Amy M. Rose; **Photo Production Manager:** Jason Allen; **Senior Art Manager:** Kelly Hendren; **Illustrations:** © Human Kinetics; **Printer:** Versa Press

We thank Long Island University in Brooklyn, New York, for assistance in providing the location for the photo and video shoot for this book.

Printed in the United States of America   10 9 8 7 6 5 4 3 2 1

The paper in this book is certified under a sustainable forestry program.

Human Kinetics
1607 N. Market Street
Champaign, IL 61820
USA

United States and International
Website: **US.HumanKinetics.com**
Email: info@hkusa.com
Phone: 1-800-747-4457

Canada
Website: **Canada.HumanKinetics.com**
Email: info@hkcanada.com

E8020

Tell us what you think!
Human Kinetics would love to hear what we can do to improve the customer experience. Use this QR code to take our brief survey.

This book is dedicated to my wife, Saveria, and son, Matteo, for the countless hours they sacrifice while I am working; to my parents, Agnes and Dennis; and to my sister, Jennifer. Saveria, I love you more than anything in this world and am so lucky to have you in my life. Matteo, you brighten my day, buddy, and keep me grounded to focus on what is really important in life. Mom and Dad, this project would not have been possible without the guidance and support you have given me throughout the years. Jen, I could not wish for a better sister; you accept me for who I am no matter what. I love you.

—MFM

I dedicate this book to my parents, Myron and Eileen, and my family and friends. Ma and Ta, thank you for your lifelong lessons and continued love, support, and encouragement, without which I could not have gotten to where I am today. To my siblings, members of my extended family, and my friends, thank you for your love, support, encouragement, and continued interest in this project and all of my work. Knowing that you are all there for me means so much more than I can say. I love you all.

And last, but definitely not least, I would like to thank Mike. Mike has been so much fun to work with; we always have a great time, no matter the project. But this time there was so much going on, both in the world and for me personally. He tried to make things easier for me as much as he could, no matter how much he had on his plate. And when he couldn't, he was, as always, patient and understanding. I couldn't ask for a better friend or partner in crime.

—CBF

We dedicate this book to the thousands of students who have helped inspire it. Their hard work, dedication, and thought-provoking questions helped solidify and transform an idea into a reality. This second edition is a true testament to their feedback. We want to wish all past, present, and future health care professionals well in their chosen careers and take a second to thank them for making a difference in their patients' lives.

Contents

Preface

Mastering palpation requires a unique blend of extensive knowledge of the underlying science and a flair for the art of its application. The psychomotor skills required are dependent on a strong knowledge of anatomy—the location and architecture of the different types of structures. The artistic component is equally important but perhaps more difficult to acquire. This component is imperative for gaining the trust of, and good rapport with, your patient. It is more dependent on an inherent "feel" than on knowledge of anatomy, in addition to experience and practice. Achieving this blend is quite a challenge and something that educators strive hard to pass along.

The purpose of this book is to assist students and health care professionals in becoming experts in surface palpation techniques. Our goal was to refine and further develop a second edition that is more comprehensive and user friendly to enhance the skills of those health care professionals who are in any of the disciplines that require palpation. This includes, but is not limited to, physical therapists, physical therapist assistants, physicians (orthopedists), physician assistants, athletic trainers, occupational therapists, chiropractors, massage therapists, and students of those fields. Throughout the book we use the term *clinician* to include all health care practitioners, and we use *patient* to cover all those on whom palpation is being performed. We are aware that these terms may not be an exact fit for everyone using this book, but we made this choice for the sake of consistency.

We wrote this book to serve as a guide to palpation skills only. While a brief review of relevant anatomy is included in the chapters on palpation skills, a thorough review of the anatomy and kinesiology concepts is a prerequisite for using this guide. We suggest that you refer back to relevant anatomy and kinesiology texts if necessary.

While a number of quality palpation texts are available on the market, we felt that as both clinical physical therapists and educators, we are in a unique position to write a guide that is user friendly and more clinically oriented. Organizationally, the book divides the human body into regions instead of joints. This serves to improve flow and simplify content throughout. Relevant bony and soft tissue structures are covered conjointly instead of independently, which will help to improve your comprehension of anatomical relationships and then carry over to improved clinical examination and treatment skills. Anatomical artwork on bony anatomy and soft tissue structures will provide you with the ability to visualize the anatomical relationships of the regional structures as you are palpating them.

Each palpation technique is presented in the form of simple bulleted step-by-step instructions. A photo accompanies the discussion of each palpation technique, allowing you to see each skill being performed in combination with the step-by-step written instructions. Please note that there are instances in which minor adjustments were made when taking the photograph in an effort to optimize the visualization of the palpation. This overall approach fosters a strong anatomical foundation, which will enhance the clarity and application of your anatomical knowledge to optimize the development of your palpation skills.

For the skills covered, we identify the optimal position or positions based on our clinical experience. Please note that other positions may be appropriate, and we encourage you to use your clinical judgment as necessary. In addition, during the clinical examination, you should consider the number of position changes required of the patient. At all times, be considerate of the comfort and modesty of your patients (draping, gowns, bolsters, and so on).

Within the chapters are notes and a feature we refer to as *Clinical Pearls*. *Notes* are brief descriptions or pointers that accompany the instructions on the specific structure being discussed. *Clinical Pearls* contain important clinically relevant information that is necessary to process and understand based on the information received from structure identification and assessment. These may or may not be supported by research—many are based on our experience as clinicians. While as a whole, the field of health care continues to move forward with evidence-based practice, we strongly believe that a substantial amount of art and finesse is required as well. We feel that this is particularly important in palpation as well as for all manual skills. We have tried to impart some of that art to you by drawing from our clinical experience and encourage you to fine-tune your skills as you gain your own experience.

At the end of each chapter is a case study describing a common regional clinical condition. This requires you to apply your newfound knowledge and skills, in combination with your previous knowledge, to perform a thorough examination and use your clinical reasoning skills to arrive at the correct diagnoses.

Updates to the Second Edition

Several updates have been made to this new edition:

- Dense anatomy text has been reworked into a bulleted format to help enhance reader comprehension.
- A new chapter on the abdomen and pelvis has been added. The visceral structures can have a profound effect on the function of the neuromusculoskeletal system. Thus, a foundational understanding

of the structure and function and accurate identification of these structures are important in aiding in the diagnosis and management of these patients.

- Anatomical overlays have been added to the palpation photos. These overlays give readers a view of the underlying anatomical detail, which helps to orient readers and aid in identification of various structures throughout the body.

- In all of the palpation chapters, soft tissues are broken into zones. This provides a regional approach to palpating structures within a body region, which helps the reader understand the relationship between structures and how they function together. In chapters 6 and 12, a key reference structure has been identified in each zone to further guide the reader in understanding structural relationships.

Online Video in HK*Propel*

New to this edition is more than 50 video clips. Watching palpation skills being done in a step-by-step format helps readers understand the nuances of difficult techniques. This is particularly attractive to those who are visual learners. Palpation techniques of these structures are supported by video:

Chapter 2
- Suprahyoids
- Infrahyoids

Chapter 3
- Superior angle of the scapula
- Acromion process
- Humerus: Greater tubercle, intertubercular groove, and lesser tubercle
- Levator scapulae
- Supraspinatus tendon
- Infraspinatus and teres minor
- Subscapularis muscle belly
- Teres major

Chapter 4
- Rib 1: Posterior approach
- Rib 2: Axilla (lateral) approach
- Pectoralis minor
- Intercostal spaces

Chapter 5
- Radial head
- Radial tuberosity

Chapter 11

- Adductor tubercle
- Pes anserine tendons
- Medial collateral ligament
- Medial meniscus
- Lateral meniscus

Chapter 12

- Talar heads
- Navicular
- Cuboid
- Lateral collateral ligament
- Fibularis longus and brevis

Throughout the text, you'll see notes like this alerting you to an online video clip: **VIDEO 4.1** ◉

To access the online video, see the card at the front of the print book for your unique HK*Propel* access code. For ebook users, reference the HK*Propel* access code instructions on the page immediately following the book cover.

Instructor Resources in HK*Propel*

Also new to this edition is a variety of resources that are available online within the instructor pack in HK*Propel*:

- *Presentation package*—The presentation package includes more than 600 slides that cover the key points from the text, including the figures, palpation technique photos, and video clips. Instructors can easily add new slides to the presentation package to suit their needs.
- *Image bank*—The image bank includes all of the figures and tables from the book, organized by chapter. These items can be added to the presentation package, student handouts, and so on.
- *Test package*—The test package includes more than 150 multiple-choice questions. These questions are available in multiple formats for a variety of instructor uses and can be used to create tests and quizzes to measure student understanding.
- Answers to the end-of-chapter review questions and answers to the case study questions are provided.

Instructor ancillaries are free to adopting instructors, including an ebook version of the text that allows instructors to add highlights, annotations, and bookmarks. Please contact your Sales Manager for details about how to access instructor resources in HK*Propel*.

"The science of healing, the art of caring" is a motto in the field of physical therapy (American Physical Therapy Association). It is one that we both strongly believe in and strive to live by. We feel that it is truly applicable to the field of health care in general. We wrote the book based on this philosophy, trying to impart the importance of both the art and the science aspects to the development of palpation skills. We hope that this is something you take to heart and apply in all areas of your practice.

Acknowledgments

The development of this book, *A Clinical Guide to Surface Palpation: The Art and Science of the Perfect Touch,* would not have been possible without the support and dedication of many individuals. We would like to thank our colleagues at Long Island University for their support throughout this process. Our fellow faculty members serve as strong role models throughout our education and careers.

A special thanks to Gregory Johnson and Dean Hazama from the Institute of Physical Art. Without them, the chapter on visceral palpation would not have come to fruition. We would also like to thank the models in the new second edition photos, Katelyn Kernoschak and Brett Shagena, as well as Kaitlin Kirker and Ayala Rosenzweig for assisting with the photo and video shoot. A big thanks to our photographer, Daniel Bergman, for his professional demeanor and endless patience throughout the photo shoot.

We also need to thank the amazing professionals at Human Kinetics. As a team, they were inspiring, helpful, and responsive and, most importantly, they maintained an open mind to the ideas we suggested as authors. Without them, this project would never have come to fruition. We would especially like to remember Josh Stone for his guidance and suggestions. Many of the additions to the second edition of the text were his suggestions. We enjoyed working with him and regret he is not able to see this project come to completion. We would also like to recognize Amanda Ewing. It was a pleasure to work with her on the first edition, and we were excited to be able to work with her on this second edition.

chapter 1

Introduction to the Art and Science of Palpation

CHAPTER OBJECTIVES

After completing this chapter, the reader will be able to do the following:

- Describe the goals of surface palpation.
- Understand the role of anatomy in surface palpation.
- Discuss the importance of surface palpation as a component of the clinical examination.
- Describe the proper technique for identifying each of the various types of tissues.
- Articulate the importance of proper body mechanics during surface palpation.

This chapter introduces important concepts that will serve as a foundation for the material covered in subsequent chapters. Most importantly, readers will understand the power of human touch and how both verbal and nonverbal communication are vital throughout the palpation process. The goals and the role of palpation are discussed, and basic guidelines for how to perform palpation of different structures are presented. The concept of proper body mechanics is introduced to emphasize safety and to improve the accuracy of surface palpation, manual skills, and rapport with patients. Throughout, it is emphasized that a thorough knowledge base of anatomy is essential for strong palpation skills.

Definition of Palpation

Palpation is derived from the Latin word *palpatio,* which in turn comes from a verb meaning "to touch." This basic definition of palpation is, however, an oversimplification of its meaning and import to health care professionals. Touch is an extremely effective tool and must not be underestimated. Humans communicate a great deal through touch. Good palpation skills are necessary for establishing patient trust, confidence, and rapport with the clinician because this is often the first time clinicians come in close physical contact with the patient. It is therefore important to have solid palpation skills. Patients can often detect when palpation skills are not strong and efficient, and this makes it difficult to establish a trusting relationship between the patient and clinician.

Palpation is the method by which the skin and subcutaneous structures (fat, fascia, muscles, ligaments, tendons, bones, and viscera) are manually identified. It is important to be mindful that there are several layers of soft tissue beneath the skin. The superficial layers consist of the epidermal and dermal layers of the skin; under these are the deeper subcutaneous fat layer, and finally, the underlying fascia (figure 1.1).[1,2] Because different structures have varying degrees of depth, it is important to consider the amount of superficial and subcutaneous tissue that lies over the particular structure being palpated. This guides the clinician in knowing how much pressure to apply to avoid being overly aggressive or too tentative.

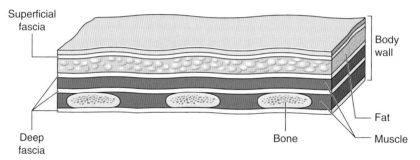

FIGURE 1.1   Layers of soft tissue.

Goals of Palpation

Palpation is a skill that is commonly used in clinical practice. Research has shown that training and experience are essential for performing accurate palpation.[3-5] Palpation can provide information about tissue integrity, degree of irritability (provocation), temperature of the affected area, swelling, and deformity.[3,4,6-13]

The information gained through palpation is compiled with the data obtained from the rest of the examination in order to arrive at the correct diagnosis. Palpation has two main goals:

1. Anatomical structure identification
2. Assessment of tissue integrity

The first goal, structure identification through anatomical palpation, is a prerequisite for the second goal of assessing tissue integrity. The primary focus of this book is to describe and provide instruction on anatomical palpation (structure identification) for the various systems of the body with a strong focus on musculoskeletal palpation. This type of palpation identifies anatomical landmarks and their relationship to other structures in the body. The book highlights how palpation of various structures provides clinicians with important clinical information, which may affect clinical decision-making. For example, tenderness to the lateral malleolus following an ankle injury, along with swelling and an inability to bear weight, should cause the clinician to recommend imaging studies of the ankle.[14]

Psychomotor Skill of Palpation

Because palpation helps establish the relationship between clinician and patient, it is imperative to develop and use strong communication skills throughout the process. This includes both verbal and nonverbal communication skills. The ability to clearly explain and make the patient comfortable with what is going to happen and to acquire consent from the patient are extremely important first steps for palpation. Simultaneously, one should pay attention to the patient's nonverbal signals such as facial expressions or hand signals. These can be signs or clues that a palpation is uncomfortable or that the patient is apprehensive about something that is being done. We encourage a slow, systematic approach during palpation to allow both a dialogue to develop between the clinician and patient and to give the brain a chance to process what the hands are feeling. Rushing through palpation techniques can lead not only to inaccurate assessment, but more importantly, can also have a negative effect on the relationship between the clinician and the patient.

Students and novice clinicians often question how much pressure should be used during palpation. Recommendations put forth regarding the degree of palpation pressure vary from 5 grams to 4 kilograms.[15-17] The difference between these two numbers is very large, and we feel that this only serves as a guideline to help clinicians and students consider the amount of pressure being applied during palpation. To clarify, we suggest considering the plane of the palpating fingers, as well as the depth of the structure. If, for example, the posterior forearm muscles are being palpated, placing the hand parallel to the muscle fibers will most likely address the skin and superficial subcutaneous layers. However, angling the fingers so they are more perpendicular to the posterior forearm muscles should increase the depth of the palpation pressure to reach deeper soft tissue structures. This is one simple way to palpate tissues at varying depths without just simply applying more pressure.

Because it is difficult to quantify the amount of pressure one is using, we suggest that it is dependent on the type of tissue being palpated and the patient's body type. As already mentioned, it is important to be mindful of the depth of the target structure, and the blanching of the nail bed can be a quick indicator for the clinician of how much pressure is being applied. For example, the medial and lateral epicondyles are extremely superficial and therefore require light pressure during palpation. This light pressure should cause only a slight, if any, blanching of the fingernails.

In contrast, during palpation of deeper structures (e.g., the psoas major) more pressure is required. In this instance, it is highly likely that more blanching of the nail bed will occur. However, we caution clinicians to notice the amount of blanching of the fingernails. Applying too much pressure during palpation may cause loss of sensitivity by the clinician to the tissue texture of the structure being palpated. Remember, if palpation pressure is excessive and the patient is apprehensive during palpation, then accurate assessment of the desired structure is extremely difficult, if not impossible. At all times, use the least amount of force required to locate and subsequently assess the structure being palpated.

Throughout the book, we recommend optimal positions for structure identification. Please understand that these are only suggestions and that other positions may also be used. Be mindful of patient positions, especially when the patient's condition may be acutely irritable because changing positions often increases symptoms. In addition, remember that certain structures in the body are deeper than others, and their palpation may be uncomfortable for the patient. We suggest palpating these structures on both sides to differentiate between normal patient responses and areas of tenderness.

- Begin on the uninvolved side to establish what the "normal" tissue feel is for that particular patient.
- This provides an additional opportunity for the patient to become more comfortable with the clinician's touch and assists with building rapport and gaining the patient's trust before moving to the involved side.

Importance of Palpation as a Component of the Examination

Palpation is a psychomotor skill and should be viewed as a component of the examination process. The examination usually includes, at the very least, a thorough history, range of motion assessment, muscle strength testing, special tests, joint mobility assessment, neurological assessment, and outcome scales. The information gleaned from the palpatory examination needs to be integrated into the remainder of the examination. This compilation of all the data gathered guides the clinician in the clinical decision-making process, establishing the diagnosis and implementing treatment strategies.

Often, students and novice clinicians struggle with the timing of palpation during the examination. While currently there is no set framework for when to conduct the palpatory part of the examination, we recommend using clinical reasoning skills to help answer this question. During the examination, it is important to pay close attention to the behavior of the symptoms reported by the patient. For example, you should make sure to question patients about symptom behavior so that you can ascertain whether the condition has been getting worse, staying the same, or improving since the initial onset of pain or injury. When a patient reports high pain levels and is extremely apprehensive of movement, this usually indicates an acute injury. A highly irritable structure is characterized by high levels of pain with movement, an increase in pain following minimal activity, and a longer period of time for pain to return to baseline levels.[18] Conversely, when a patient reports lower levels of pain and is less apprehensive about movement, this is usually indicative of a condition in the subacute or chronic phase of healing.[18] According to Maitland, one of the main objectives of the examination process is to assess the degree of irritability.[18] This information can be used to help determine the sequence of the examination process.

After trauma to the musculoskeletal system, structures typically progress through three phases of tissue healing.

1. The *inflammatory process* is characterized by redness, heat, swelling, and pain. The goal of the *inflammatory phase* is to remove dead cells from the site of injury and prevent infection from occurring. This phase lasts approximately 7 days and sets the stage for the remainder of the healing process.

2. The *repair phase* is characterized by migration of fibroblasts to the site of the wound to continue tissue healing.[19,20] The most important part of this phase is collagen formation to give the wound tensile strength. This phase lasts from 3 to 20 days.

3. The *remodeling phase* is characterized by scar formation and conversion of type III collagen to type I collagen, the main type found in connective tissue. This phase begins around day 10 and continues until the tissue has returned to preinjury strength.

It is important to remember that these phases are not mutually exclusive of one another and that significant overlap occurs throughout the process.[19,20]

Palpation can sometimes irritate tissues, which may affect the accuracy of the information gathered from the remaining portions of the examination (range of motion, muscle testing, and so on). The information from the patient history should tell the clinician the degree of irritability present. This guides the clinician as to whether palpation should be performed at the beginning or the end of the examination. Because this determination requires continuous clinical decision-making, it can be difficult for students and novice clinicians. Therefore, in our opinion, a general rule of thumb can be helpful—that palpation belongs at the end of the examination. This provides clinicians with a standardized point in the examination to conduct palpation and lessens the chance that palpation will irritate tissues.

Role of Anatomy in Palpation

Before placing hands on patients, it is necessary to have a thorough understanding of anatomy. The following are simple tips to help in the development of palpation skills.

- Visualize the structure or structures to be palpated before attempting to locate them on the patient.
- Keep in mind the depth of a particular structure. This will give some indication of how much pressure to exert during the palpation.
- Think about and visualize where and to what the target structure attaches. Keep in mind surrounding tissues and the relationships that the structures have with each other.
- Knowledge of contractile versus noncontractile tissues can be used to enhance the identification of various structures throughout the musculoskeletal system. Consider whether the target structure has a main action that can help make the palpation easier. This applies particularly to skeletal muscles that can contract and relax, making identification easier.
- Above all, be patient, and do not get frustrated. Just because the structure being palpated cannot be identified does not mean that the patient cannot feel the palpation of the structure. While always important, in this case, it is especially important to have an ongoing dialogue to allow the patient to report what he or she is feeling. Take your time, grade your force, and give your brain a chance to process the different tissue textures.

These simple steps will provide structure and guidance during palpation. Each chapter highlights clinical anatomy that is pertinent to the palpations covered. Relevant anatomical structures are discussed in the text. In addition, there are tables that cover origins, insertions, innervations, blood supply, and muscle actions.

To set the framework for the remainder of the book, basic anatomy needs to be reviewed. It is important to remember the concept of anatomical neutral. This is the position to which all anatomical landmarks are referenced (figure 1.2) and is the position used to describe relationships between different anatomical structures by all health care professionals. For a listing and examples of the terms for anatomical relationships, see table 1.1.[21]

Palpation of Different Structures

The following is a brief overview of the various structures that are covered throughout the book. In this section, we discuss the basics of the techniques

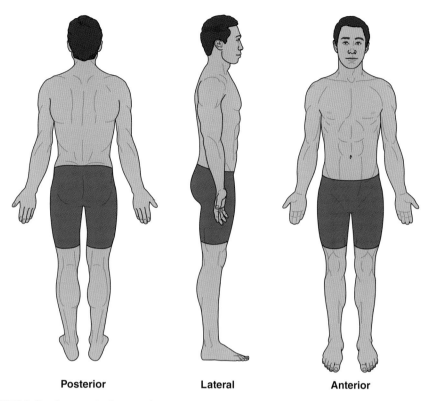

| Posterior | Lateral | Anterior |

FIGURE 1.2 Anatomical neutral.

Table 1.1 Anatomical Relationship Terms

Term	Meaning	Example
Anterior	In front of; front of the body	Umbilicus is anterior to colon
Posterior	Behind; back of the body	Trapezius is posterior to rhomboids
Superior	Above; toward the head	Nose is superior to mouth
Inferior	Below; toward the feet	Umbilicus is inferior to sternum
Medial	Toward the midline of the body	Digit 5 is medial to digit 1
Lateral	Farther from the midline of the body	Radius is lateral to ulna
Proximal	Higher up on a limb	Shoulder is proximal to elbow
Distal	Lower down on a limb	Hand is distal to elbow
Superficial	Closer to the surface of the skin	Biceps is superficial to brachialis
Deep	Farther away from the surface of the skin	Piriformis is deep to gluteus maximus

and the interpretation of the information yielded by the assessment. In addition, we provide the reader with tips on the depth of the tissue and how that can change the amount of pressure and hand positioning that is necessary.

Skin

The skin is the most superficial, and hence the first, structure encountered during palpation. Because this organ is extremely superficial, only gentle pressure is required to assess the skin during palpation. As previously mentioned, this requires the clinician to keep the palpating hand and fingers more parallel to the surface of the skin. Palpation of the skin can provide information about temperature, edema, tissue mobility, hydration, and trophic changes.[8]

Temperature

The dorsum of the hand contains many free nerve endings, which are particularly sensitive to changes in skin temperature. Thus, the dorsum of the hand is used to assess for changes in skin temperature, indicating the degree of inflammation, which will assist the clinician in deciding both when to palpate during the examination and how much pressure to use. Only light touch is required for the clinician to accurately assess the skin temperature.

Edema

Several types of edema exist, but this book discusses musculoskeletal swelling only, specifically joint effusion. To examine for swelling, light pressure is applied to the skin to assess for potential rebounding of fluid into the tissue, which may indicate the presence of edema. A specific test known as the stroke test has been developed to assess knee joint effusion. The clinician begins below the joint line on the medial aspect of the knee and applies a gentle upward stroke to the level of the suprapatellar pouch two or three times. With the other hand, the clinician applies a gentle downward force along the lateral aspect of the patella. The clinician then looks for a wave of fluid along the medial aspect of the patella.[22] A study has demonstrated this test to be a reliable method for assessing knee joint effusion.[23]

Tissue Mobility

The four main tissue types in the body are epithelial, connective (bone, ligaments, tendons), muscle, and nervous.[19] While all of these tissue types are encountered during palpation, the majority of this book focuses on connective tissue, muscle tissue, and nervous tissue. General tissue mobility is assessed to determine whether adhesions are present between the skin and underlying subcutaneous tissues.[24] Normal tissue is usually soft and mobile and should move equally in all directions. In the presence of pathology or injury, tissues may feel hard, tender to the touch, ropey, or crunchy. General tissue mobility can be assessed by a combination of the skin gliding test, finger sliding test, and skin rolling test.[24]

- The skin gliding test is performed to assess the ability of the skin to glide on the underlying soft tissues. The clinician places a hand on the skin and gently attempts to slide the skin on the underlying soft tissue structures.

- The finger sliding test is used to assess the ability of the fingers to slide across the skin. In the absence of pathology, the fingers should be able to slide across the skin with little resistance to movement. During injury, pathology, or dehydration, the clinician feels increased resistance.

- The skin rolling test is performed by approximating the skin between the thumb and either the second or third digit as one moves across the region being assessed (figure 1.3). This test evaluates the ability of the skin to be lifted from underlying soft tissue structures and usually yields the most information.

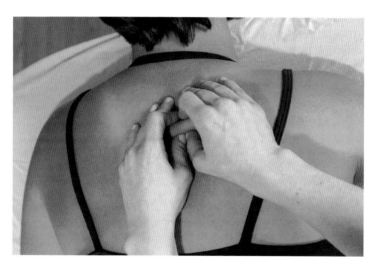

FIGURE 1.3 Skin rolling.

Hydration

Assessment of the skin can provide baseline information regarding the overall hydration status of the patient. Clinicians should assess for the presence of symptoms of hypo- and hyperhidrosis. Scaly, cracking skin is potentially a sign of dehydration or hypohidrosis, and the clinician must investigate the potential causes.

Trophic Changes

Clinicians need to assess for skin integrity changes. These can include, but are not limited to, shiny skin, excessive hair, hair loss, and even the potential for soft tissue swelling. These can be signs of local or systemic disease and need to be investigated accordingly.

Bones

There are approximately 206 bones in the human body. Palpation of bony structures can yield valuable information, such as potential structural defects, irritation of the bone itself, or irritation of the soft tissue attaching to the bone. In addition, bony landmarks are also frequently used to help orient the clinician when palpating other regional tissues. During bony palpation, the fingertips should be perpendicular to the structure being palpated. This minimizes movement of the soft tissues (skin, fascia, and so on) that are superficial to the structure being identified. In some instances, the bony landmark protrudes from the surrounding soft tissues and is therefore easily identified. In these cases, minimal pressure is necessary, and the fingertip-to-structure angle is less important.

Muscles

The body is composed of more than 600 skeletal muscles, not all of which are accessible for palpation. The pressure used to palpate the desired structure depends on the depth of the target muscle. For example, the upper trapezius is a commonly palpated superficial muscle of the upper quadrant, and minimal pressure is needed. If excessive pressure is applied, the levator scapulae may be the muscle that is palpated instead.

The size of muscles is highly variable. When palpating muscles, one should consider the size of the muscle belly. This serves to guide how many fingers to use for the palpation. When a larger muscle belly is being palpated, such as the quadriceps femoris, multiple fingers should be used. Conversely, when a smaller muscle is being palpated, such as the teres minor, the number of fingers should be minimized to eliminate the risk of palpating adjacent muscles. To verify accurate palpation of the desired muscle belly, have the patient alternately contract and relax the muscle. If the contraction cannot be felt, consider reassessing finger placement. Remember that certain muscles may be more easily identified near their proximal attachment (origin), while others may be better identified near the distal attachment (insertion).

Tendons

Tendons are among the soft tissue structures that most frequently present with local pathology, such as tendinitis or tendinosis.[25,26] They are composed of connective tissue, specifically type I collagen, and are found at the ends of muscles attaching to bony landmarks.[19] Because tendons have a smaller surface area than most muscle bellies, the number of fingers used to palpate tendons should be kept to a minimum (one or two). For more superficial tendons, it may be sufficient to use the tip of the finger along the tendon border. For deeper tendons, use the pads of the fingers directly over where the tendon is expected to be. The patient should then be instructed to alternately contract and relax the muscle, which will put tension on the tendon, helping to verify structure identification.

Some tendons are rather superficial (e.g., the Achilles tendon) and therefore require minimal pressure to assess for tendon texture, integrity, tenderness, or signs of inflammation. Other tendons in the musculoskeletal system (e.g., the subscapularis tendon) are deeper and require greater pressure to assess tendon status accurately. Consider palpating tendons perpendicular to their tissue orientation (i.e., muscle fiber direction); this allows for better assessment of structural defects, areas of inflammation, or tenderness.

Ligaments

Ligaments are another type of connective tissue. They connect bone to bone and usually prevent excessive motion at a particular joint.[27] Ligaments are noncontractile tissue and increase the passive stability of the joint.[28] Similar to tendons, certain ligaments are more superficial, thus rendering them easily accessible for palpation; the lateral collateral ligament of the knee is an example. Other ligaments in the musculoskeletal system are deeper and more difficult to palpate (if they are palpable at all), such as the posterior talofibular ligament. As with tendons, we recommend palpation of ligaments perpendicular to their fiber orientation. This can aid in assessing for possible disruption of ligament integrity.

Nerves

Palpation of nerves as part of the examination process continues to become more common in clinical practice. Some nerves, such as the inferior and superior gluteal nerves, cannot be palpated directly. Other nerves, such as the ulnar and common fibular nerves, are more superficial and thus easily accessible.

Again, palpate with the pads of the fingers perpendicular to the structure. A moderate amount of pressure should be used, because often not enough force is provided to identify the nerve accurately. Because of their solidity, nerves have a firm consistency.

Similar to other structures in the musculoskeletal system, nerves change in length based on the forces applied to them. Patients often present clinically with signs and symptoms consistent with nerve irritation. Because many nerves cannot be directly assessed in their resting position, gentle tension placed on the nerve may improve the ability to accurately identify the structure in question. In some cases of nerve injury (e.g., axonotmesis), placing tension on the nerve to improve accuracy of palpation may be contraindicated.[29]

Blood Vessels

While one of the goals of surface palpation is to accurately identify various structures throughout the body, palpation of blood vessels is unique. In contrast to the situation with the structures previously discussed, the main goal in the assessment of blood vessels is to identify the presence or absence of distal pulses throughout the extremities, not the structure itself. The assessment of pulses throughout the extremities and trunk is, at times, an extremely important part of the examination process. Frequently, following trauma or surgery, assessment of distal pulses is imperative. While some arteries in the body are impossible to palpate (e.g., the vertebral artery), others are superficial and thus easily accessible (e.g., brachial, radial, and femoral). A thorough understanding of anatomy is mandatory to assess for pulses throughout the extremities.

The pulse should be objectively assessed as normal, heightened, diminished, or absent.[30] To enhance the accuracy of blood vessel palpation, perform the following:

- Palpate using minimal pressure with the pad of one or pads of two fingers.
- The thumb (digit 1) should not be used to palpate blood vessels; instead, the index and middle fingers should be used to properly evaluate the pulse.
- Deeper pressure may occlude the vessel and increase the difficulty of assessment.
- Make every effort to place as little tension on the surrounding superficial tissues as possible. For example, to identify the brachial artery accurately, instruct the patient to relax as much as possible, and place the patient's forearm in a position of elbow flexion. This will place the muscles of the anterior arm on slack and increase the likelihood that palpation will be accurate.

Bursae

Several bursae throughout the musculoskeletal system may need assessment during the examination. While in most cases a bursa cannot be palpated as a unique structure, there are times when pressure over a bursa will elicit tenderness, thus providing valuable information to be used during the clinical decision-making process. For example, the subdeltoid bursa lies between the deltoid and rotator cuff tendons. This structure cannot be palpated independently of the surrounding tissues. However, in the case of subdeltoid bursitis, localized pain and tenderness may be found and, in combination with other components of the examination, allow for a more accurate diagnosis.

During palpation of bursae, we suggest using the pads of two or three fingers over the involved structure in a slow, systematic fashion. It is our opinion that bursa palpation is an example of a case in which the order of palpation can make a significant difference to examination findings. Most patients presenting with acute bursitis are in a great deal of pain. Palpating the bursa before performing the remainder of the examination can irritate the structure, possibly rendering the results of other components of the examination unreliable.

Capsules

Most joints in the musculoskeletal system possess a joint capsule that contributes to passive joint stability. Similar to some other musculoskeletal tissues, some capsules cannot be palpated directly. Other capsules, such as those surrounding the elbow and knee joints, are more superficial and easily palpable. Following injury or surgery, it is common for the capsules of the musculoskeletal system to become inflamed. When compared to what is found in the uninvolved extremity, swelling and subsequent capsular distension may be observed.

Palpate the capsule in a slow systematic fashion, feeling for any movement of fluid or other signs of inflammation. The number of fingers used depends on the size of the joint. For example, the elbow joint is smaller than the knee joint, and fewer fingers should be used to assess the capsule and surrounding tissues accurately.

Plica

Some joints in the musculoskeletal system present with synovial folds called plicae. At times, these can be found in the facet joints of the spine, as well as along both the medial and lateral aspects of the knee. The plicae present in the facet joints are impossible to palpate. However, the plicae in the knee are more easily palpable, especially in the event of trauma or irritation to the knee joint, when they can become inflamed and enlarged.

Plicae should be palpated with firm pressure, using the pads of two fingers. It is imperative that palpation be done in a slow systematic manner so that the structure is not completely missed or passed over during the palpatory exam. Sometimes during palpation, joint position may need to be altered to further expose the plica.

Viscera

The visceral organs are vital players in the various body systems that allow the human body to function as a cohesive unit. Healthy body systems, including, but not limited to, the digestive system, the respiratory system, the reproductive system, and the circulatory system are vital to optimal function of the movement system that clinicians play a role in rehabilitating. It is important for clinicians to be able to identify the visceral organs and discern them from musculoskeletal structures using palpation. In addition, clinicians should apply their findings to rule out sinister pathology of the various body systems to determine whether the patient's impairments and pain are arising from musculoskeletal origin. When appropriate, clinicians may find it beneficial to address decreased mobility of such structures to improve the patient's overall quality of life. To palpate the viscera, follow these guidelines:

- Palpate in a slow, systematic fashion.
- Avoid abrupt movement into deeper tissues; this often causes guarding and apprehension in the patient.
- Initially make broad and gentle, but firm, contact with both hands before narrowing to palpate smaller, more specific structures with one or two fingers.

Body Mechanics

The body mechanics of the practicing clinician is an extremely important concept. It not only protects the clinician from potential injury but also aides in proper positioning between the patient and clinician to improve structure identification and treatment. Proper body mechanics will not only help the clinician work more efficiently but also aid the clinician in applying the appropriate force during examination and treatment. It is important to be constantly mindful of the stresses being put on your body. Always strive to be as efficient as possible (e.g., using gravity, using larger muscle groups, aligning the forearm when applying force) when performing techniques, and minimize trying to "muscle through it." The following are techniques to consider for manual assessment and intervention.

- It is important to make sure the height of the table is correct. This allows for appropriate application of desired forces. For example, a downwardly directed force is one of the most frequently used, and one needs to make sure that force is perpendicular to the tissue. Often, students and novice clinicians place the table too high, which leads to inefficient application of forces in addition to poor movement patterns on the part of the clinician (e.g., hiking the shoulder, too much elbow flexion). This often results in excessive firing of muscles, which will cause fatigue during treatment. Conversely, if the table is too low, there is a tendency to adopt a position of lumbar spine flexion (as opposed to neutral), putting the clinician at increased risk of developing low back pain.

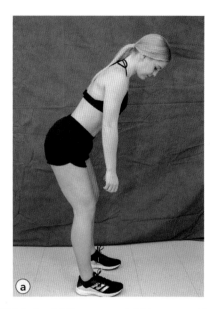 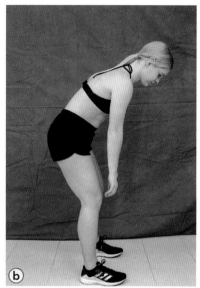

FIGURE 1.4 *(a)* Correct and *(b)* incorrect hip hinge.

- It is important to understand the concept of a hip hinge and its role in a healthy back. Proper hip flexion rather than thoracolumbar flexion should be maintained (figure 1.4). The lumbar spine should be in a natural lordotic position. Excessive or insufficient lordosis can create excessive forces through the lumbar spine, which may increase the likelihood of injury.

- Be cognizant of foot position. A staggered stance is often optimal because it increases the clinician's base of support and provides increased stability to the lower half of the body, optimizing alignment of the upper extremities for force application. Additionally, foot direction (neutral or externally rotated) is key to aligning the base of support with the force vector.

- Position the head, neck, and scapula in a neutral position. Often, clinicians work in a poor position, with the head forward, scapular elevation and protraction, and excessive neck flexion. This position not only makes it more difficult to appropriately apply force, but it can also cause excessive fatigue and pain to the treating clinician. Stacking the joints of the spine in a neutral column distributes forces to the sturdy vertebral column rather than to soft tissues.

- The most important tools are the hands. Clinicians must take care of them. During all palpation and manual therapy techniques, clinicians must avoid hyperextending their fingers during force application. This can lead to excessive compressive forces to the small joints of the hands (especially the first carpometacarpal joint) and may lead to early joint breakdown.

PALPATION CLINICAL PEARLS

- Most importantly, patients must first know how much you care.
- Remember to respect patient modesty and comfort and *always* obtain informed consent before beginning palpation.
- Touch is an extremely important aspect of the physical examination process. It helps foster the development of the patient–clinician relationship.
- Patient trust is imperative to their ability to avoid guarding the region being palpated.
- Firm but gentle hands enhance structure identification and also place the patient at ease.
- You must be aware of what your hands feel like from the perspective of the patient. Nails must be kept trimmed and smooth. The skin of the fingers and palms of the hands must also be kept soft and smooth.
- A thorough understanding of anatomy is essential for accurate palpation.
- Think about the structure you are trying to palpate and how that particular structure can be more easily identified.
- Always begin the palpation examination with superficial structures that can help orient you.

Conclusion

Throughout this first chapter, we have attempted to provide the background information a clinician needs to become skillful in palpation. Palpation is important and necessary as part of the clinical examination process and for ongoing patient care. Remember that practicing palpation improves psychomotor skills, but that clinicians must also devote ample time to metacognition and clinical decision-making skills.

CHAPTER REVIEW QUESTIONS

1. What are the two main goals of surface palpation?
2. What are the main tissue types in the body?
3. What are the three types of tests used to assess skin mobility?
4. What is the most important clinical pearl for surface palpation?
5. What are the three phases of tissue healing?
6. According to Maitland, what is one of the main objectives of the physical examination?
7. What are the important anatomical tips to consider when palpating?

chapter **2**

Skull and Face

CHAPTER OBJECTIVES

After completing this chapter, the reader will be able to do the following:

- Identify the key bony anatomical structures of the skull and face.
- Identify and describe the soft tissue anatomy of the skull and face, including muscles, ligaments, nerves, arteries, and veins.
- Identify on bony or skeletal models the origins and insertions of the muscles of the skull and face in order to aid in understanding osteokinematic action and surface palpation.
- Palpate structures of the orofacial region.
- Integrate surface palpation findings to aid in the differential diagnosis of a patient with orofacial pain.

Although the skull and face is not one of the more commonly treated regions of the body, a thorough knowledge of the underlying anatomy, physiology, blood supply, and nerve supply is necessary for accurate assessment of these structures. While dentists and physicians treat the majority of orofacial pathologies (e.g., fractures, bony anomalies, and occlusion disorders), the most important joint in this region, the temporomandibular joint (TMJ), is often treated by physical therapists and other rehabilitation specialists. Temporomandibular joint or orofacial pain is a common occurrence, with approximately one-third of all patients experiencing persistent symptoms.[1-3]

Functions of the Skull and Face

One of the most important functions of the skull and face is the protection of vital structures. The skull can be divided into two distinct regions known as the neurocranium and the facial skeleton.

- The neurocranium is composed of eight bones and is responsible for protecting the underlying brain and cranial meninges.
- The facial skeleton is composed of 14 bones and is responsible for giving architectural structure to the region, which provides a base for muscle and ligament attachments. This complex, efficient system gives shape to the face, helps with functions of mastication and vocalization, and partially forms the sockets of the eyes and fossa of the TMJ.

Bony Anatomy

Together, the neurocranium and the facial skeleton are composed of 22 bones. The neurocranium consists of the frontal, parietal, temporal, occipital, sphenoid, and ethmoid bones (figure 2.1). The roof of the neurocranium is referred to as the calvaria, which has three sutures that connect the bones of the skull into a single complex by forming syndesmotic joints, which are immobile because of tough fibrous connective tissue.[4]

- The coronal suture connects the frontal bone to the parietal bone.
- The sagittal suture connects both parietal bones.
- The lambdoid suture connects the parietal bones to the occipital bone.

The large frontal bone is best seen from an anterior view of the skull. The eye orbits are the biggest feature of the frontal bone. The orbital rim is composed of six bones. The outer rim is composed of the frontal, zygomatic, and maxilla bones, while the inner orbital rim is made up of the lacrimal, sphenoid, and ethmoid bones.[4]

On the lateral aspect of the skull (figure 2.2) are the parietal bones. It is quite evident from a lateral view that the frontal bone does not project too far posteriorly, and the parietal bones occupy most of the surface area of the skull. Also visible on the lateral view is the zygomatic arch, which is formed by the temporal process of the zygomatic bone and the zygomatic process of the temporal bone.

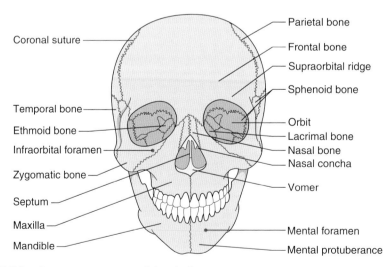

FIGURE 2.1   Anterior structures of the skull.

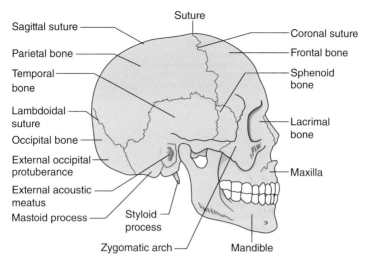

Suture
Sagittal suture
Coronal suture
Parietal bone
Frontal bone
Temporal bone
Sphenoid bone
Lambdoidal suture
Lacrimal bone
Occipital bone
External occipital protuberance
Maxilla
External acoustic meatus
Mastoid process
Styloid process
Zygomatic arch
Mandible

FIGURE 2.2   Lateral structures of the skull.

The temporal bone has several important anatomical landmarks, such as the temporal fossa, which forms part of the TMJ, and the mastoid process, which serves as an attachment for several muscles as well as an important landmark in the identification of the transverse processes of the first cervical vertebra (atlas).[4] Posteriorly is the large occipital bone, which also has important anatomical landmarks: the external occipital protuberance, the superior and inferior nuchal lines, and the foramen magnum, where the spinal cord begins. While only the external occipital protuberance is directly palpable, all these landmarks serve as attachments for posterior cervical spine musculature.[4] The external occipital protuberance is an important anatomical landmark for describing how to palpate the spinous process of C2.

The facial skeleton contains many small bones that are not all easily palpable. However, the zygomatic arches, nasal bones, orbital rims, and the mandible are easily palpable and serve as important anatomical landmarks that can aid you during the palpatory examination. While the bones of the facial skeleton are small and immobile as a whole, the mandible is a large and easily palpable bone. The mandible (figure 2.3) is composed of an upright portion called the ramus and a horizontal portion called the body, which are joined together at the mandibular angle. On the superior aspect of the mandible is the condylar process, which is subdivided into the head and neck. This condyle articulates with the temporal bone to form the TMJ.[4]

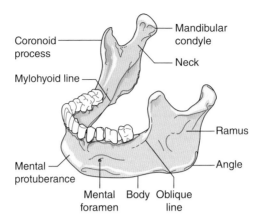

FIGURE 2.3 Structures of the mandible.

The hyoid bone is located in the anterior aspect of the neck near the third cervical vertebral level. This bone functions to keep the airway open and also serves as an attachment for neck muscles. Additionally, it is one of the few bones that does not articulate with any other bone but has soft tissue attachments to surrounding bones.[4]

Soft Tissue Anatomy

Four muscles are directly involved with movements of the TMJ (figure 2.4). The temporalis and masseter muscles are more superficial and easily palpable. The medial and lateral pterygoid muscles are much deeper and, at times, require intraoral palpation for accurate identification and treatment. Collectively, these four muscles are involved with opening and closing the mouth.[4] The TMJ has an articular disc that is between the temporal fossa and the mandibular condyle. This disc serves to increase the congruency of the TMJ. Of particular importance is the role of the superior lateral pterygoid muscle, which functions to eccentrically control the articular disc during mouth closing.[5,6]

Other muscles, the suprahyoids and infrahyoids (figure 2.5), also have an indirect effect on the TMJ.[4]

- The suprahyoids consist of the geniohyoid, mylohyoid, stylohyoid, and the digastric muscles, which all perform elevation of the hyoid bone.
- The infrahyoids consist of the sternohyoid, sternothyroid, thyrohyoid, and omohyoid muscles, which all depress the hyoid bone.

While these muscles cannot directly move the TMJ, certain postural deviations, such as forward head posture, can affect the resting length of these muscles, thereby changing the forces acting on the TMJ.[7]

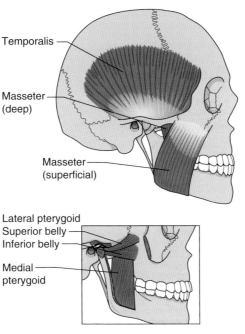

FIGURE 2.4 Superficial and deep muscles of the temporomandibular joint.

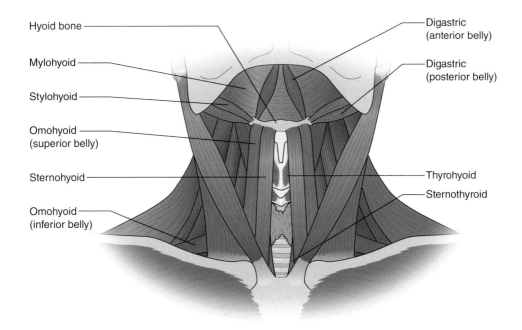

FIGURE 2.5 Hyoid bone with suprahyoids and infrahyoids.

In addition to the muscles, other soft tissues surround the TMJ. This joint, similar to other joints in the musculoskeletal system, has a joint capsule with ligaments. These structures work in combination with the muscles of the TMJ to increase stability during movement. The most important ligament stabilizing the TMJ is the lateral ligament. This ligament runs from the zygomatic arch and neck of the mandible to the lateral pole of the mandibular condyle (figure 2.6). It is responsible for stabilizing the lateral side of the capsule and guiding the condyle during movement.[7,8]

Posterior to the mandibular condyle is the articular disc with its retrodiscal tissues. This is extremely important for normal biomechanics of the TMJ and should be in continuous contact with the mandibular condyle during mouth opening and closing.[7,8] The disc is well innervated with pain fibers and may become a source of pain, as well as limit TMJ opening when a dislocation is present.[2,8,9]

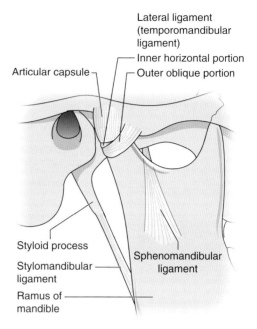

FIGURE 2.6 Ligaments of the temporomandibular joint.

Neurovascular Anatomy

Several important arteries and nerves are located in the skull and face region. To understand these structures, it is important to consider where they originate. Three main branches arise from the aortic arch.[4]

- Arising from the left side of the arch are the left subclavian artery and left common carotid artery.

- Arising from the right side is an additional branch called the right brachiocephalic trunk, which then divides into the right subclavian and right common carotid arteries.

In this chapter we discuss the common carotid artery only. The common carotid artery runs superiorly, and at approximately the superior border of the thyroid cartilage it divides into the internal and external carotid arteries (figure 2.7).

- The internal carotid artery runs superiorly into the brain and then branches into the middle and anterior cerebral arteries on both sides.[4]

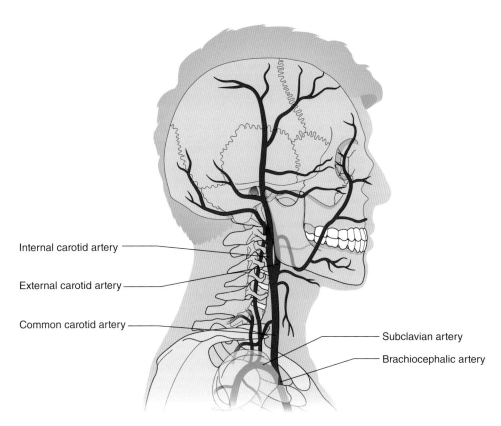

FIGURE 2.7   Arteries of the head, neck, and face.

Internal carotid artery

External carotid artery

Common carotid artery

Subclavian artery

Brachiocephalic artery

- The external carotid artery is responsible for the blood supply of the face and scalp. In the neck, this artery lies anterior to the sternocleidomastoid in the carotid sheath.[4]

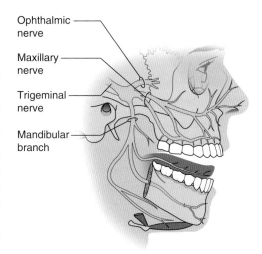

Ophthalmic nerve

Maxillary nerve

Trigeminal nerve

Mandibular branch

FIGURE 2.8   Trigeminal nerve.

The skull and face are well innervated with nerve fibers. The various layers of the scalp are innervated by the trigeminal nerve (cranial nerve V), as well as the C2 and C3 nerve roots, which are part of the cervical plexus.[4] The facial region is exclusively supplied by the trigeminal nerve (figure 2.8). This is a mixed cranial nerve with both motor and sensory branches. The sensory branches (ophthalmic, maxillary, and mandibular) are responsible for providing sensation to the facial region. The motor function of this nerve is responsible for innervating the muscles of mastication as well as the TMJ.[4]

Structural Inspection

- Observation of the skull and face should be performed with the patient sitting and the clinician assessing from the anterior, lateral, and posterior aspects.

- Structural deviations or abnormalities should be documented and considered in context with the rest of the physical examination.

- Particular attention should be paid to lacerations, ecchymosis, or other bruising, which may be a sign of active or prior trauma, as well as other facial or cervical asymmetries that may contribute to abnormal movement of the TMJ.

- The clinician should also observe the TMJ, which lies directly anterior to the external auditory meatus. This is difficult because there are no obvious superficial bony contours to this joint. For this reason, the clinician should assess the TMJ during movement (opening and closing) to assess for signs of possible movement dysfunction or deviations.

External Occipital Protuberance

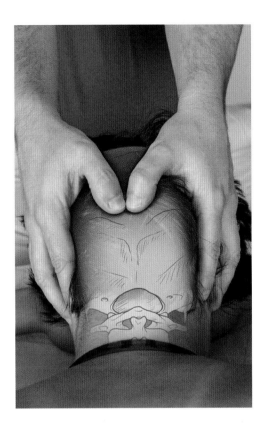

Positions
- Patient: prone or seated
- Clinician: sitting at the head of the table or standing behind the patient

Instructions
- If the patient is prone, place the patient's upper cervical spine in slight flexion.
- Palpate the top of the head with two or three fingers.
- Move your fingers in an inferior and posterior direction until palpating a rounded protuberance.

Note
This is one of the origins of the trapezius muscle and will also help orient you for palpation of the spinous processes of the cervical vertebrae.

Orbital Rim

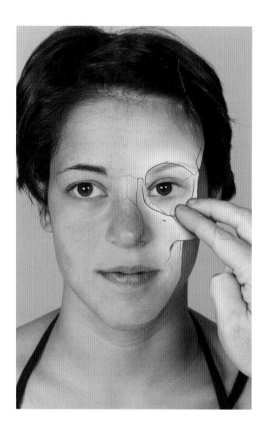

Positions

- Patient: sitting
- Clinician: standing in front of and slightly lateral to the patient, on the side being palpated

Instructions

- Place the patient's head and neck in a neutral position.
- Begin to palpate just below the eye socket with two fingers and move circumferentially around the entire orbital rim.

Nasal Bone

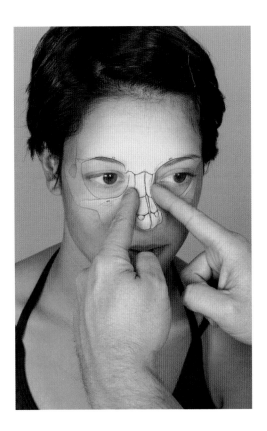

Positions

- Patient: sitting
- Clinician: standing, directly facing the patient

Instructions

- Place the patient's head and neck in a neutral position.
- Begin to palpate at the bridge of the nose with two fingers, one on each side.
- Move inferiorly until the nasal bone–cartilage junction is felt.

Zygomatic Arch

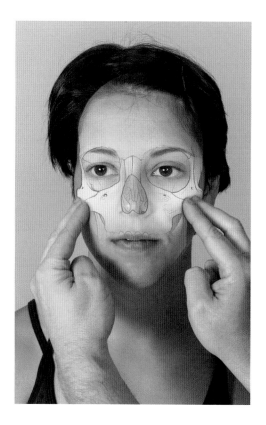

Positions

- Patient: sitting
- Clinician: standing, directly facing the patient

Instructions

- Place the patient's head and neck in a neutral position.
- Approximately halfway down and just lateral to the nose, begin to palpate with the pads of two fingers on each side.
- Proceed with firm pressure from medial to lateral, following the zygomatic arch on both sides.

Mastoid Process

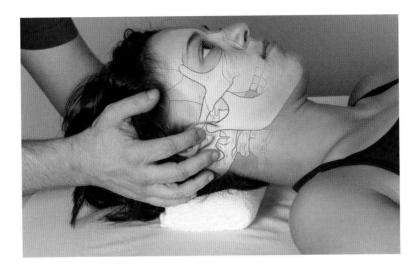

Positions
- Patient: supine
- Clinician: sitting at the patient's head

Instructions
- Place the patient's head and neck in slight flexion, and place a towel under the external occipital protuberance. This will provide support and keep the head and neck in flexion.
- Locate the external auditory meatus on both sides (ear canal) with two fingers.
- While moving the earlobe with one finger, palpate the mastoid process, a bony prominence, with the other.
- The mastoid process is directly posterior to the external auditory meatus.

Note
This structure is extremely important because it serves as the initial landmark for palpating the transverse processes of the atlas (C1).

Mandibular Condyle

Positions

- Patient: sitting
- Clinician: standing, directly facing the patient

Instructions

- Place the patient's head and neck in a neutral position.
- Locate the external auditory meatus (ear canal) on both sides.
- Palpate directly anterior to the ear canals using the pads of both second digits.
- The mandibular condyle is the bony prominence that is directly anterior to the external auditory meatus.
- Palpate the condyle moving under your finger as the patient opens and closes the mouth.
- Alternately, the clinician can palpate the condyle from inside the ear canal by placing either the index finger or digit 5 in the external auditory meatus and pressing anteriorly.

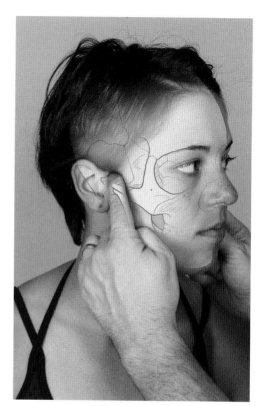

CLINICAL PEARL

Clicking may be a symptom of TMJ dysfunction, such as internal derangement of the disc (dislocation). However, the accuracy of this isolated symptom for ruling in TMJ dysfunction is not well supported in the literature.[2,3,9] We suggest combining this symptom with the subjective complaints of pain and the remainder of the clinical examination for a more accurate diagnosis.

Mastoid Process

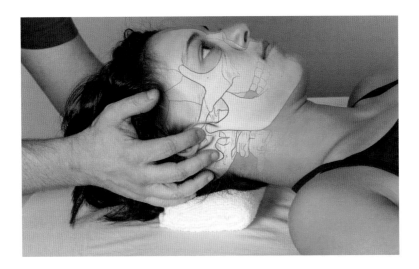

Positions

- Patient: supine
- Clinician: sitting at the patient's head

Instructions

- Place the patient's head and neck in slight flexion, and place a towel under the external occipital protuberance. This will provide support and keep the head and neck in flexion.
- Locate the external auditory meatus on both sides (ear canal) with two fingers.
- While moving the earlobe with one finger, palpate the mastoid process, a bony prominence, with the other.
- The mastoid process is directly posterior to the external auditory meatus.

Note

This structure is extremely important because it serves as the initial landmark for palpating the transverse processes of the atlas (C1).

Mandibular Condyle

Positions
- Patient: sitting
- Clinician: standing, directly facing the patient

Instructions
- Place the patient's head and neck in a neutral position.
- Locate the external auditory meatus (ear canal) on both sides.
- Palpate directly anterior to the ear canals using the pads of both second digits.
- The mandibular condyle is the bony prominence that is directly anterior to the external auditory meatus.
- Palpate the condyle moving under your finger as the patient opens and closes the mouth.
- Alternately, the clinician can palpate the condyle from inside the ear canal by placing either the index finger or digit 5 in the external auditory meatus and pressing anteriorly.

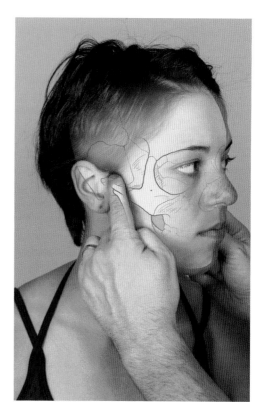

CLINICAL PEARL
Clicking may be a symptom of TMJ dysfunction, such as internal derangement of the disc (dislocation). However, the accuracy of this isolated symptom for ruling in TMJ dysfunction is not well supported in the literature.[2,3,9] We suggest combining this symptom with the subjective complaints of pain and the remainder of the clinical examination for a more accurate diagnosis.

Mandibular Angle

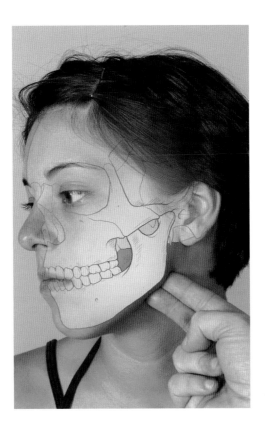

Positions
- Patient: sitting or supine
- Clinician: standing in front of and slightly lateral to the patient, on the side being palpated

Instructions
- Place the patient's head and neck in slight rotation away from the side being palpated.
- Using the pads of two fingers, palpate the mandibular condyle and move your fingers inferiorly and slightly anterior to the edge of the mandible.
- A curved bony prominence will be felt under your fingers. The mandibular angle is where the ramus and body of the mandible join.

Note
Just inferior and posterior to the mandibular angle is the submandibular gland.[2,4] This is an extremely sensitive structure that can become uncomfortable for the patient during this palpation. Caution should be used to avoid irritating this structure during palpation.

Hyoid Bone

Positions

- Patient: sitting
- Clinician: standing, directly facing the patient

Instructions

- Place the patient's head and neck in a neutral position.
- With the thumb and index finger spread approximately 1 inch (2.5 centimeters) apart, palpate the anterior neck region at the level of the C3 vertebra (larynx, or voice box).
- You should be able to palpate both sides of the hyoid bone.
- To confirm palpation, ask the patient to swallow and feel the movement of the hyoid bone under your fingers.

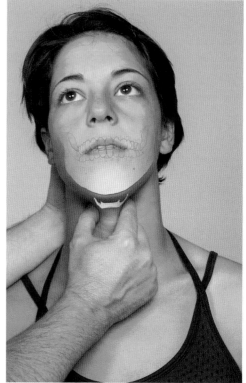

Notes

- This is a sensitive area for patients, and you should use as little force as possible (minimal blanching of your fingernails) during the palpation. Before beginning this palpation, be sure to thoroughly explain the procedure and get consent from the patient. We suggest continuous attention be paid to the patient's nonverbal signals.
- Use the pads of both second digits on their respective sides when using the hyoid bone to orient yourself when palpating the suprahyoid and infrahyoid muscles.

Muscles Acting on the TMJ and Hyoid Bone

Muscle	Origin	Insertion	Innervation	Blood supply	Action
SUPRAHYOIDS					
Mylohyoid	Mandible	Body of hyoid bone	Branch of trigeminal nerve	Branches of lingual and facial arteries	Elevation of the hyoid bone, depression of the mandible
Geniohyoid	Mandible	Anterior surface body of hyoid bone	Hypoglossal nerve	Branch of lingual artery	Elevation of the hyoid bone, depression of the mandible
Stylohyoid	Posterior border styloid process of temporal bone	Body of hyoid bone	Facial nerve	Branches of facial and occipital arteries	Elevation and retraction of the hyoid bone
Digastric	*Anterior belly:* digastric fossa of mandible *Posterior belly:* mastoid notch of temporal bone	Body of hyoid bone	*Anterior belly:* branch of trigeminal nerve *Posterior belly:* facial nerve	*Anterior belly:* branches of submental artery *Posterior belly:* branches of posterior auricular and occipital arteries	Elevation of the hyoid bone and depression of the mandible
INFRAHYOIDS					
Sternohyoid	Posterior surface of manubrium and medial end of clavicle	Medial aspect lower border body of hyoid bone	Ansa cervicalis (C1-C3)	Branches of superior thyroid and lingual arteries	Depression of the hyoid bone
Omohyoid	Superior border of scapula	Body of hyoid bone	Ansa cervicalis (C1-C3)	Branches of lingual and superior thyroid arteries	Depression of the hyoid bone
Sternothyroid	Posterior aspect of manubrium and first costal cartilage	Thyroid cartilage	Ansa cervicalis (C1-C3)	Branch of superior thyroid artery	Depression of the hyoid bone
Thyrohyoid	Thyroid cartilage	Body and greater horn of hyoid bone	Hypoglossal nerve (cranial nerve XII)	Branch of superior thyroid artery	Depression of the hyoid bone

> continued

MUSCLES ACTING ON THE TMJ AND HYOID BONE   > *continued*

Muscle	Origin	Insertion	Innervation	Blood supply	Action
TMJ MUSCLES					
Masseter	Zygomatic arch	Coronoid process and ramus of mandible	Branch of trigeminal nerve (mandibular nerve)	Transverse facial artery and branch of maxillary and facial arteries	Elevation and protrusion of the mandible; deep fibers: retraction of the mandible
Temporalis	Floor of temporal fossa	Coronoid process and ramus of mandible	Branch of trigeminal nerve (mandibular nerve)	Superficial temporal and maxillary arteries	Elevation of the mandible; posterior fibers: retraction of the mandible
Medial pterygoid	Lateral pterygoid plate	Medial surface of ramus and angle of mandible	Branch of trigeminal nerve (mandibular nerve)	Facial and maxillary arteries	*Bilaterally:* elevation and protrusion of the mandible *Unilaterally:* contralateral lateral excursion
Lateral pterygoid	*Superior head:* greater wing of sphenoid *Inferior head:* lateral pterygoid plate	Mandible, joint capsule and disc of TMJ	Branch of trigeminal nerve (mandibular nerve)	Branches of maxillary artery	*Bilaterally:* protrusion of the mandible *Unilaterally:* contralateral lateral excursion *Superior head:* eccentric control of disc during TMJ closing *Inferior head:* depression of the mandible

Zone I: Hyoid Muscles

Suprahyoids

Positions

- Patient: supine
- Clinician: sitting at the head of the table

Instructions

- Place the patient's head and neck in a neutral position.
- Palpate the hyoid bone using the pads of both second digits.
- Gently palpate immediately above the hyoid bone using the pads of digits 2 and 3 of both hands.
- Move the fingers from medial to lateral to assess all the suprahyoids.

Note

This is a sensitive area, and you should use as little force as possible (minimal blanching of your fingernails) during the palpation. Before beginning this palpation, be sure

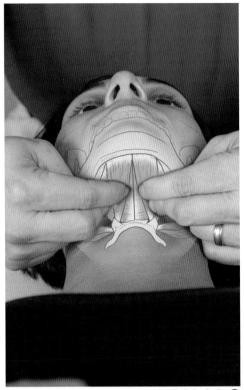

VIDEO 2.1 ▶

to thoroughly explain the procedure and get consent from the patient. We suggest a continuous dialogue between the clinician and the patient during this palpation, with particular attention paid to the patient's nonverbal signals. Keep in mind that while we are showing the palpation of the suprahyoids as a group, you should make every attempt to isolate each individual muscle based on anatomical location.

Infrahyoids

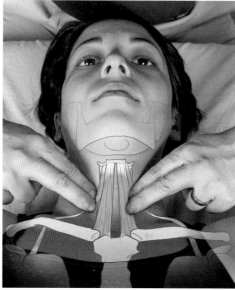

VIDEO 2.2 ▶

Positions
- Patient: supine
- Clinician: sitting at the head of the table

Instructions
- Place the patient's head and neck in a neutral position.
- Palpate the hyoid bone using the pads of both second digits.
- Begin to gently palpate immediately below the hyoid bone using the pads of digits 2 and 3 of both hands.
- Move the fingers from medial to lateral to assess all the infrahyoids.

Note
This is a sensitive area, and you should use as little force as possible (minimal blanching of your fingernails) during the palpation. Before beginning this palpation, be sure to thoroughly explain the procedure and get consent from the patient. We suggest a continuous dialogue between the clinician and the patient during this palpation, with particular attention paid to the patient's nonverbal signals. Keep in mind that while we are showing the palpation of the infrahyoids as a group, you should make every attempt to isolate each individual muscle based on anatomical location.

Zone II: TMJ Muscles

Masseter

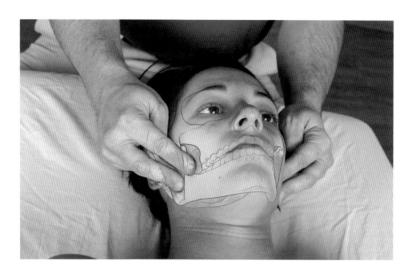

Positions
- Patient: supine
- Clinician: sitting at the head of the table

Instructions
- Place the patient's head and neck in a neutral position.
- Bilaterally, palpate inferior to the zygomatic arch, using the pads of two or three fingers.
- To confirm palpation, have the patient bite down. You should feel the muscle contract under your fingers.

Temporalis

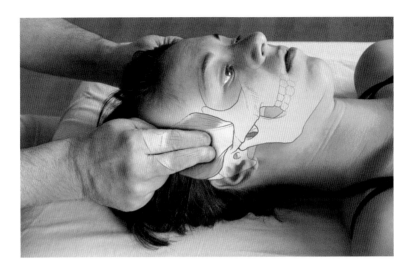

Positions
- Patient: supine
- Clinician: sitting at the head of the table

Instructions
- Place the patient's head and neck in a neutral position.
- Bilaterally, palpate the temporal bones superior to the ear, using the pads of two or three fingers.
- To confirm palpation, have the patient bite down. You should feel the muscle contract under your fingers.

Medial Pterygoid

Intraoral

Note

Before attempting intraoral palpation, the clinician should review nonverbal signs of communication with the patient to establish hand signals to indicate the palpation is uncomfortable.

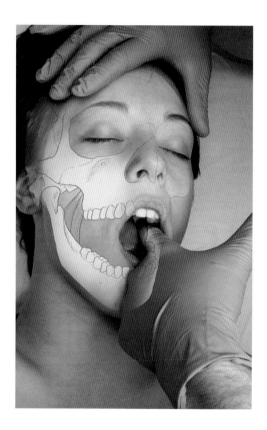

Positions
- Patient: supine
- Clinician: standing next to the head of the patient

Instructions
- Wearing gloves, place the second digit posterior to the last molar on the lower jaw.
- Push against the inside of the cheek in a posterior–lateral direction.
- To confirm palpation, have the patient perform lateral excursion to the contralateral side. You should feel a small contraction under your fingers.

> continued

MEDIAL PTERYGOID > *continued*

Extraoral

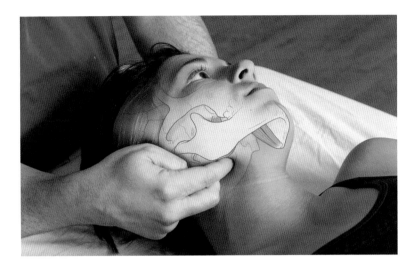

Positions
- Patient: supine
- Clinician: sitting at the head of the table

Instructions
- Palpate the angle of the mandible with the pads of the second and third digits.
- Hook the fingers around to the medial surface of the mandibular angle.
- To confirm palpation, have the patient bite down. You should feel a small contraction under your fingers.

Lateral Pterygoid

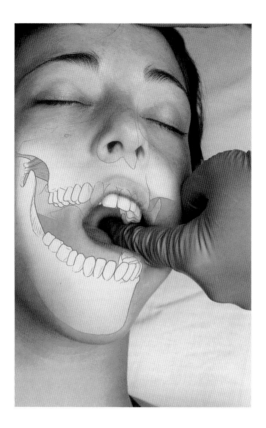

Positions
- Patient: supine
- Clinician: standing next to the head of the patient

Instructions
- Wearing gloves, place the second digit lateral and posterior to the last molar on the upper jaw.
- Apply pressure superiorly and posteriorly into the small space formed by the inside of the cheek and the mandibular condyle.
- To confirm palpation, have the patient perform lateral excursion to the contralateral side. You should feel a small contraction under the fingers.

Note
These palpations can be performed with the clinician standing either contralateral or ipsilateral to the side being palpated. In addition, the intraoral palpations are preferred for these muscles. Extraoral palpation should be performed only if the patient is unable to open the mouth enough to allow proper performance or if the patient is uncomfortable with the clinician's hands in his or her mouth.

Case Study

History

A 35-year-old female presents to your clinic reporting progressive right TMJ pain. She states that the pain began 4 weeks ago after having dental work done, during which her mouth was kept in an open position for 2 hours. She reports calling the dentist, who advised her to apply ice and take Motrin for pain relief. Over the past month, the pain has gotten worse, and it is now interfering with eating, sleeping, and working. She states that the pain is just anterior to her ear canal and radiates to the right cheek. She also reports that she is experiencing intermittent headaches three or four times a week. She reports no clicking with opening or closing of her mouth. She is an administrative assistant for a law firm and works between 40 and 50 hours per week. She is married with no children.

- Based on the subjective information alone, what are the three most likely diagnoses?

Examination

Past medical history	Unremarkable
Medication	Motrin
Observation	Increased scapular winging, forward head posture, increased thoracic kyphosis
Active range of motion	Cervical spine within normal limits, pain at end-range flexion, temporomandibular opening 0 to 20 millimeters with pain and deviation to the right
Passive range of motion	Same as above
Manual muscle testing	Serratus anterior, middle trapezius, and lower trapezius = 4–/5 Deep neck flexors (longus colli and capitis)—poor endurance
Special tests	Negative Spurling's test Negative distraction test Negative craniocervical rotation test
Other	Hypomobility of right TMJ Normal neurological screen

- Based on the subjective and objective information together, what are the two most likely diagnoses? Give your rationale for eliminating the third diagnosis.
- What structures should you palpate on this patient based on your differential diagnoses?

- Given all the information presented, what would you expect to find upon palpation of those structures?

Case Solution and Discussion

Potential Diagnoses Based on History
- Anterior disc displacement with reduction
- Cervicogenic headaches
- TMJ soft tissue dysfunction

Potential Diagnoses Based on History and Examination
- Cervicogenic headaches
- TMJ soft tissue dysfunction

Anterior disc displacement with reduction: This diagnosis can be eliminated due to the lack of subjective reports of clicking and the lack of palpable or audible clicking during range of motion testing.

Structures to Be Palpated
- Masseter
- Temporalis
- Pterygoids
- Suboccipital muscles
- Sternocleidomastoid
- Mandibular condyle (with mouth opening and closing)
- Transverse processes of C1

Palpation Findings
- Tenderness to palpation of the masseter, temporalis, and suboccipital muscles and the sternocleidomastoid
- Exquisite tenderness to palpation of the right medial pterygoid
- Tenderness to palpation of the mandibular condyle and transverse processes of C1

Clinical Reasoning
- Cervicogenic headache: The forward head posture and suboccipital muscle spasm combined with the reports of intermittent headaches and poor endurance of the deep neck flexor muscles can be indicative of cervicogenic headaches. However, the negative craniocervical flexion test and normal cervical spine active and passive ranges of motion allow this diagnosis to be ruled out.
- TMJ soft tissue dysfunction: The prolonged dental work, subjective reports of pain, and limited active range of motion suggest a TMJ

dysfunction. The absence of clicking allows a disc dysfunction to be ruled out, while right mandibular deviation with opening of the mouth suggests a hypomobile right TMJ leading to subsequent muscle spasm.

Case Study Questions

1. What information do the palpation findings of the case give the clinician? How can this information be incorporated in the clinical decision-making process?
2. Think about how the examination findings (subjective and objective) lead to the differential diagnosis. What might you do differently?
3. If there was also a cervicogenic headache component to this case, how might this change the examination or treatment for this patient?

CHAPTER REVIEW QUESTIONS

1. What are the bones that comprise the neurocranium?
2. Name the important anatomical landmarks of the mandible.
3. What muscles are part of the suprahyoid group?
4. What muscles are part of the infrahyoid group?
5. What artery is responsible for bringing blood supply to the face?
6. What nerve is responsible for innervating the face?
7. What are the muscles of mastication? Which ones are superficial, and which are deep?

Superficial Back and Shoulder Complex

After completing this chapter, the reader will be able to do the following:

- Identify the key bony anatomical structures of the shoulder girdle complex.
- Identify and describe the soft tissues of the shoulder girdle complex, including muscles, ligaments, nerves, arteries, and veins.
- Identify on bony and skeletal models the origins and insertions of the rotator cuff and scapulothoracic muscles in order to aid in understanding osteokinematic action and surface palpation.
- Draw and discuss the parts of the brachial plexus.
- Palpate structures of the shoulder girdle.
- Integrate surface palpation findings to aid in the differential diagnosis of a patient with shoulder pain.

The shoulder girdle is frequently a source of pain and disability. Research has suggested that shoulder pain is common in the population, affecting approximately 16% to 21% of individuals.[1,2] The integrated ligaments, capsules, muscles, nerves, and vascular structures of this complex anatomical region can be a source of pain and functional limitations for many.[1,2]

Functions of the Shoulder Girdle Complex

The main function of the shoulder girdle and its associated soft tissues is proper placement of the hand in space.[3] This is possible because the shoulder girdle permits motion in all three cardinal planes. It is important to consider the amount of mobility available in the shoulder girdle. While mobility is important for people to accomplish functional tasks in everyday life, it also renders the shoulder girdle, specifically the glenohumeral joint, inherently unstable. It is for this reason that the joint's associated muscles are extremely important for dynamic stability during functional activities. Without the synchronous complex interaction of the bones, muscles, and ligaments in this region, people may become susceptible to a variety of pathologies causing pain and functional limitations in daily life.

Bony Anatomy

The shoulder complex is composed of the scapula, humerus, clavicle, and rib cage. The scapula (figure 3.1) is a broad, flat bone that sits on the rib cage between the second and seventh ribs.

- The anterior aspect of the scapula, the subscapular fossa, is concave.
- Posteriorly, the scapula is convex, with the spine of the scapula located at approximately the T4 vertebral level. The spine of the scapula separates the supraspinous fossa from the infraspinous fossa.[4]

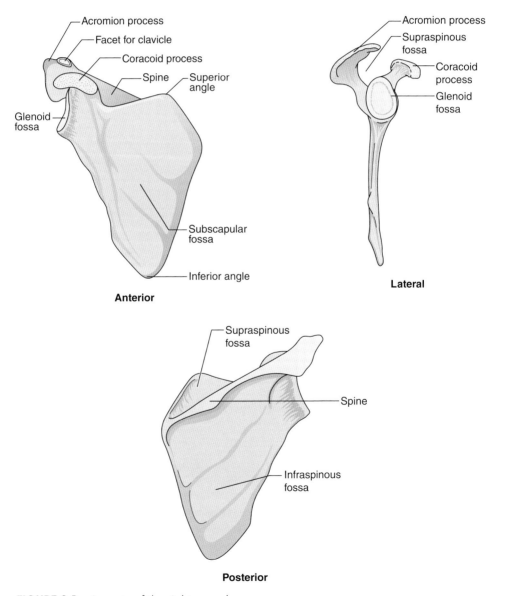

FIGURE 3.1 Aspects of the right scapula.

- At the lateral end of the spine of the scapula is the acromion process, which articulates with the clavicle (see figure 4.4), a curved bone that connects the axial skeleton to the appendicular skeleton and functions to transmit forces to (and from) the upper extremity.[3]

Superiorly on the scapula is the superior angle, located at approximately the T2 vertebral level, as well as the suprascapular notch. Located inferiorly is the inferior angle of the scapula, which is located at approximately the T7 vertebral level. The inferior angle of the scapula is often used for orientation, especially with helping to locate the lateral and medial borders of the scapula. The medial border, also called the vertebral border, is in close proximity to the spinous processes of the first seven thoracic vertebrae. Located laterally on the scapula is the glenoid fossa, a concave depression where the humeral head articulates to form the glenohumeral joint.[4]

In addition to the humeral head, the humerus has several other important landmarks (figure 3.2).

- Inferior to the humeral head is the anatomical neck of the humerus, which is an intra-articular structure.
- Below this are the surgical neck (extra-articular), greater tubercle, lesser tubercle, and the intertubercular (or bicipital) groove.[4]

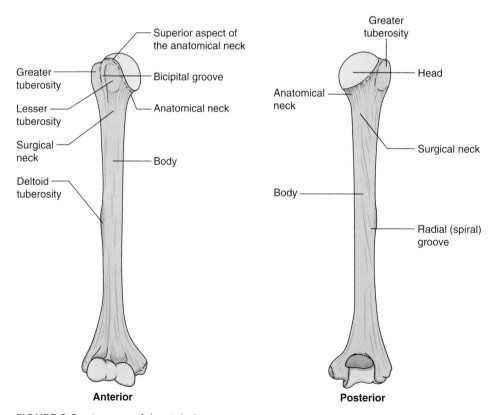

FIGURE 3.2 Aspects of the right humerus.

- On the midshaft of the anterior humerus is the deltoid tuberosity. This is where the deltoid muscle inserts.

- On the midshaft of the posterior humerus is the radial (or spiral) groove. The radial nerve wraps around the humerus through the spiral groove, while the axillary nerve wraps around the surgical neck of the humerus. Fractures of these bony landmarks can present with concomitant nerve damage.[4,5]

It should be pointed out that there is a functional relationship between the cervicothoracic spine and shoulder girdle. Many superficial and intermediate muscles of the cervical and thoracic spine have distal attachments on the clavicle, scapula, and humerus, and therefore move the scapula or humerus during overhead activities. While this chapter does not provide a detailed description of the bony landmarks of the cervical and thoracic spine, we encourage you to remember that there is a close relationship between the shoulder complex and proximal spinal anatomy that you should take into consideration during the examination of patients with shoulder pain.

The shoulder girdle consists of four joints:

- Glenohumeral joint (GHJ)
- Scapulothoracic joint (STJ)
- Acromioclavicular joint (ACJ)
- Sternoclavicular joint (SCJ)

The largest and most mobile of these joints is the GHJ. While many consider this joint the most important, we want to impress on you the importance of assessing the other joints as thoroughly and completely as possible. Full overhead motion is dependent on synchronized motion of all these joints. During the examination it is important to assess all the joints of the shoulder so you can ascertain the source of the problem. This will guide your clinical decision-making for choosing interventions that are specific for each joint involved.

The GHJ is a ball and socket joint that permits motion in the sagittal, frontal, and transverse planes. Due to the anatomic and kinesiologic design of the GHJ, its bony congruency is not enough to maintain the humeral head in the glenoid fossa.[3] The GHJ works together with the STJ, a functional joint between the scapula and rib cage, to produce full shoulder elevation. This concept is called scapulohumeral rhythm and is extremely important to assess during a shoulder examination. The scapula upwardly rotates so that people can perform shoulder flexion and abduction to 180°.

It is necessary for the ACJ and SCJ to work together for proper shoulder movement. The ACJ is a planar joint that is formed by the distal end of the clavicle and the acromion process, with an articular disc to increase joint congruency. The SCJ is a saddle joint that is formed by the medial end of the clavicle and the manubrium of the sternum, which also has an articular disc to increase joint congruency. Both of these joints produce osteokinematic (bone movement) and arthrokinematic (joint movement) motions to achieve full shoulder elevation. The SCJ is primarily responsible for STJ motion during the early phases of shoulder elevation, while the ACJ is responsible for allowing STJ motion during the later phases of shoulder elevation.[3]

Soft Tissue Anatomy

Several muscles that have important roles in coordinated movement surround the shoulder complex. These muscles can be divided into the axioscapular and scapulohumeral muscle groups.

- The axioscapular group (figure 3.3) consists of the trapezius, rhomboids, levator scapulae, and latissimus dorsi, which can all, depending on their anatomical attachments, move the scapula, the cervical spine, or both.
  - These muscles can be further broken down into superficial (trapezius and latissimus dorsi) and intermediate (levator scapulae and rhomboids) back muscles. The superficial muscles are easily palpable; whereas the deeper, intermediate muscles are more difficult to isolate.[4]
  - Knowing the different layers of these muscles can help you better appreciate the amount of force needed during palpation. These muscles, along with the rotator cuff muscles, serve to produce dynamic stability during functional activities.
- The scapulohumeral group runs from the scapula to the humerus. The larger and more superficial of these muscles are the deltoid and teres major, which are responsible for producing larger movements of the humerus.
- The deeper and smaller of these muscles are collectively known as the rotator cuff muscles.
  - The rotator cuff consists of four muscles: the supraspinatus, infraspinatus, teres minor, and subscapularis (figure 3.4).

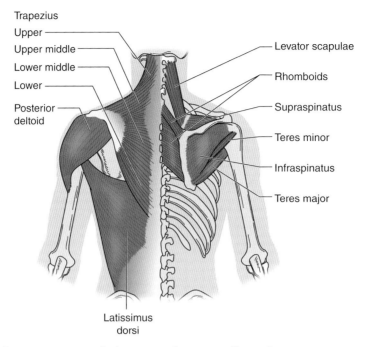

FIGURE 3.3   Posterior scapulothoracic and rotator cuff muscles.

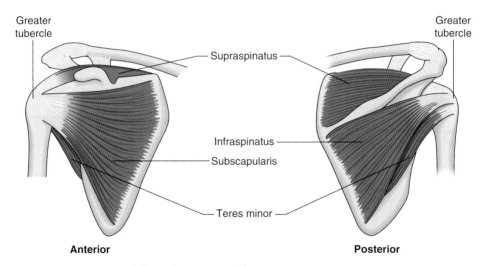

FIGURE 3.4   Aspects of the right rotator cuff.

- The supraspinatus, infraspinatus, and teres minor are all posteriorly located on the scapula, while the subscapularis occupies the subscapular fossa along the anterior side of the scapula.[4]
- Collectively, these are classified as local stabilizing muscles and function to increase dynamic stability of the shoulder joint.[3,4]

On the posterior aspect of the shoulder is the quadrangular space. The quadrangular space has four borders:[4]

- The superior border of the quadrangular space is the teres minor.
- The inferior border is the teres major.
- The medial border is the long head of the triceps.
- The lateral border is the surgical neck of the humerus.

Passing through the quadrangular space are the axillary nerve and posterior circumflex humeral artery (see figure 4.6). After passing through the quadrangular space, the axillary nerve is responsible for innervating the deltoid, teres minor, and the skin on the superior lateral aspect of the shoulder (superior lateral brachial cutaneous nerve).[4]

The joints of the shoulder also have several other soft tissue structures that increase passive stability, especially during overhead motion. The passive structures of the GHJ are the glenoid labrum, the capsule, and several ligaments.

- The labrum is a fibrocartilaginous tissue that adds both mechanical and proprioceptive stability. It functions to deepen the glenoid fossa and increase surface area for the articulating humeral head.

- The ligaments of the GHJ can be divided into intrinsic and extrinsic ligaments. The intrinsic ligaments attach to the joint capsule and include the superior, middle, and inferior glenohumeral ligaments as well as the coracohumeral ligament (figure 3.5).[4] These ligaments function to provide passive stability during different positions of shoulder abduction and external rotation.[3,6]

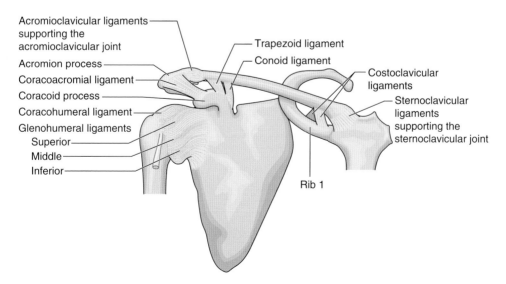

FIGURE 3.5 Ligaments of the shoulder complex.

- The only extrinsic ligament of the GHJ is the coracoacromial ligament, which attaches from the coracoid process to the acromion process, forming the coracoacromial arch, or space. Passing under this arch are the supraspinatus tendon, the long head of the biceps, and the subdeltoid bursa.

In healthy people, the height of the coracoacromial arch measures only 1 centimeter (0.4 inch), thereby increasing the chance for compression or impingement of the structures passing under the arch.[7] The subdeltoid bursa is responsible for preventing friction between the superficial deltoid and the deeper rotator cuff tendons.[3]

Both the ACJ and the SCJ also have ligaments that help provide passive stability. The ACJ is stabilized by both the acromioclavicular and coraco-clavicular ligaments, while the SCJ has the costoclavicular and sterno-clavicular ligaments (see figure 3.5). In addition, both joints contain an articular disc that functions to increase the congruency of these joints.[4] All these structures, along with the joint capsules, provide passive stability.

Neurovascular Anatomy

As mentioned in chapter 2, the right subclavian artery is a branch of the brachiocephalic trunk, and the left subclavian artery comes directly off the aortic arch (see figure 2.7). These arteries are located in the same positions anatomically and follow identical paths on the two sides of the body.

- The subclavian artery runs posterior to the clavicle and becomes the axillary artery at the border of the first rib (figure 3.6).

- The axillary artery has several branches that are responsible for providing blood supply to the shoulder region. This artery travels in the axilla, where it lies posterior to the medial and lateral cords of the brachial plexus (chapter 4). The axillary artery travels as far down as the inferior border of the teres major, where it becomes the brachial artery.[4]

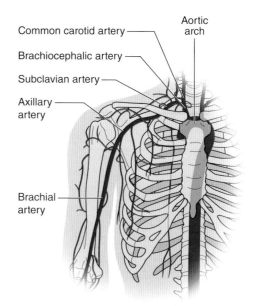

Common carotid artery

Aortic arch

Brachiocephalic artery

Subclavian artery

Axillary artery

Brachial artery

FIGURE 3.6 Subclavian, axillary, and brachial arteries.

In the shoulder region, two nerves, the suprascapular nerve and the axillary nerve, arise from the brachial plexus and are of particular importance (figure 3.7).

- The suprascapular nerve branches off the superior trunk of the plexus. It is responsible for innervating the supraspinatus and infraspinatus muscles. This nerve travels through the suprascapular notch and may become entrapped or compressed in the notch, thereby causing supraspinatus and infraspinatus muscle atrophy.[4,8]

- The axillary nerve is a branch of the posterior cord of the brachial plexus. It then passes through the quadrangular space and is responsible for innervating the deltoid, the teres minor, and the skin on the superior lateral aspect of the shoulder.[4]

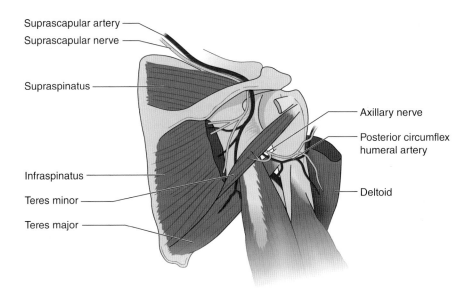

FIGURE 3.7 Quadrangular space with arteries and nerves of the shoulder.

Structural Inspection

- The clinician should first observe the patient walking into the examining room. This will allow the clinician to assess for deviations from the normal reciprocal arm swing pattern that occurs during gait. If the clinician observes guarded movement in one upper extremity during gait, it may be an indication of poor movement quality, pain, weakness, loss of motion, nerve injury, or a combination of these.

- If appropriate, the clinician should next observe as the patient removes any clothing necessary for the examination. This provides valuable information that can be immediately used to structure and prioritize the remainder of the examination.

- Observation of the patient in a static position from the anterior, posterior, and lateral views will give the clinician an opportunity to assess for scapular and humeral head position, as well as the overall position of the rib cage and thoracic spine.

- Clinicians should also assess for atrophy from one side to the other, paying particular attention to the deltoid and the regions above and below the spine of the scapula for possible findings suggestive of axillary or suprascapular nerve dysfunction, respectively.

- When assessing from the anterior view, the clinician should start by observing the clavicles bilaterally. These are easily observable and can provide information regarding the position of the entire shoulder girdle.

- Asymmetries of the entire shoulder girdle (particularly elevated or depressed scapula) should then be assessed from the posterior view to confirm findings.

- All observations should subsequently be integrated with the remainder of the examination findings.

Medial Border of the Scapula

Positions

- Patient: seated
- Clinician: standing behind the patient, on the side being palpated

Instructions

- Place the patient's hand behind the back, making the medial scapular border more prominent.
- Palpate along the medial border from a superior to inferior direction using two or three fingers.
- The medial border of the scapula is approximately 2 inches (5 centimeters) lateral from the spinous processes of the thoracic spine.

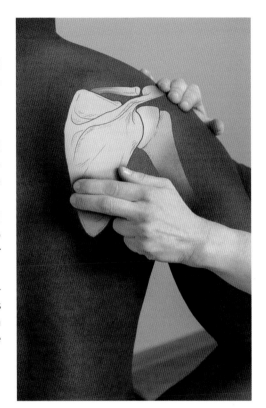

CLINICAL PEARL

The medial border of the scapula may become more prominent with weakness of the serratus anterior or damage to the long thoracic nerve.[9] This is called scapular winging (see the photo) and may be present in patients with shoulder pathology such as subacromial impingement syndrome and rotator cuff tears.[10]

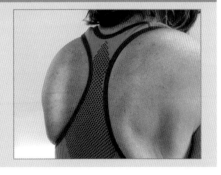

Superior Angle of the Scapula

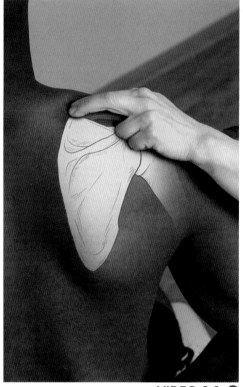

VIDEO 3.1 ▶

Positions
- Patient: seated
- Clinician: standing behind the patient, on the side being palpated

Instructions
- Place the patient's hand behind the back, making the medial scapular border more prominent.
- Palpate along the medial border using two fingers until the most superior aspect is reached and a bony prominence is felt under your fingers.

Inferior Angle of the Scapula

Positions

- Patient: seated
- Clinician: standing behind the patient, on the side being palpated

Instructions

- Place the patient's hand behind the back, making the medial scapular border more prominent.
- Palpate along the medial border using two fingers until the most inferior aspect is reached and a curved bony prominence is felt under your fingers.

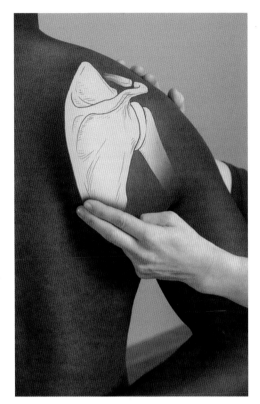

CLINICAL PEARL

The inferior angle is often used to assess scapulohumeral rhythm and eccentric scapular control by the trapezius and serratus anterior muscles.[3] In patients presenting with subacromial impingement and rotator cuff tears, eccentric control of these muscles is extremely important for producing coordinated, smooth, and efficient movement of the shoulder girdle complex.[1,10] During overhead motion, you should assess for several types of scapular dysfunction, including, but not limited to, scapular winging, scapular tipping, and scapular elevation.[11]

Lateral Border of the Scapula

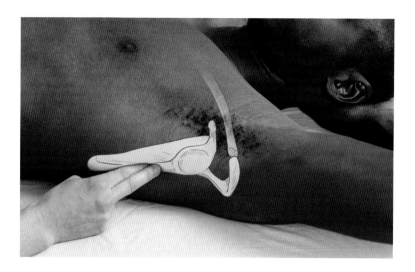

Positions

- Patient: supine
- Clinician: sitting to the side of the patient, on the side being palpated

Instructions

- Place the patient's hand behind the head (with the shoulder in flexion, abduction, and external rotation), making the lateral scapular border more prominent.
- Palpate along the lateral border from a superior to inferior direction using two or three fingers.

CLINICAL PEARL

The soft tissue around the lateral scapular border can become tender and short (tight) with prolonged guarding or shoulder immobilization.

Spine of the Scapula

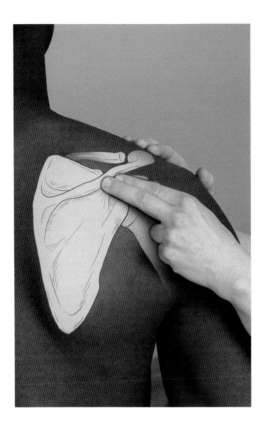

Positions
- Patient: seated
- Clinician: standing behind patient, on the side being palpated

Instructions
- Place the patient's hand behind the back, making the medial scapular border more prominent.
- Palpate along the medial border from an inferior to superior direction.
- Approximately three-fourths of the way up (T4 vertebral level), a bony ridge will be palpable.
- Palpate along the spine of the scapula by moving two fingers from medial to lateral.

Acromion Process

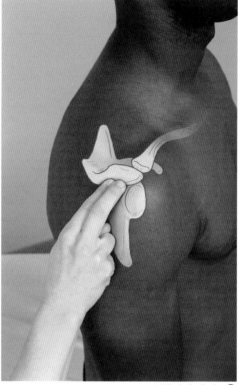

VIDEO 3.2 ▶

Positions
- Patient: seated
- Clinician: standing on the side and slightly posterior to the shoulder being palpated

Instructions
- Place the patient's hand on the anterior–lateral aspect of the iliac crest.
- Palpate the spine of the scapula.
- Follow along the spine of the scapula, from medial to lateral using two fingers, until it joins with the acromion process.
- Palpate the posterior, lateral, and anterior aspects of the acromion process.

Coracoid Process

Positions

- Patient: seated
- Clinician: standing facing the patient, slightly lateral to the shoulder being palpated

Instructions

- Using two fingers, palpate the lateral aspect of the clavicle.
- At the most distal aspect (concave segment), move slightly inferiorly and apply force in a posterior–lateral direction toward the humeral head.
- A bony prominence should be felt under your fingers.

Note

Several soft tissues attach to the coracoid process (short head of the biceps brachii, coracobrachialis, pectoralis minor, and the coracoacromial ligament) and thus may make this palpation uncomfortable for patients. We encourage you to compare the amount of tenderness to the opposite, uninvolved extremity during the examination process to differentiate between normal tenderness and possible pathology. You may also alter the position of the upper extremity to account for patient comfort.

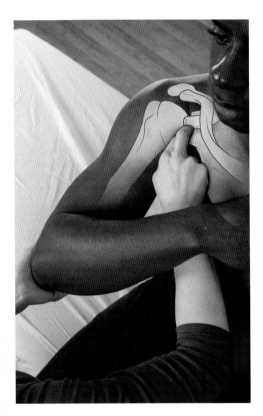

Greater Tubercle of the Humerus

Positions

- Patient: seated
- Clinician: standing to the side of and slightly posterior to the patient

Instructions

- Place the patient's hand on the thigh.
- Palpate the lateral border of the acromion.
- Move two fingers inferiorly approximately one finger-width and palpate the greater tubercle. There should be a slight step-off between the lateral end of the acromion and the greater tubercle of the humerus.
- To confirm the palpation, have the patient alternately internally and externally rotate the shoulder while you feel for movement of the greater tubercle.

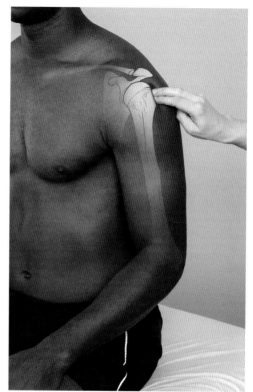

VIDEO 3.3 ▶

CLINICAL PEARL

If tenderness is assessed at the greater tubercle of the humerus following trauma to the shoulder, you should consider referring the patient to a physician to rule out possible fractures or rotator cuff tears.

Intertubercular Groove of the Humerus

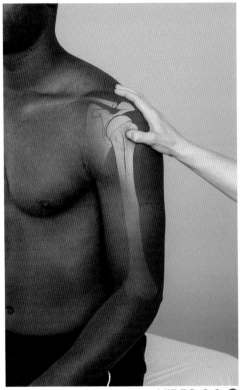

VIDEO 3.3 ▶

Positions
- Patient: seated
- Clinician: standing to the side of the patient, on the side being palpated

Instructions
- Place the patient's hand on the thigh.
- Palpate the greater tubercle of the humerus with digit 1.
- Move one fingerwidth medially and anteriorly to palpate the intertubercular groove.
- The long head of the biceps brachii lies within the intertubercular groove. When palpating the long head of the biceps, internally and externally rotate the humerus. You should feel it move under your fingers.
- The intertubercular (bicipital) groove is more easily palpated with the shoulder in external rotation.

Lesser Tubercle of the Humerus

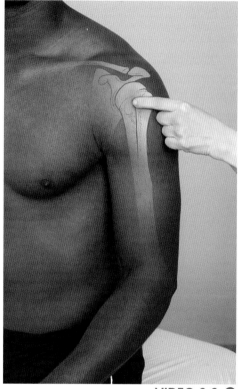

VIDEO 3.3 ▶

Positions
- Patient: seated
- Clinician: standing to the side of the patient, on the side being palpated

Instructions
- Place the patient's hand on the thigh.
- Palpate the intertubercular groove of the humerus with digit 2.
- Move slightly anteriorly and medially to palpate the lesser tubercle.

Note
The lesser tuberosity is at the level of the coracoid process.

Deltoid Tuberosity

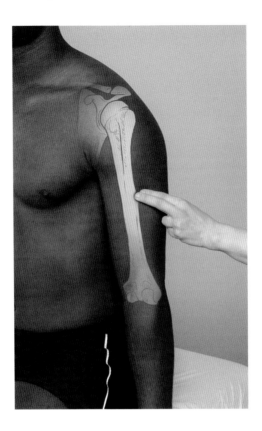

Positions
- Patient: seated
- Clinician: standing to the side of and slightly posterior to the patient, on the side being palpated

Instructions
- Place the patient's hand on the waist.
- Palpate the lateral aspect of the acromion process using two fingers.
- Move your fingers inferiorly approximately 2 to 2.5 inches (5 to 6.4 centimeters).
- You should feel a small bony projection along the midshaft of the anterior lateral humerus.
- To confirm palpation, have the patient abduct the shoulder. You should feel the deltoid contract at the distal attachment.
- Ask the patient to relax so that you can accurately feel the deltoid tuberosity.

Muscles of the Superficial Back and Shoulder

Muscle	Origin	Insertion	Innervation	Blood supply	Action
AXIOSCAPULAR					
Trapezius	External occipital protuberance, superior nuchal line, ligamentum nuchae, spinous processes of C7 to T12	Acromion process, spine of the scapula, lateral one-third of the posterior aspect of the clavicle	Spinal accessory nerve (cranial nerve IX, C3-C4)	Transverse cervical artery, dorsal scapular artery	Upward scapular rotation, ipsilateral side bending, contralateral rotation of the neck *Upper fibers:* elevation of the scapula *Lower fibers:* depression of the scapula *Middle fibers:* retraction of the scapula
Latissimus dorsi	Iliac crest, lower three or four ribs, thoracolumbar fascia, spinous processes T7 to T12, inferior angle of the scapula	Floor of the intertubercular groove of the humerus	Thoracodorsal nerve (C6-C8)	Thoracodorsal artery	Shoulder extension, internal rotation, and adduction
Rhomboids	Spinous processes of C7 to T5	Medial border of the scapula	Dorsal scapular nerve (C5)	Dorsal scapular artery	Scapular retraction and downward rotation
Levator scapulae	Posterior tubercles, transverse processes of C1 to C4	Superior angle of the scapula into the medial border	Dorsal scapular nerve (C5)	Dorsal scapular artery, transverse cervical artery	Elevation of the scapula, downward scapular rotation, ipsilateral side-bending, and rotation of the neck

Muscle	Origin	Insertion	Innervation	Blood supply	Action
SCAPULOHUMERAL					
Deltoid	Acromion process, spine of the scapula, lateral one-third of the anterior aspect of the clavicle	Deltoid tuberosity of the humerus	Axillary nerve (C5-C6)	Posterior circumflex humeral artery, branch of thoraco-acromial artery	*Anterior fibers:* flexion and internal rotation of the shoulder *Posterior fibers:* extension and external rotation of the shoulder *Middle fibers:* abduction of the shoulder
Supraspinatus	Supraspinous fossa of the scapula	Superior facet of the greater tubercle of the humerus	Suprascapular nerve (C5-C6)	Suprascapular artery	Shoulder abduction
Infraspinatus	Infraspinous fossa of the scapula	Middle facet of the greater tubercle of the humerus	Suprascapular nerve (C5-C6)	Suprascapular artery	Shoulder external rotation
Teres minor	Lateral border of the scapula	Inferior facet of the greater tubercle of the humerus	Axillary nerve (C5-C6)	Circumflex scapular artery	Shoulder external rotation and adduction
Subscapularis	Subscapular fossa	Lesser tubercle of the humerus	Upper and lower subscapular nerve (C5-C7)	Subscapular artery, lateral thoracic artery	Shoulder internal rotation and adduction
Teres major	Inferior angle of the scapula	Intertubercular groove of the humerus	Lower subscapular nerve (C6-C8)	Circumflex scapular artery	Shoulder internal rotation and adduction

Zone I: Axioscapular Muscles

Trapezius

Positions

- Patient: prone
- Clinician: standing to the side of the patient, on the side being palpated

Instructions

- Locate the external occipital protuberance and place the pads of four fingers on the upper fibers of the trapezius, just inferior and slightly lateral to the protuberance.

- Use one hand to palpate the upper fibers of the trapezius, while the other hand palpates the middle and lower fibers.

- To confirm palpation of the upper fibers of the trapezius, have the patient elevate the scapula. You should feel the muscle contract under your fingers.

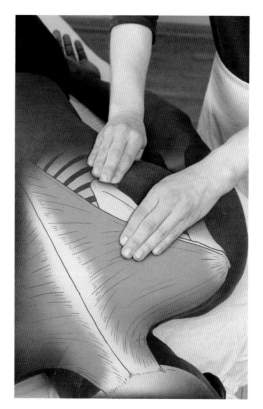

- To confirm palpation of the middle and lower fibers of the trapezius, have the patient retract and depress the scapula, respectively. You should feel the muscle contract under your fingers.

CLINICAL PEARL

The upper trapezius often becomes short (tight), and the middle and lower fibers of the trapezius become long and weak, contributing to certain shoulder pathologies such as subacromial impingement syndrome and rotator cuff tears.[10]

Latissimus Dorsi

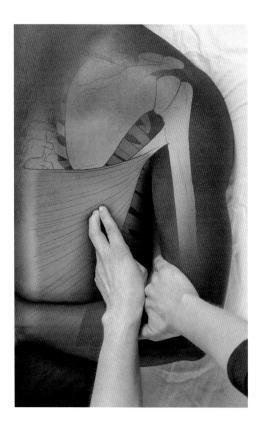

Positions
- Patient: prone, with the dorsal aspect of the patient's hand resting in the small of the back
- Clinician: sitting to the side of the patient, on the side being palpated

Instructions
- Palpate along the posterior–lateral trunk from the iliac crest up to the lateral scapular border using two or three fingers.
- To confirm palpation, have the patient perform resisted extension and adduction of the arm by providing manual resistance at the posterior–medial elbow (right hand pictured). You should feel a large contraction under your fingers (left hand pictured).

Rhomboids

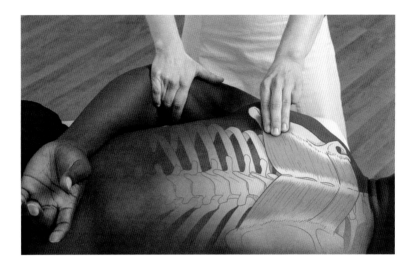

Positions

- Patient: prone, with the dorsal aspect of the hand resting in the small of the back
- Clinician: standing slightly behind and lateral to the side being palpated

Instructions

- Palpate the medial border of the scapula.
- Move the pads of two or three fingers medially until palpating soft tissue.
- To confirm palpation, have the patient retract the scapula while you provide resistance at the posterior–medial elbow (right hand pictured). You should feel the muscle contract under your fingers (left hand pictured).

Note

Placing the hand in the small of the back downwardly rotates the scapula, thereby inhibiting the trapezius, making palpation of the rhomboid easier.

Levator Scapulae

Positions

- Patient: sitting, with the dorsal aspect of the hand resting in the small of the back
- Clinician: standing slightly behind the patient, on the side being palpated

Instructions

- Palpate the superior angle of the scapula using two fingers.
- With firm pressure, feel for the insertion of the levator scapulae.
- To confirm palpation, have the patient slowly elevate the scapula. You should feel a small contraction under your fingers.

Notes

- This position of the hand behind the back will inhibit the trapezius muscle and make

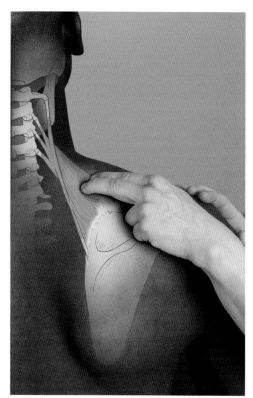

VIDEO 3.4 ▶

palpation of the levator scapulae more accurate. Follow this muscle up into the posterior cervical triangle where it will no longer be covered by the trapezius.

- A slow elevation of the scapula will be performed by the levator scapulae, while a rapid elevation of the scapula is more likely to be elicited by a contraction of the upper trapezius.

Zone II: Scapulohumeral Muscles

Deltoid

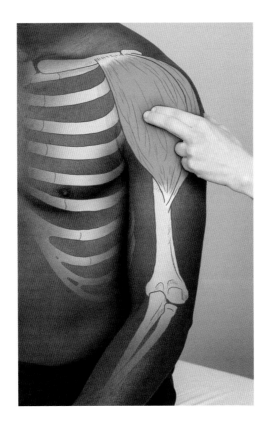

Positions
- Patient: sitting
- Clinician: standing to the side of the patient, on the side being palpated

Instructions
- Palpate the contour of the shoulder.
- Palpate the origin of the anterior, middle, and posterior fibers of the deltoid using two or three fingers. Start anteriorly, move laterally, and then posteriorly to assess all three parts of the deltoid.
- Follow the fibers inferiorly as the muscle inserts on the deltoid tuberosity of the humerus.
- To confirm palpation, have the patient perform resisted shoulder flexion (anterior deltoid), resisted shoulder abduction (middle deltoid), and resisted shoulder extension (posterior deltoid). You should feel a large contraction under your fingers.

Supraspinatus

Positions

- Patient: sitting with the dorsal aspect of the hand resting in the small of the back
- Clinician: standing behind the patient, on the side being palpated

Muscle Belly

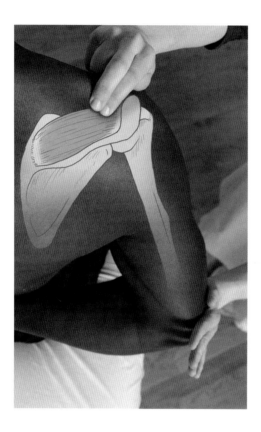

Instructions

- Palpate the spine of the scapula from medial to lateral.
- Close to the posterior aspect of the acromion process, move two fingers superiorly into a small depression, which is the supraspinous fossa.
- To confirm palpation, have the patient perform resisted shoulder abduction (right hand pictured). You should feel a small contraction under your fingers (left hand pictured).

> continued

Tendon

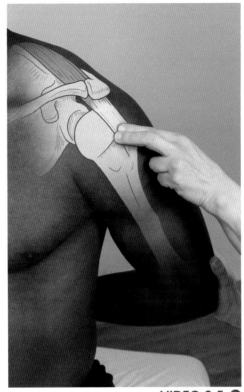

VIDEO 3.5 ▶

Instructions
- Palpate the anterior aspect of the acromion process.
- Drop one fingerwidth below the anterior aspect of the acromion process and palpate the supraspinatus tendon on its way to the greater tubercle using two fingers.
- To confirm palpation, have the patient perform resisted shoulder abduction (right hand pictured). You should feel a small contraction under your fingers (left hand pictured).

CLINICAL PEARL

Gaining better access to the supraspinatus tendon by moving the larger deltoid muscle out of the way (by having the dorsal aspect of the hand in the small of the back) increases the accuracy of the palpation.[12] This can assist clinicians during treatment when performing cross-friction massage of the musculotendinous and tenoperiosteal aspects of the supraspinatus.

Soft Tissues

Infraspinatus and Teres Minor

Positions

- Patient: prone on elbows
- Clinician: standing to the side of the patient, on the side being palpated

Instructions

- Have the patient shift his or her weight to the side being palpated.
- Palpate the spine of the scapula from medial to lateral.
- Identify the lateral aspect of the acromion using two fingers.
- Move inferiorly to palpate the greater tubercle.
- Move your fingers one finger-width down to palpate the tendons of the infraspinatus and teres minor. To palpate the muscle bellies, move your fingers medially below the spine of the scapula.

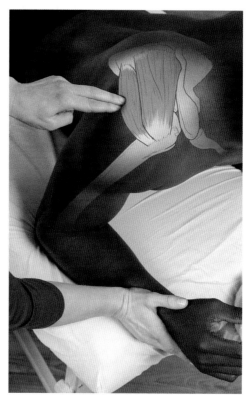

VIDEO 3.6 ▸

- To confirm palpation, have the patient perform resisted shoulder external rotation (right hand pictured). You should feel the contraction under your fingers (left hand pictured).

CLINICAL PEARL

This position will allow better access to the tendons of the posterior rotator cuff muscles.[12] These tendons are often involved clinically in pathologies such as rotator cuff tears, subacromial impingement, and rotator cuff tendinitis or tendinosis, and may require palpation and subsequent soft tissue mobilization.[13,14]

Subscapularis

Positions
- Patient: supine, with the shoulder in abduction (i.e., hand on anterior superior iliac spine)
- Clinician: sitting to the side of the patient, on the side being palpated

Muscle Belly

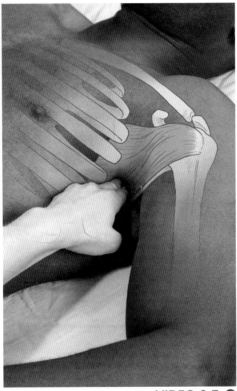

VIDEO 3.7 ▶

Instructions
- Palpate the lateral border of the scapula using two or three fingers.
- Move anterior to the lateral border until soft tissue is felt—this is the subscapular fossa.
- To confirm palpation, have the patient perform resisted shoulder internal rotation. You should feel a large contraction under your fingers.

Tendon

Instructions

- Making a diamond with your first and second digits bilaterally, place your hands on the patient with your second digits cupping over the superior aspect of the shoulder.
- With your thumbs, palpate the superior aspect of the axilla.
- Slowly applying firm pressure, apply force in a superior direction until palpating the subscapularis tendon.
- To confirm palpation, have the patient perform resisted shoulder internal rotation. You should feel a small contraction (similar to a guitar string) under your fingers.

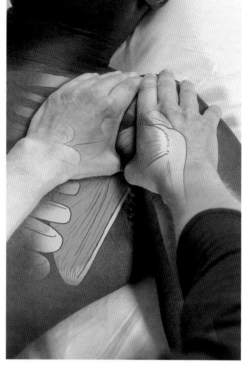

Notes

- Because this is a very deep structure, it may be uncomfortable for the patient during palpation, and good communication skills are extremely important during this palpation technique.
- With the hand resting on the waist, the shoulder is placed in the scapular position to allow better access to the muscle.

CLINICAL PEARL

When performing palpation of the subscapularis tendon, it is important to remember that the brachial plexus and axillary artery are located in close proximity to the tendon. The patient should be educated on the possibility of feeling numbness or tingling (or both) in the hand and on the importance of communicating this to the clinician so adjustments to the palpation technique can be made if necessary. It is our opinion that this specific subscapularis tendon palpation technique is extremely important as a treatment intervention for patients who have been in a sling for a period of time, in which the shoulder is immobilized in internal rotation and adduction. Often these patients have limitations of shoulder external rotation. Accurate palpation of the tendon will allow you to perform soft tissue mobilization when indicated, which may decrease pain, increase blood flow, and improve tissue extensibility.[1,3,12]

Teres Major

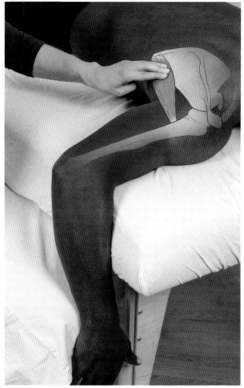

VIDEO 3.8 ▶

Positions

- Patient: prone, with the arm off the table in 90° of abduction resting on the clinician's knee or thigh
- Clinician: sitting next to the patient, on the side being palpated

Instructions

- Palpate the inferior angle of the scapula.
- Move three fingers from medial to lateral, assessing along the border of the teres major.
- To confirm palpation, have the patient perform resisted shoulder internal rotation. You should feel the muscle contract under your fingers.

Zone III: Subacromial and Subdeltoid Bursa

Subacromial Space

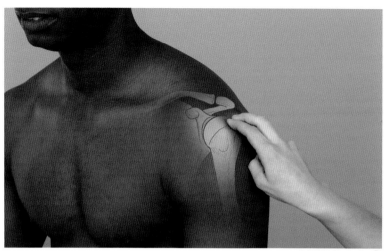

VIDEO 3.2 ▶

Positions
- Patient: seated
- Clinician: standing facing the patient, slightly lateral to the shoulder being palpated

Instructions
- Place the patient's hand on the waist.
- Palpate the acromion process.
- Move two fingers to the lateral-most aspect of the acromion.
- Move your fingers about a half to one fingerwidth inferior and lateral to the acromion, stepping off the lateral ridge until a gap is felt.
- Slowly follow along the subacromial space in both a posterior and anterior direction.

CLINICAL PEARL

Palpation of the subacromial space can provide information about the subacromial and subdeltoid bursa. Bursae are usually difficult to palpate, as indicated in chapter 1. However, when they are irritated and become filled with fluid, they often swell and may become more easily palpable. Palpating just below the anterior and lateral aspects of the acromion process will place the clinician's fingers (two) in the best possible location to assess the bursa.

Case Study

History

An 18-year-old male high school pitcher presents to your clinic complaining of right shoulder pain. The patient reports that the symptoms began 3 weeks ago after practice. He states that he saw the trainer at school, who iced his shoulder. He reports that the intensity of the pain has increased over the last 3 weeks, with a decrease in symptom onset time during throwing. He states that the pain is over the posterior and lateral aspect of his right shoulder. Symptoms are temporarily relieved with ice and over-the-counter anti-inflammatory medication. He is right hand dominant, lives at home with his parents, and works part time in a sporting goods store. He is the starting pitcher for the school team. They practice five times a week for 2 hours and have a game once a week. The patient starts a game once every 5 days.

- Based on only the information from the history, what are the three most likely diagnoses?

Examination

Past medical history	Unremarkable
Medication	Aleve
Observation	Increased scapular winging, forward head posture, increased thoracic kyphosis
Active range of motion	Right shoulder flexion = 0° to 160°, abduction = 0° to 160°, internal rotation = 0° to 50°, external rotation = 0° to 125°
Passive range of motion	Right shoulder within normal limits, except external rotation = 0° to 132°
Manual muscle testing	Within normal limits, except right external rotation = 3+/5 (secondary to pain), serratus anterior and middle and lower trapezius = 4−/5
Special tests	Negative Neer's test Negative Hawkins–Kennedy test Negative Yocum's test Negative labral tests (crank, O'Brien's, biceps load II) Positive internal rotation resisted strength test Positive relocation test Negative internal and external rotation lag signs
Other	Pain at end-range active and passive external rotation Pain at late cocking and deceleration phases of pitching Altered scapulohumeral rhythm (early upward rotation with flexion and abduction) Poor eccentric scapular control

- Based on the subjective and objective information together, what are the two most likely diagnoses? Give your rationale for eliminating the third diagnosis.
- What structures should you palpate on this patient based on your differential diagnoses?
- Given all the information presented, what would you expect to find upon palpation of those structures?

Case Solution and Discussion

Potential Diagnoses Based on History
- Impingement syndrome
- Labral tear
- Rotator cuff tear

Potential Diagnoses Based on History and Examination
- Labral tear
- Posterior impingement syndrome

Rotator cuff tear: This diagnosis can be eliminated due to the lack of a specific incident. Given the patient's age, a tear would most likely be caused by a traumatic incident. In addition, negative internal and external rotation lag signs, as well as no weakness with abduction strength testing, makes this diagnosis unlikely.

Structures to Be Palpated
- Trapezius
- Levator scapulae
- Long head of biceps
- Subscapularis
- C7 to T1 spinous and transverse processes
- Supraspinatus
- Infraspinatus and teres minor

Palpation Findings
- Tenderness to palpation of right upper, middle, and lower trapezius and levator scapulae
- Tenderness to palpation of right infraspinatus, teres minor, subscapularis, and long head of biceps

Clinical Reasoning
- Impingement syndrome: There are two types of impingement syndrome; subacromial impingement is the more common one, in which

the rotator cuff tendons get impinged under the coracoacromial arch. The other one, posterior (or internal) impingement, occurs when there is an anterior translation of the humeral head, and the articular surface of the supraspinatus and infraspinatus is irritated by their compression between the humeral head and glenoid labrum. This is common in overhead athletes, especially younger ones. Because this patient is a pitcher, he is in the group that is prone to posterior impingement. His younger age, reports of posterior and lateral shoulder pain, pain occurring in the late cocking and deceleration phases of pitching, negative special tests for subacromial impingement, positive relocation test, pain with passive external rotation, weak and tender external rotators and scapular muscles, altered scapulohumeral rhythm, and poor eccentric scapular control all indicate posterior impingement syndrome.

- Labral tear: The weakness and tenderness to palpation of the rotator cuff muscles, the altered scapulohumeral rhythm, and pain at the end range of external rotation and passive range of motion can be indicative of a labral tear. While this is common in overhead pitchers, no report of clicking and the negative special tests rule it out.

Case Study Questions

1. What information do the palpation findings of the case give the clinician? How can this information be incorporated in the clinical decision-making process?

2. Think about how the examination findings (subjective and objective) lead to the differential diagnosis. What might you do differently?

3. Think about the long-term outcome for this patient. Is surgical intervention necessary? Explain your answer.

CHAPTER REVIEW QUESTIONS

1. Name the four rotator cuff muscles. Which are anterior and which are posterior?

2. What structure sits in the intertubercular groove?

3. What is the difference between the anatomical and surgical necks of the humerus?

4. At what vertebral level are the spine of the scapula and the inferior angle of the scapula?

5. Name the three branches off the aortic arch.

6. What are the borders of the quadrangular space?

chapter **4**

Pectoral and Axillary Regions

CHAPTER OBJECTIVES

After completing this chapter, the reader will be able to do the following:

- Identify the key bony anatomical structures of the axillary and pectoral regions.
- Identify the borders of the axilla.
- Describe and draw the brachial plexus.
- Identify and describe the soft tissue anatomy of the axillary and pectoral regions, including muscles, ligaments, nerves, arteries, and veins.
- Identify on bony or skeletal models the origins and insertions of the muscles of the axillary and pectoral regions in order to aid in understanding osteokinematic action and surface palpation.
- Palpate structures of the axillary and pectoral regions.
- Integrate surface palpation findings to aid in the differential diagnosis of a patient with anterior chest or shoulder girdle pain or both.

The pectoral region and axilla are areas often examined and treated in patients with upper quarter or cervical dysfunction. It is important to be mindful of the vital vascular and neural structures that are related to this anatomical region. The brachial plexus as well as the axillary artery and its branches can produce signs, symptoms, or dysfunction that may be independent of any shoulder girdle or cervical dysfunction. This knowledge will assist you in making an accurate diagnosis. During palpation of this region, you should carefully educate your patients to communicate discomfort or symptoms that may indicate irritation to any of the vascular or neural structures present in this anatomical region.

Functions of the Pectoral Region

One of the most important functions of this anatomical region is the protection of the underlying thoracic viscera, most importantly the heart and lungs. In addition, the rib cage is not a rigid structure, and proper movement is necessary for rib cage expansion and contraction during breathing. This anatomical region, in conjunction with the shoulder girdle, creates a bridge between the axial and appendicular skeleton. Without proper stability of this area, mobility of the upper extremity may be lost or impaired.

Bony Anatomy

The pectoral region is composed of the sternum, rib cage, clavicles, and shoulder girdles (discussed in chapter 3). The sternum is a flat bone that has three parts: the manubrium, body, and xiphoid process (figure 4.1).

- The superior portion of the sternum is the manubrium, which serves as an important landmark for the identification of two other anatomical structures: the jugular notch and the sternal angle.
- The jugular notch is directly superior to the manubrium.
- The sternal angle is directly inferior to the manubrium. The sternal angle is between the manubrium and the body and is palpable in some individuals.[1]

The ribs are long, curved bones that form most of the thoracic cage (figure 4.2). There are 12 pairs of ribs on each side of the thoracic cage that articulate with their respective costal cartilage before finally attaching to the sternum at different points.

- Rib 1 attaches to the manubrium of the sternum.
- Rib 2 attaches to the sternal angle.
- Ribs 3, 4, 5, 6, and 7 attach to the body of the sternum.

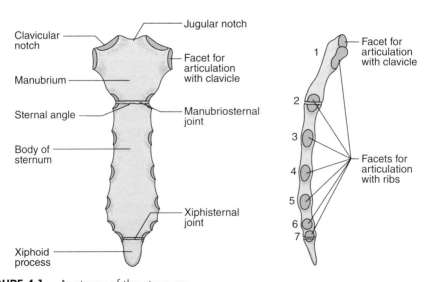

FIGURE 4.1 Anatomy of the sternum.

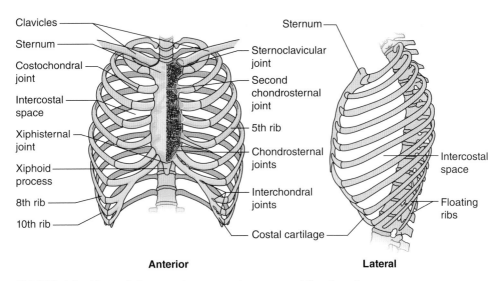

FIGURE 4.2 View of rib cage demonstrating true and floating ribs.

- Ribs 8, 9, and 10 do not have an attachment to the sternum, but rather attach to the rib above.
- Ribs 11 and 12 have no anterior attachment at all and thus are called floating ribs.

Posteriorly, the ribs each attach to a vertebra in the thoracic spine at the vertebral body (costovertebral joint) and the transverse process (costotransverse joint).[1] Between each rib is an intercostal space. These intercostal spaces serve as important anatomical landmarks during auscultation of the heart and lung sounds.

Posteriorly, each rib has a head, a neck, and an articular tubercle (figure 4.3). The head and articular tubercle of each rib articulates with a thoracic

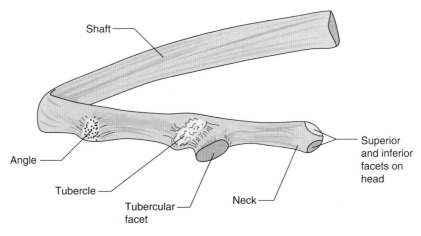

FIGURE 4.3 Typical rib.

vertebra to form the costovertebral and costotransverse joints.[1] These are both synovial joints that are capable of movement during ventilation and associated movements of the thoracic spine and are therefore stabilized with ligaments.[1,2] Ribs 11 and 12 do not have a costotransverse joint.[1,2]

At the superior portion of the thoracic cage are the clavicles (figure 4.4). These are long curved bones that connect the axial skeleton to the appendicular skeleton. The medial portion of the clavicle is convex anteriorly, making it easily palpable, while the lateral third of the clavicle is concave anteriorly, making it somewhat more difficult to palpate. The lateral end of the clavicle is called the acromial end and articulates with the acromion process to form the acromioclavicular joint (ACJ). The medial end of the clavicle is called the sternal end and articulates with the manubrium at the clavicular notch, to form the sternoclavicular joint (SCJ).[1] Superior and slightly posterior to the clavicle is the supraclavicular triangle. This triangle is formed by the clavicle anteriorly, the trapezius posteriorly, and the acromion process laterally.[1] Inside this triangle is where the first rib can be palpated from the posterior aspect.

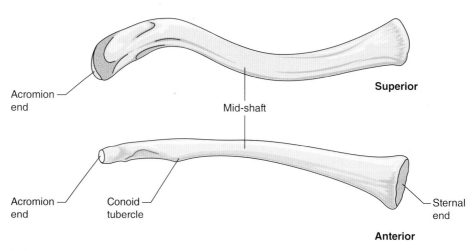

Acromion end

Mid-shaft

Superior

Acromion end

Conoid tubercle

Sternal end

Anterior

FIGURE 4.4 Views of the clavicle.

Soft Tissue Anatomy

Four muscles are located in the pectoral and axillary regions: the pectoralis major, the pectoralis minor, the serratus anterior, and the subclavius muscles (figure 4.5). The first three produce movements of the humerus and scapula, while the subclavius is responsible for increasing stability

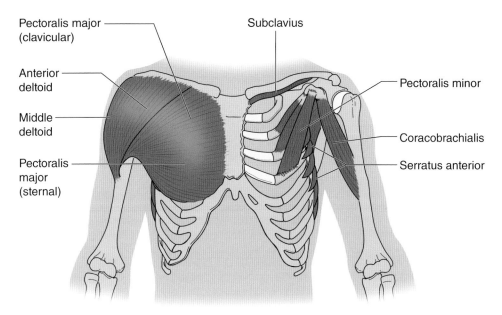

Pectoralis major
(clavicular)

Subclavius

Anterior
deltoid

Pectoralis minor

Middle
deltoid

Coracobrachialis

Pectoralis
major
(sternal)

Serratus anterior

FIGURE 4.5   Muscles of the anterior shoulder and axillary regions.

to the lateral aspect of the clavicle.[1] The largest of these muscles is the pectoralis major. It has three heads—the clavicular head, sternocostal head, and abdominal head—and is located directly under the skin on the anterior aspect of the thorax. Between the pectoralis major and the deltoid is the deltopectoral groove, where the cephalic vein travels. Deep to the pectoralis major and covered in fascia is the pectoralis minor muscle.[1] The serratus anterior occupies the anterior, lateral aspect of the rib cage, and the subclavius is located directly inferior to the clavicle.[1]

Three of the four muscles in this region form the borders of the axilla. The axilla has four borders.

- The anterior border is formed by the pectoralis major and pectoralis minor (figure 4.5).
- The posterior border is formed by the latissimus dorsi, subscapularis, and teres major (see figures 3.3 and 3.4). The posterior border of the axilla is where the quadrangular space can be found (see chapter 3).
- The medial border is the serratus anterior.
- The lateral border is the intertubercular groove of the humerus.

Several anatomical structures are located deep in the axilla (figure 4.6). These are the axillary artery and vein, the cords of the brachial plexus, and the long thoracic nerve, which innervates the serratus anterior muscle.[1]

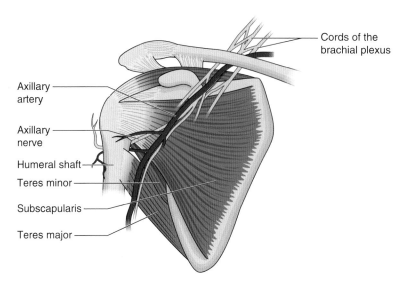

FIGURE 4.6 Neurovascular structures of the axilla.

Neurovascular Anatomy

Several important neurovascular structures in the axilla are responsible for providing both blood supply and innervation to the upper extremity. The axillary artery, which is the continuation of the subclavian artery, starts at the lateral aspect of the first rib and has three parts (figure 4.7).

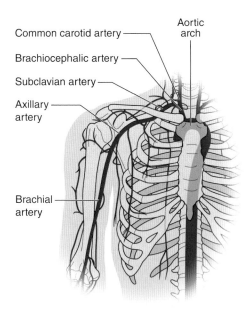

FIGURE 4.7 Arteries of the pectoral region.

- The first part runs from the lateral aspect of the first rib to the pectoralis minor.
- The second part runs posterior to the pectoralis minor.
- The third part travels from the pectoralis minor to the teres major.

The axillary artery and its branches are responsible for providing blood supply to the structures of the axilla, as well as the glenohumeral joint (GHJ).[1] The second part of the axillary artery is of particular importance because the cords of the brachial plexus are named with reference to this part of the artery. For example, the medial cord of the brachial plexus lies medial to the axillary artery, while the lateral cord of the brachial plexus lies lateral to the axillary artery. Anterior to the medial and lateral cords of the brachial plexus is the axillary vein.

The brachial plexus is formed from the ventral rami of the C5 to T1 nerve roots (figure 4.8). It is divided into different parts: roots, trunks, divisions, cords, and terminal branches.

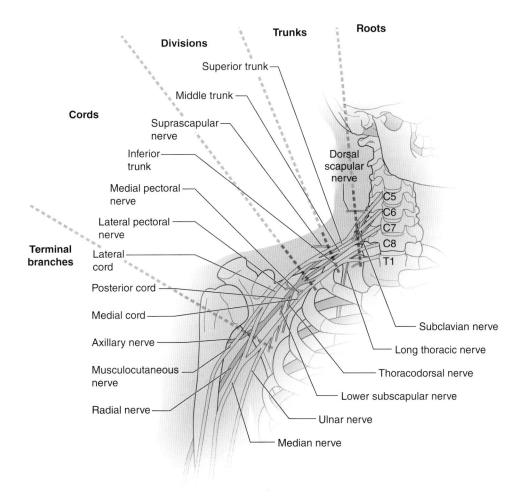

FIGURE 4.8 The brachial plexus.

- The roots of the brachial plexus (C5-T1) give rise to two nerves: the dorsal scapular nerve and the long thoracic nerve.[1]
- The roots of the plexus then combine to form the superior trunk (C5-C6), the middle trunk (C7), and the inferior trunk (C8-T1).
  - The superior trunk gives rise to two nerves, the suprascapular nerve and the nerve to the subclavius.
- Each trunk then divides to give three anterior divisions and three posterior divisions.
- These divisions reunite to form the lateral cord (C5-C7), the medial cord (C8-T1), and the posterior cord (C5-T1). Seven nerves come from the cords of the brachial plexus.
  - The lateral pectoral nerve comes from the lateral cord.
  - The medial pectoral nerve as well as the medial cutaneous nerve of the arm and the medial cutaneous nerve of the forearm come from the medial cord.
  - The upper, middle (thoracodorsal), and lower subscapular nerves come from the posterior cord.[1]
- Each cord then splits into two terminal branches.
  - The lateral cord splits into the musculocutaneous nerve and the lateral portion of the median nerve.
  - The medial cord splits into the ulnar nerve and the medial portion of the median nerve.
  - The posterior cord splits into the axillary nerve and radial nerve.

These nerves are responsible for innervating all muscles of the upper extremity.[1]

Structural Inspection

- Observation of the pectoral region and rib cage can be performed with the patient either sitting or standing.
- The sitting position may provide the clinician with information about the position of the spine and pectoral region when the lower extremities are not bearing weight.
- We encourage clinicians to assess the position of the pectoral region and rib cage with the patient both sitting and standing.
- One of the more important aspects to assess is the position of the rib cage relative to the pelvis.[3] While the Kendall classification system of posture has been the long-standing reference for many allied health professionals, it does not consider this relationship of the rib cage relative to the pelvis.[4] The relationship between the rib cage and pelvis

can provide information on how the spine and other structures accept load during functional activities. Clinicians should consider using the Saliba postural classification system[3] to determine the vertical alignment between the thorax and the pelvis.

- In addition, clinicians should assess for scapular movement that may be occurring while observing movement of the rib cage. Optimal movement is characterized by the scapula moving independently of the rib cage. Often, people are unable to do this and develop sub-optimal movement patterns during scapular exercises or functional activities. Please refer to chapter 3 for a more detailed discussion of scapular position and posture.

Sternal End of Clavicle

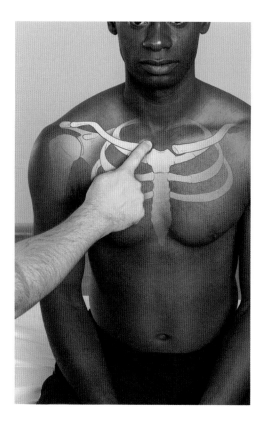

Positions

- Patient: sitting or supine
- Clinician: standing, facing the patient

Instructions

- Palpate along the medial one-third of the clavicle up to the jugular notch using one finger.
- Move laterally about one fingerwidth to palpate the medial end of the clavicle. You should feel a sharp bony prominence under your finger.

CLINICAL PEARL

Fractures of the medial one-third of the clavicle, which can include the sternal end, are not common in clinical practice.[5,6] However, possible neurovascular injury to the subclavian artery or brachial plexus needs to be evaluated during the examination via assessment of distal sensation in the medial, ulnar, and radial nerves as well as the brachial and radial pulses.

Acromial End of Clavicle

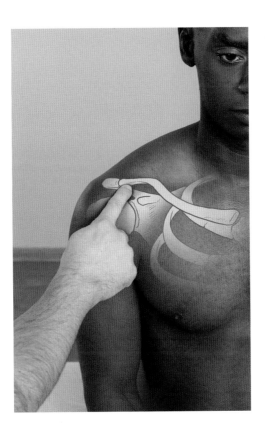

Positions

- Patient: sitting or supine
- Clinician: standing, facing the patient

Instructions

- Palpate the sternal end of the clavicle.
- Move one finger laterally along the shaft of the clavicle until reaching the acromion process (ACJ).
- Move medially one fingerwidth to palpate the acromial end of the clavicle.

CLINICAL PEARL

Fractures of the acromial end (distal one-third of the clavicle) account for a small percentage of clavicular fractures.[6,7] Possible complications include disruption of the ACJ, which if not surgically stabilized can lead to early degenerative changes in the joint. During palpation you may feel crepitus or an asymmetry at the ACJ.

Jugular Notch

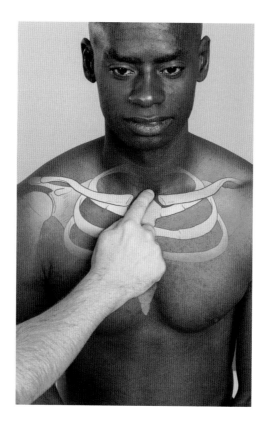

Positions

- Patient: sitting or supine
- Clinician: standing, facing the patient

Instructions

- Palpate the sternal end of the clavicle.
- Move one finger medially about one-half fingerwidth to palpate the jugular notch. You should feel a soft indentation under your finger.

Note

Palpate gently because the trachea is superficial in this area.

Manubrium

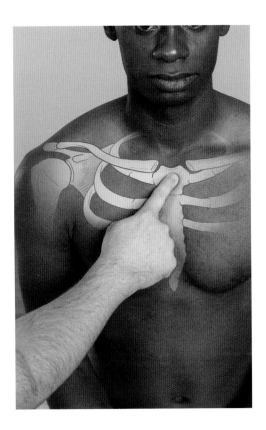

Positions
- Patient: sitting or supine
- Clinician: standing, facing the patient

Instructions
- Palpate the jugular notch.
- Move one finger inferiorly 1 to 2 inches (2.5 to 5 centimeters) to palpate the manubrium. You should feel a flat bone under your finger.

Sternal Angle

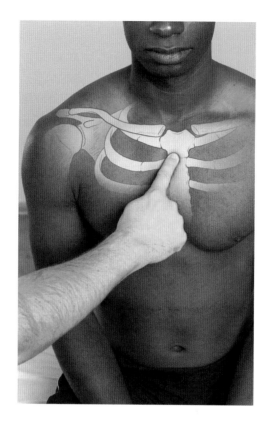

Positions
- Patient: sitting or supine
- Clinician: standing, facing the patient

Instructions
- Palpate the manubrium.
- Move inferiorly along the manubrium until a bony ridge is felt.

Note
The second rib articulates with the sternal angle.

Body of the Sternum

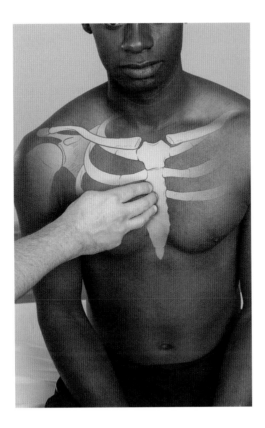

Positions

- Patient: sitting or supine
- Clinician: standing, facing the patient

Instructions

- Palpate the sternal angle.
- Move inferiorly to palpate the entire length of the body of the sternum using three fingers (approximately 5 inches, or 13 centimeters). You should feel a flat bone under your fingers.

Xiphoid Process

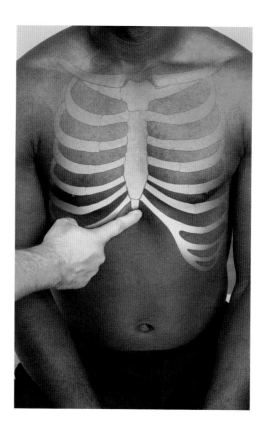

Positions

- Patient: sitting or supine
- Clinician: standing, facing the patient

Instructions

- Palpate the body of the sternum.
- Using one finger, move inferiorly to the point at which the lowermost ribs articulate with the sternum. You should feel a pointed structure under your finger.

Rib 1

Anterior Approach

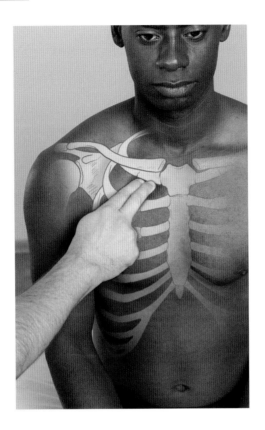

Positions
- Patient: sitting or supine
- Clinician: standing, facing the patient

Instructions
- Palpate the inferior surface of the sternal end of the clavicle.
- Using two fingers, move inferiorly and laterally to palpate the first rib under the clavicle.

> continued

Posterior Approach

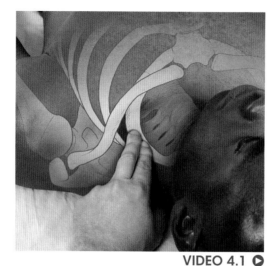

VIDEO 4.1 ▶

Positions
- Patient: supine
- Clinician: sitting or standing at the head of the patient

Instructions
- Palpate the clavicle anteriorly.
- Move two fingers posteriorly into the supraclavicular triangle.
- Using the pads of digits 2 and 3, apply force inferiorly (deep) to palpate the posterior border of the first rib. You should be posterior to the clavicle and anterior to the trapezius.

Note
Upon inspiration, the first rib should move superiorly into your finger.

CLINICAL PEARL

The first rib can become elevated or hypomobile secondary to a short anterior or middle scalene, causing cervical or thoracic spine pain or upper extremity symptoms (or both) on the involved side. The mobilization or manipulation to correct an elevated first rib is performed using the posterior approach. The cervical rotation lateral flexion (CRLF) test has been developed to assess for first-rib dysfunction.[8]

Rib 2

Anterior Approach

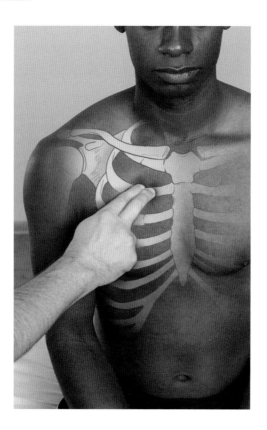

Positions
- Patient: sitting or supine
- Clinician: standing, facing the patient

Instructions
- Palpate the sternal angle.
- Using two fingers, move laterally to palpate along the entire border of rib 2.

> continued

RIB 2 > *continued*

Axilla (Lateral) Approach

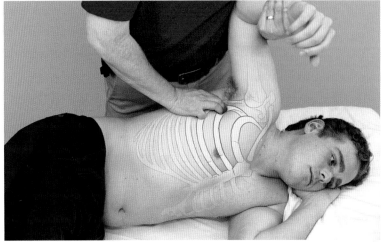

VIDEO 4.2 ▶

Positions
- Patient: supine or side-lying
- Clinician: sitting or standing

Instructions
- Cradling the patient's upper extremity, passively place it in a position of scaption (halfway between the sagittal and frontal planes).
- With the other hand, use two or three fingers to palpate the subscapularis along the posterior border of the axilla.
- Slide your fingers anteriorly to the medial border of the axilla (serratus anterior).
- From superficial to deep, apply gentle but firm inferior pressure to palpate the superior aspect of rib 2 by hooking on the superior aspect of the bone. You should feel a curved bone under your fingers.

CLINICAL PEARL
Mobility of the second rib should be assessed in people with cervicothoracic and shoulder pain. Hypomobility can lead to irritation of the radial nerve, which may cause nerve-like symptoms such as tingling, prickling, and creeping (paresthesia) in the posterior aspect of the arm and forearm and in the dorsum of the hand.

Rib 12

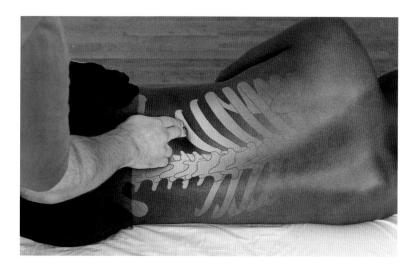

Positions

- Patient: sitting or side-lying
- Clinician: standing on the side being palpated or behind the patient

Instructions

- Palpate the inferior angle of the scapula.
- Move medially to palpate the T7 spinous process.
- Move inferiorly until the T12 spinous process.
- Using the pads of digits 2 and 3, move laterally to palpate the length of the 12th rib. You should feel a curved bone under your fingers.

Muscles of the Pectoral and Axillary Regions

Muscle	Origin	Insertion	Innervation	Blood supply	Action
Pectoralis major	*Clavicular head:* anterior aspect of the clavicle *Sternocostal head:* sternum and superior six costal cartilages *Abdominal head:* fascia of the external abdominal oblique	Lateral lip of the intertubercular groove of the humerus	Medial and lateral pectoral nerves (C5-C8)	Pectoral branch of thoraco-acromial artery, perforating branches of internal thoracic artery	Shoulder internal rotation and horizontal adduction *Clavicular head:* shoulder flexion *Sternocostal head:* shoulder extension
Pectoralis minor	Lateral aspect of ribs 3 to 5	Coracoid process	Medial pectoral nerve (C8-T1)	Pectoral branch of thoraco-acromial artery, superior and lateral thoracic arteries	Assistance in protraction and downward rotation of the scapula
Serratus anterior	Lateral aspect of ribs 1 to 8	Medial border of the scapula	Long thoracic nerve (C5-C7)	Lateral thoracic artery	Upward rotation of scapula and protraction
Subclavius	Lateral, inferior aspect of rib 1	Inferior aspect of clavicle	Nerve to subclavius (C5-C6)	Clavicular branch of thoracoacromial artery	Prevention of lateral displacement of the clavicle

Zone I: Anterior Border of the Axilla

Pectoralis Major

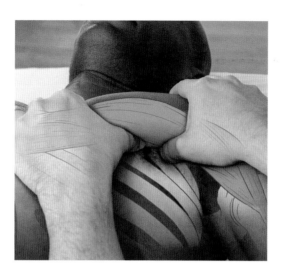

Positions
- Patient: supine
- Clinician: sitting, facing the patient, on the side being palpated

Instructions
- Place the patient's hand on the waist so the elbow is flexed to 90°.
- Using both thumbs, lift the lateral aspect of the pectoralis major and cup digits 2 to 5 over the anterior aspect in order to palpate the clavicular origin of the muscle (pictured).
- To palpate the origin of the sternocostal head, move your fingers inferiorly (not pictured).
- To confirm palpation, have the patient perform resisted shoulder horizontal adduction. You should feel a large muscle contraction under your fingers. Follow the fibers laterally as the muscle inserts on the humerus.

Pectoralis Minor

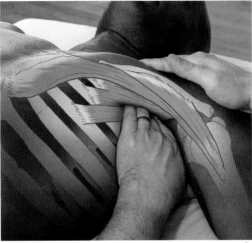

VIDEO 4.3 ▶

Positions
- Patient: supine
- Clinician: sitting, facing the patient, on the side being palpated

Instructions
- Place the patient's hand on the waist so the elbow is flexed to 90°.
- With one hand, palpate along the lateral border of the pectoralis major (right hand pictured).
- Slide three or four fingers under the pectoralis major to palpate the superior–lateral aspect of ribs 3 to 5 (left hand pictured).
- Use the other hand to passively shorten the pectoralis major over the palpating hand.
- To confirm palpation and isolate the pectoralis minor, have the patient tip the shoulder forward to anteriorly tilt the scapula. You should feel a subtle contraction under your fingers.

CLINICAL PEARL

The pectoralis minor inserts on the coracoid process, and when tight, can anteriorly tilt the scapula, thereby decreasing the diameter of the coracoacromial space.[9] Although the supporting literature is inconclusive, some evidence suggests that a tight pectoralis minor can contribute to subacromial impingement syndrome.[10-12]

Zone II: Medial Border of the Axilla

Serratus Anterior

Positions

- Patient: sitting
- Clinician: standing, slightly behind the patient and on the side being palpated

Instructions

- Place the patient's shoulder in 90° of flexion.
- With one hand, palpate along the anterior–lateral thorax from ribs 1 to 8 using three or four fingers.
- To confirm palpation and to isolate the serratus anterior, have the patient protract the scapula.

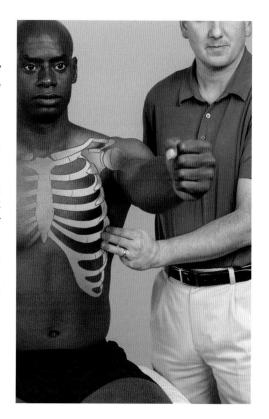

CLINICAL PEARL

The serratus anterior is innervated by the long thoracic nerve. Damage to this nerve or weakness in the muscle can result in winging of the scapula (see following photo). This muscle is important because it works with the rotator cuff muscles to produce coordinated scapulohumeral rhythm.[2] The serratus anterior works synergistically with the upper and lower trapezius to produce

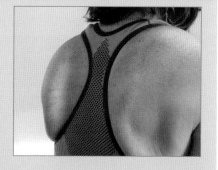

upward rotation of the scapula so the shoulder complex can achieve 180° of elevation.[2]

Zone III: Anterior Aspect of the Rib Cage

Subclavius

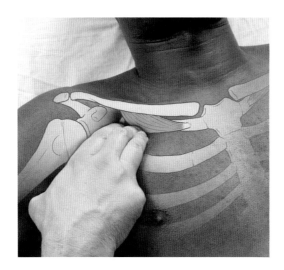

Positions

- Patient: supine
- Clinician: sitting, facing the patient, on the side being palpated

Instructions

- Place the patient's hand on the waist so the elbow is flexed to 90°.
- Palpate the middle third of the clavicle.
- Move three fingers inferiorly to palpate the subclavius muscle.

Note

This area may be sensitive and tender to palpation for many individuals because there are several soft tissue structures around the inferior border of the clavicle. Palpate in a slow fashion, gently adding greater pressure.

Intercostal Spaces

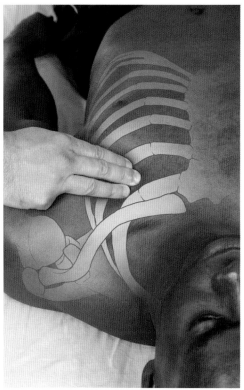

VIDEO 4.4 ▶

Positions
- Patient: sitting or supine
- Clinician: standing, facing the patient

Instructions
- Palpate the manubrium of the sternum and move laterally about one or two fingerwidths.
- Using a three-finger approach, the third digit should be in the intercostal space, with the second and fourth digits on the rib above and below, respectively.

Note
The fourth intercostal space is approximately at the level of the nipple.

Case Study

History

A 50-year-old male presents to your clinic with complaints of right anterior clavicle and pectoral pain after having been tackled 2 days ago in a weekend football game. He immediately felt pain over his anterior rib cage and shoulder on the right and noticed swelling over his right pectoralis major. He was unable to fully lift his right arm because of pain. He reported no loss of consciousness and no numbness or tingling, and radiographs at the hospital were negative. He is a paralegal, married with two children, and enjoys playing football on the weekends.

- Based on this information only, what are the three most likely diagnoses?

Examination

Past medical history	Unremarkable
Medication	Aleve
Observation	Decreased willingness to move the right arm, with arm held against thorax Ecchymosis over right anterior chest
Active range of motion	Right shoulder flexion = 0° to 113°, abduction = 0° to 112°, internal rotation = 0° to 60°, external rotation = 0° to 54°
Passive range of motion	Same as for active
Manual muscle testing	Within normal limits, except right shoulder flexion, internal rotation, and horizontal adduction = 3+/5 (secondary to pain)
Special tests	Negative acromioclavicular shear test Negative passive horizontal adduction test
Other	Normal neurological and vascular exam

- Based on the subjective and objective information together, what are the two most likely diagnoses? Give your rationale for eliminating the third diagnosis.
- What structures should you palpate on this patient based on your differential diagnoses?
- Given all the information presented, what would you expect to find upon palpation of those structures?

Case Solution and Discussion

Potential Diagnoses Based on History

- Acromioclavicular joint separation
- Clavicular fracture
- Pectoralis major contusion

Potential Diagnoses Based on History and Examination

- Clavicular fracture
- Pectoralis major contusion

Acromioclavicular joint separation: This diagnosis can be ruled out because of the negative acromioclavicular shear test and passive horizontal adduction test as well as the absence of tenderness to palpation over the ACJ and the negative radiograph.

Structures to Be Palpated

- Clavicle
- Pectoralis major
- Pectoralis minor
- Long head of biceps
- Subscapularis
- Acromioclavicular joint
- Rib 1
- Rib 2

Palpation Findings

- Tenderness to palpation throughout pectoralis major
- Mild tenderness to palpation of pectoralis minor
- Tenderness to palpation of ribs 1 and 2

Clinical Reasoning

- Clavicular fracture: The mechanism of injury, ecchymosis over the anterior chest, and reluctance of the patient to move the arm can all be indicative of a clavicular fracture. However, the lack of tenderness of the clavicle, negative acromioclavicular shear test, lack of gross structural deformity, and negative radiograph allow this diagnosis to be ruled out.
- Pectoralis major contusion: The mechanism of injury, bruising over the anterior chest, reluctance of the patient to move the arm, weakness of the motions produced by the pectoralis major, and tenderness to palpation of the pectoralis major and ribs 1 and 2 all indicate a pectoralis major contusion.

Case Study Questions

1. What information do the palpation findings of the case give the clinician? How can this information be incorporated in the clinical decision-making process?

2. Think about how the examination findings (subjective and objective) lead to the differential diagnosis. What might you do differently?

3. If the patient were not responding and developed an increase in pain with the development of crepitus along the clavicle and ACJ, how would you respond?

CHAPTER REVIEW QUESTIONS

1. Identify the structures that comprise the four borders of the axilla.

2. Describe blood supply to the proximal upper extremity.

3. What are the three trunks of the brachial plexus and their nerve roots?

4. Name the three cords of the brachial plexus and the nerves that come off each of the cords.

5. Which nerve innervates the serratus anterior? What is the clinical significance of damage to this nerve?

6. What key structure sits in the deltopectoral groove?

chapter 5

Elbow and Forearm

After completing this chapter, the reader will be able to do the following:

- Describe the key bony anatomical structures of the elbow and forearm.
- Identify and describe the soft tissue anatomy of the elbow and forearm, including muscles, ligaments, nerves, arteries, and veins.
- Differentiate the layers of muscles in the arm and forearm.
- Identify the borders of the cubital fossa and the structures located within it.
- Identify on bony or skeletal models the origins and insertions of the muscles of the arm and forearm in order to aid in understanding osteokinematic action and surface palpation.
- Palpate structures of the elbow and forearm.
- Integrate surface palpation findings to aid in the differential diagnosis of a patient with elbow or forearm pain.

The joints of the elbow and forearm represent the middle joints of the upper extremity. The elbow and forearm consist of articulations between the distal humerus and proximal radius and ulna. Three joints are located in the elbow and forearm: the humeroulnar, humeroradial, and proximal radioulnar joints. The ulnar nerve runs superficially along the medial aspect of the elbow joint and can be easily irritated because of its location.

Functions of the Elbow and Forearm

The elbow and forearm are partially responsible for positioning the hand in space for most functional activities and often work in conjunction with the shoulder girdle for optimal positioning of the upper extremity.[1] The bones of the forearm, the radius and ulna, function to transmit forces proximally to the humerus.[1] In addition, these bones help form the proximal and distal radioulnar joints, which permit forearm pronation and supination. This, combined with the elbow's ability to perform flexion and extension, results in a large amount of movement with which to accomplish a variety of functional activities.

Bony Anatomy

The elbow and forearm are formed by three bones: the humerus, radius, and ulna. On the distal aspect of the humerus are the medial and lateral supracondylar ridges (figure 5.1). Distal to these anatomical landmarks are the medial and lateral epicondyles. These anatomical landmarks are important because several muscles and ligaments attach to them.

- The lateral epicondyle serves as the attachment for the common extensor tendon as well as the radial (lateral) collateral ligament.
- The medial epicondyle serves as the attachment for the ulnar (medial) collateral ligament in addition to the common flexor tendon.

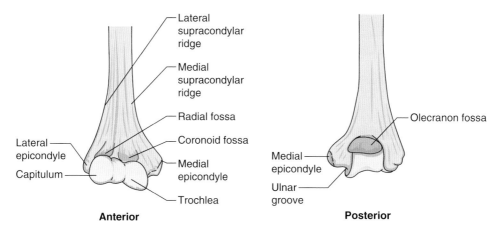

FIGURE 5.1 Views of the humerus.

Just posterior to the medial epicondyle is a small depression, the cubital tunnel, where the ulnar nerve is located. The distal articulating condyles of the humerus are called the capitulum and trochlea. The capitulum is located laterally and the trochlea medially. Above the condyles of the humerus are three fossae:

- Radial fossa
- Coronoid fossa
- Olecranon fossa

The radial and coronoid fossae are located on the anterior aspect, while the olecranon fossa is located posteriorly (figure 5.1). The olecranon process articulates with the olecranon fossa in elbow extension.[2]

The forearm consists of two bones: the radius and ulna (figure 5.2). The ulna, which is located on the medial side of the forearm, is the stronger of the two bones. The proximal ulna has several anatomical landmarks. The ulna tuberosity and coronoid process are located anteriorly, with the olecranon process located posteriorly. On the proximal lateral aspect of the ulna is the radial notch, which articulates with the radial head to form the proximal radioulnar joint. The radius is the bone that occupies the lateral aspect of the forearm. The proximal radius has a head, neck, and tuberosity. It articulates medially with the ulna and proximally with the humerus.[2]

The elbow and forearm are composed of three joints: the humeroulnar, humeroradial, and proximal radioulnar joints, all of which are enclosed in a single joint capsule. The humeroulnar joint is a hinge joint formed by the trochlea of the humerus and the trochlear notch of the ulna. The humeroradial joint, formed by the capitulum of the humerus and the radial head, functions both as a hinge joint and as a pivot joint. Together these two joints permit elbow flexion and extension. The proximal radioulnar joint is formed by the radial head and radial notch of the ulna. It is the movement at this joint, as well as at the humeroradial and distal radioulnar joints, that allows for forearm pronation and supination.[1]

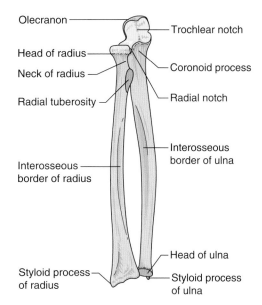

FIGURE 5.2 Anterior aspect of the right ulna and radius.

Soft Tissue Anatomy

Several groups of muscles surround the elbow and forearm.

- Anteriorly, the elbow flexors consist of the biceps brachii, brachialis, and brachioradialis.
- Posteriorly, the triceps brachii and anconeus compose the elbow extensor group (figure 5.3).
- The medial elbow is covered by the flexor–pronator group of muscles.
- The lateral elbow is occupied by the extensor–supinator group of muscles.

Anatomically, these muscle groups are separated into layers, and knowing the relative depth of these muscles during palpation is an important consideration so that proper force can be applied for structure identification.

The posterior forearm is divided into two layers:

- The superficial layer contains the brachioradialis, extensor carpi radialis longus, extensor carpi radialis brevis, extensor digitorum, extensor digiti minimi, and extensor carpi ulnaris (figure 5.4, superficial).

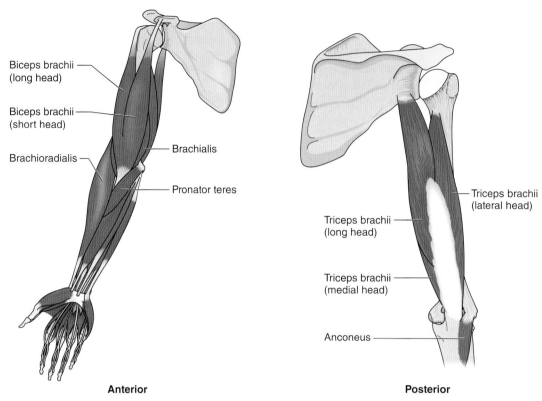

Anterior

Posterior

FIGURE 5.3 Muscles of the arm.

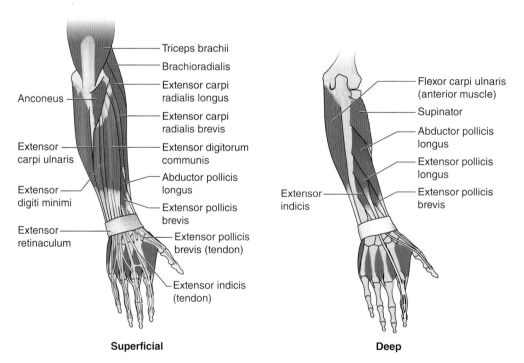

Superficial

Deep

FIGURE 5.4 Posterior forearm muscles.

- The deep layer is composed of the supinator, abductor pollicis longus, extensor pollicis brevis, extensor pollicis longus, and the extensor indicis (figure 5.4, deep).

All muscles of the posterior forearm are innervated by the radial nerve.[2]

The anterior forearm muscles are broken into superficial, intermediate, and deep layers (figure 5.5).

- The superficial layer consists of the pronator teres, flexor carpi radialis, palmaris longus, and flexor carpi ulnaris.
- The intermediate layer consists of the flexor digitorum superficialis.
- The deepest layer consists of the flexor digitorum profundus, the flexor pollicis longus, and the pronator quadratus.

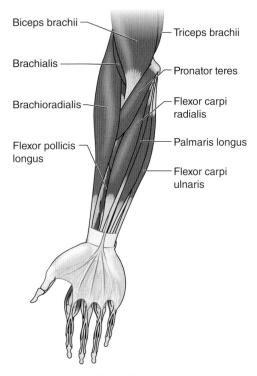

Superficial

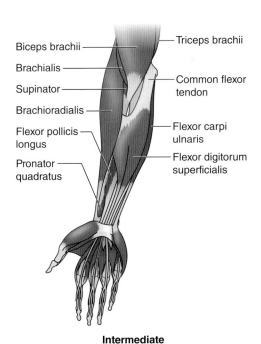

Intermediate

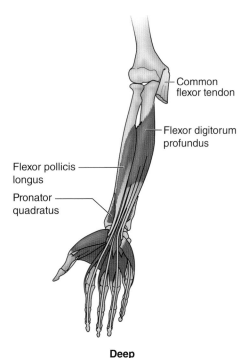

Deep

FIGURE 5.5 Anterior forearm muscles.

It should be pointed out that certain anatomy textbooks consider the anterior forearm in four layers, which the primary author of this text would agree with. This is because the pronator quadratus is located deep to the flexor pollicis longus and flexor digitorum profundus.

These muscles produce movement of the elbow, forearm, wrist, and hand and provide dynamic stability to all these joints. The anterior forearm muscles are innervated by the median or ulnar nerve or both.[2]

The muscles surrounding the elbow and forearm form a bordered space known as the cubital fossa. This triangular-shaped depression has a medial border, a lateral border, and a base.

- The medial border is the pronator teres.
- The lateral border is the brachioradialis.
- The base is an imaginary line between the medial and lateral epicondyles.

The floor of the cubital fossa is the brachialis muscle, which lies directly over the elbow joint. The cubital fossa contains the biceps tendon, radial nerve, median nerve, and brachial artery.[2]

In addition to the muscles crossing the elbow joint, the capsule and several ligaments add passive stability to these joints (figure 5.6).

- The medial and lateral aspects of the elbow are reinforced by the ulnar (medial) collateral ligament and the radial (lateral) collateral ligament, respectively.[1,2]
  - The ulnar collateral ligament runs from the medial epicondyle of the humerus to the coronoid process of the ulna and resists valgus (abduction) forces
  - The radial collateral ligament runs from the lateral epicondyle of the humerus to the radial head and resists varus (adduction) forces.[1,3-5]

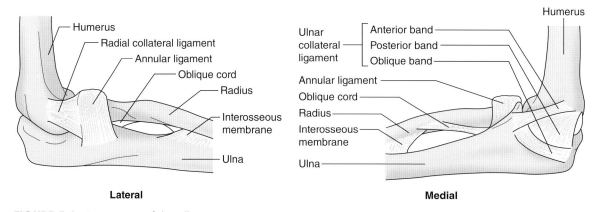

Lateral

Medial

FIGURE 5.6   Ligaments of the elbow.

- The proximal radioulnar joint is reinforced by the thick annular ligament. This ligament is responsible for holding the radial head in the radial notch of the ulna during pronation and supination of the forearm.[1,2]

Neurovascular Anatomy

The brachial artery, a continuation of the axillary artery, is superficial as it runs down the distal, medial aspect of the arm, and a pulse can be taken here (figure 5.7). In the arm, the brachial artery is medial to the median nerve, but this relationship changes in the cubital fossa where the brachial artery becomes lateral to the median nerve. Just distal to the cubital fossa, the brachial artery splits into the radial and ulnar arteries.[2] The brachial artery is important to palpate because it serves as the auscultation point during blood pressure assessment.

While several nerves cross the elbow joint (median, musculocutaneous, radial, and ulnar), the ulnar nerve is the most superficial and easily palpable (figure 5.8). This nerve arises from the medial cord of the brachial

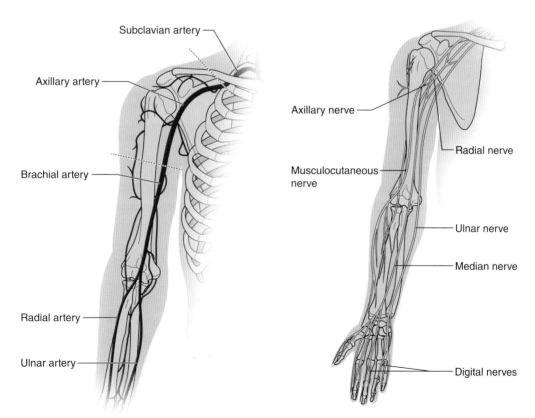

FIGURE 5.7 Major arteries of the upper extremity.

FIGURE 5.8 Major nerves of the upper extremity.

119

plexus and then heads posteriorly to run alongside the long head of the triceps. It then pierces the intermuscular septum and travels posterior to the medial epicondyle of the humerus.[2] The median nerve, arising from both the medial and lateral cords of the brachial plexus, runs down the anterior arm into the cubital fossa, where it lies medial to the brachial artery. Both the ulnar and median nerves travel down the upper arm without innervating any muscles. The musculocutaneous nerve coming from the lateral cord of the brachial plexus runs down the anterior arm and is responsible for innervating the biceps brachii, brachialis, and coracobrachialis muscles. Finally, the radial nerve, a branch of the posterior cord of the brachial plexus, runs down the lateral aspect of the triceps, which it innervates, before piercing the intermuscular septum. It then runs between the brachialis and brachioradialis muscles.[2]

Structural Inspection

- When examining the elbow and forearm region, the bony alignment between the distal humerus and proximal radius and ulna should be assessed.

- Clinicians should make particular note of the carrying angle. Normal alignment of the elbow results in slight cubital valgus, which should be measured. A normal carrying angle should be between 5° and 15°.[1] A decrease in the normal carrying angle will result in cubital varus. Excessive cubital valgus may be linked to ulnar nerve neuropathy.

- Clinicians should assess for a large collection of swelling around the posterior elbow, which can be suggestive of olecranon bursitis. These patients may present with the elbow in 30° to 45° of flexion to accommodate the accumulation of fluid.

- Regardless of the pathology in question, patients presenting with a loss of either active or passive (or both) elbow extension will require aggressive treatment to restore a loss of elbow extension.

- A loss of elbow flexion will present with difficulty completing functional activities such as eating, dressing, and grooming.

- Clinicians should assess muscle tone along the anterior and posterior aspects of the arm and of the muscles originating from the common extensor and flexor tendons.

- As always, compare bilaterally to assess for atrophy or other differences.

Lateral Supracondylar Ridge

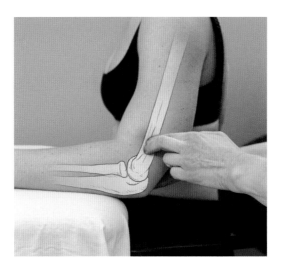

Positions
- Patient: sitting
- Clinician: sitting, facing the patient, on the side being palpated

Instructions
- Place the patient's elbow in 90° of flexion.
- Palpate the deltoid tuberosity along the lateral aspect of the midhumerus.
- Using two fingers, move your fingers in an inferior direction until a bony prominence is felt.

Note
The lateral supracondylar ridge is much longer and more prominent than the medial supracondylar ridge.

Lateral Epicondyle

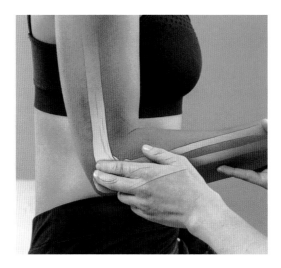

Positions
- Patient: sitting
- Clinician: sitting, facing the patient, on the side being palpated

Instructions
- Place the patient's elbow in 90° of flexion.
- Using two fingers, palpate along the lateral aspect of the elbow until a bony prominence is felt.

CLINICAL PEARL
The lateral epicondyle is the attachment of the common extensor tendon. Individuals with lateral epicondylalgia (tennis elbow) present with exquisite tenderness over the lateral epicondyle. Lateral epicondylalgia is now considered more of a tendinosis than a true tendinitis. Joint hypomobility in the cervical or thoracic spine (or both), weakness in the scapular muscles, or poor alignment can lead to abnormal forces down the kinetic chain, causing this condition.[6]

Capitulum

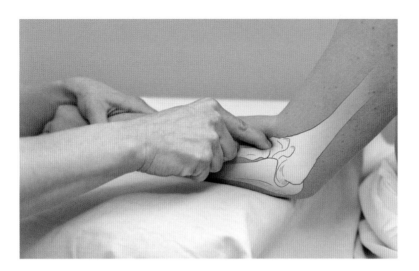

Positions

- Patient: sitting
- Clinician: sitting, facing the patient, on the side being palpated

Instructions

- Place the patient's elbow in 90° of flexion with the forearm in a neutral position.
- Palpate the lateral epicondyle.
- Move one or two fingers slightly distally and medially to palpate the capitulum.

Medial Epicondyle

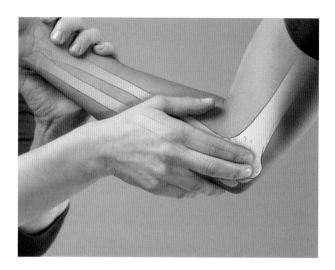

Positions

- Patient: sitting
- Clinician: sitting, facing the patient, on the side being palpated

Instructions

- Place the patient's elbow in 90° of flexion.
- Using one or two fingers, palpate along the medial aspect of the elbow until a bony prominence is felt.

CLINICAL PEARL

The medial epicondyle is the attachment for the common flexor tendon. Individuals with medial epicondylalgia (golfer's elbow) present with exquisite tenderness over the medial epicondyle. This should be assessed and treated similarly to lateral epicondylalgia.

Trochlea

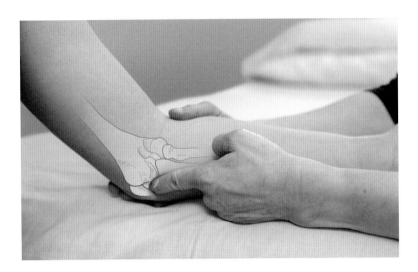

Positions

- Patient: sitting
- Clinician: sitting, facing the patient, on the side being palpated

Instructions

- Place the patient's elbow in 90° of flexion with the forearm in a neutral position.
- Palpate the medial epicondyle.
- Move one or two fingers slightly distally and laterally to palpate the trochlea.

Medial Supracondylar Ridge

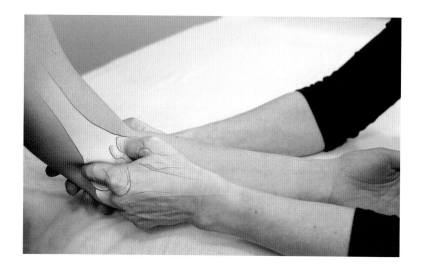

Positions

- Patient: sitting
- Clinician: sitting, facing the patient, on the side being palpated

Instructions

- Place the patient's elbow in 90° of flexion.
- Palpate the medial epicondyle.
- Move two fingers proximally until a short bony ridge is felt.

Note

Keep in mind that the medial supracondylar ridge is less prominent and more difficult to palpate.

Olecranon Process

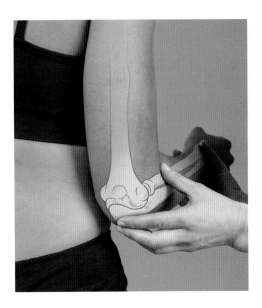

Positions
- Patient: sitting
- Clinician: standing, facing the patient, on the side being palpated

Instructions
- Place the patient's elbow in 90° of flexion, bringing the olecranon process out of the olecranon fossa.
- Using two fingers, palpate the prominent process on the posterior aspect of the proximal ulna.

Radial Head

Positions

- Patient: sitting
- Clinician: standing, facing the patient, on the side being palpated

Instructions

- Place the patient's elbow in 90° of flexion.
- Palpate the lateral epicondyle.
- Using the pads of digits 1, 2, and 3 (pincer grasp), move your fingers approximately 1 inch (2.5 centimeters) distally and medially to palpate the radial head (left hand pictured).

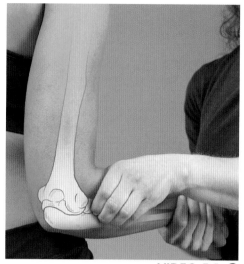

VIDEO 5.1 ▶

- To confirm the palpation, have the patient pronate and supinate the forearm. You will feel the radial head spin under your fingers.

Notes

- This structure is embedded deep within the posterior forearm muscles, and you must use a fair amount of pressure for this palpation.
- As an alternative, the radial head can be palpated from the lateral aspect of the forearm. This is done by palpating the lateral epicondyle, moving slightly distally and anteriorly, and feeling it spin under your fingers as the patient pronates and supinates (not pictured). This method may be especially useful when there is a large amount of forearm soft tissue bulk (as in the second photo).
- The pincer grasp is used when trying to palpate two sides of the same structure.

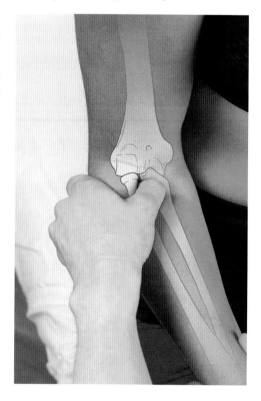

Radial Tuberosity

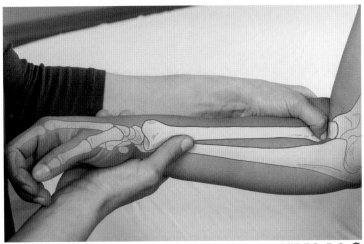

VIDEO 5.2 ▶

Positions
- Patient: sitting
- Clinician: standing, facing the patient, on the side being palpated

Instructions
- Place the patient's elbow in 90° of flexion, with the forearm in supination.
- Have the patient contract the biceps muscle by resisting elbow flexion (and supination).
- Palpate the biceps tendon in the cubital fossa using your thumb.
- Have the patient relax, and slowly apply more pressure to palpate the radial tuberosity.
- To confirm palpation, have the patient pronate and supinate so you can feel the tuberosity moving under your fingers.

Note
This can be uncomfortable for the patient, so apply slow, firm pressure to accurately assess this structure.

Humeral Shaft

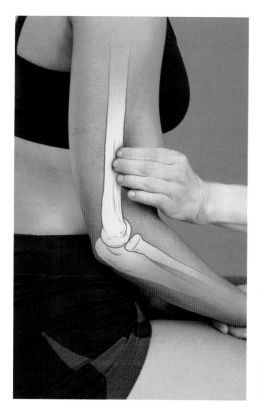
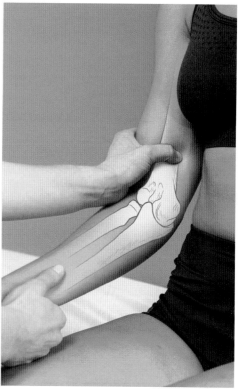

Positions

- Patient: sitting
- Clinician: standing, facing the patient, on the side being palpated

Instructions

- Palpate the deltoid tuberosity.
- Using the pads of digits 1, 2, and 3 (pincer grasp), move your fingers distally to palpate the distal shaft of the humerus.
- In addition, using the pads of digits 2 and 3 or using the thumb, palpate the proximal shaft of the humerus.
- You will need to palpate the anterior, medial, lateral, and posterior aspects individually.

Radial Shaft

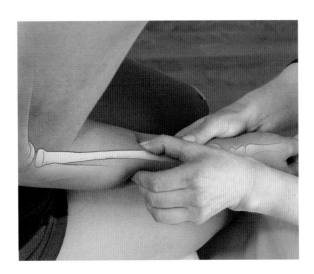

Positions

- Patient: sitting
- Clinician: standing, facing the patient, on the side being palpated

Instructions

- Palpate the radial head.
- Using a pincer grasp, move your fingers distally to palpate the entire shaft of the radius.

Ulnar Shaft

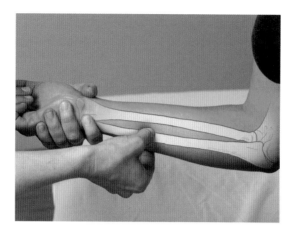

Positions

- Patient: sitting
- Clinician: standing, facing the patient, on the side being palpated

Instructions

- Palpate the medial epicondyle.
- Using a pincer grasp, move your fingers distally and slightly posteriorly to identify the proximal shaft of the ulna.
- Continue moving your fingers distally to palpate the entire shaft of the ulna.

Muscles of the Anterior and Posterior Arm and Forearm

Muscle	Origin	Insertion	Innervation	Blood supply	Action
ARM					
Biceps brachii	*Long head:* supraglenoid tubercle of the scapula *Short head:* coracoid process of scapula	Radial tuberosity, fascia of the forearm through bicipital aponeurosis	Musculocutaneous nerve (C5-C6)	Muscular branches of brachial artery	Forearm supination and elbow flexion *Long head:* shoulder flexion and abduction
Brachialis	Distal one-fourth of the anterior humerus	Coronoid process and tuberosity of the ulna	Musculocutaneous nerve (C5-C7)	Radial recurrent artery, muscular branches of the brachial artery	Elbow flexion
Coracobrachialis	Coracoid process of the scapula	Anterior, medial aspect of the distal humerus	Musculocutaneous nerve (C5-C6)	Muscular branches of brachial artery	Shoulder flexion and adduction
Triceps brachii	*Long head:* infraglenoid tubercle of the scapula *Lateral head:* posterior aspect of the humerus superior to the radial groove *Medial head:* posterior aspect of the humerus inferior to the radial groove	Olecranon process of the ulna	Radial nerve (C6-C8)	Profunda brachial artery	Elbow extension *Long head:* shoulder extension
Anconeus	Lateral epicondyle of the humerus	Posterior proximal aspect of the ulna, lateral surface of the olecranon	Radial nerve (C7-C8)	Profunda brachial artery	Assistance with elbow extension, assistance with stabilization of the lateral aspect of the elbow
POSTERIOR FOREARM (TWO LAYERS)					
Brachioradialis (superficial layer)	Proximal two-thirds of the lateral supracondylar ridge of the humerus	Distal, lateral aspect of the radius just proximal to the styloid process	Radial nerve (C6-C8)	Radial recurrent artery	Elbow flexion and assistance with forearm supination

> continued

Soft Tissues

Muscle	Origin	Insertion	Innervation	Blood supply	Action
POSTERIOR FOREARM (TWO LAYERS) *continued*					
Extensor carpi radialis longus (superficial layer)	Distal one-third of the lateral supracondylar ridge of the humerus	Posterior aspect of metacarpal 2	Radial nerve (C6-C8)	Radial and radial recurrent arteries	Wrist extension and radial deviation
Extensor carpi radialis brevis (superficial layer)	Lateral epicondyle of the humerus (common extensor tendon)	Posterior aspect of metacarpal 3	Radial nerve (C6-C8)	Radial and radial recurrent arteries	Wrist extension and radial deviation
Extensor digitorum (superficial layer)	Lateral epicondyle of the humerus (common extensor tendon)	Middle and distal phalanges of digits 2 to 5 (extensor expansions)	Posterior interosseous nerve (C7-C8)	Posterior interosseous artery	Extension of the metacarpopha-langeal (MCP) joints of digits 2 to 5
Extensor digiti minimi (superficial layer)	Lateral epicondyle of the humerus (common extensor tendon)	Extensor expansion of digit 5	Posterior interosseous nerve (C7-C8)	Posterior interosseous artery	Extension of the fifth MCP joint
Extensor carpi ulnaris (superficial layer)	Lateral epicondyle of the humerus (common extensor tendon) and the posterior border of the ulna	Fifth metacarpal	Radial nerve (C6-C7)	Posterior interosseous artery	Wrist extension and ulnar deviation
Supinator (deep layer)	Lateral epicondyle of the humerus, radial collateral ligament, annular ligament, supinator fossa, and crest of ulna	Anterior, posterior, and lateral aspects of the proximal radius	Radial nerve (C5-C6)	Radial recurrent and posterior interosseous artery	Forearm supination
Abductor pollicis longus (deep layer)	Posterior surface of the radius, ulna, and interosseous membrane	Base of metacarpal 1	Posterior interosseous nerve (C7-C8)	Posterior interosseous artery	Abduction of the first car-pometacarpal (CMC) joint

Muscle	Origin	Insertion	Innervation	Blood supply	Action
Extensor pollicis brevis (deep layer)	Posterior surface of the radius and interosseous membrane	Base of the proximal phalanx of the thumb	Posterior interosseous nerve (C7-C8)	Posterior interosseous artery	Extension of the first MCP joint
Extensor pollicis longus (deep layer)	Posterior surface of the middle one-third of the ulna and interosseous membrane	Base of the distal phalanx of the thumb	Posterior interosseous nerve (C7-C8)	Posterior interosseous artery	Extension of MCP and inter-phalangeal joint of the first digit
Extensor indicis (deep layer)	Posterior aspect of the ulna and interosseous membrane	Extensor expansion of the second digit	Posterior interosseous nerve (C7-C8)	Posterior interosseous artery	Extension of the second MCP joint

ANTERIOR FOREARM (FOUR LAYERS)

Muscle	Origin	Insertion	Innervation	Blood supply	Action
Pronator teres (layer 1)	*Humeral head:* medial epicondyle of the humerus (common flexor tendon) *Ulnar head:* coronoid process of the ulna	Proximal, lateral surface of the radius	Median nerve (C6-C7)	Anterior ulnar recurrent artery	Forearm pronation and assistance with elbow flexion
Flexor carpi radialis (layer 1)	Medial epicondyle of the humerus (common flexor tendon)	Base of metacarpals 2 and 3	Median nerve (C6-C7)	Radial artery	Wrist flexion and radial deviation
Palmaris longus (layer 1)	Medial epicondyle of the humerus (common flexor tendon)	Palmar aponeurosis and flexor retinaculum	Median nerve (C7-T1)	Posterior recurrent ulnar artery	Wrist flexion
Flexor carpi ulnaris (layer 1)	*Humeral head:* medial epicondyle of the humerus (common flexor tendon) *Ulnar head:* olecranon and posterior border of the ulna	Base of metacarpal 5, hook of the hamate, and the pisiform bone	Ulnar nerve (C7-C8)	Posterior ulnar recurrent artery	Wrist flexion and ulnar deviation

> continued

135

Muscle	Origin	Insertion	Innervation	Blood supply	Action
ANTERIOR FOREARM (FOUR LAYERS) *continued*					
Flexor digitorum superficialis (layer 2)	*Humeroulnar head:* medial epicondyle of the humerus (common flexor tendon) and the coronoid process of the ulna *Radial head:* proximal one-half of the radius	Bases of the anterior middle phalanges of digits 2 to 5	Median nerve (C7-C8)	Ulnar and radial arteries	Flexion of the proximal inter-phalangeal (PIP) joints of digits 2 to 5
Flexor digitorum profundus (layer 3)	Proximal three-fourths of the anterior surface of the ulna and interosseous membrane	Bases of the anterior distal phalanges of digits 2 to 5	Tendon 1 and 2 median nerve, tendon 3 and 4 ulnar nerve (C8-T1)	Anterior interosseous artery	Flexion of the distal interpha-langeal (DIP) joints of digits 2 to 5
Flexor pollicis longus (layer 3)	Anterior aspect of the radius and interosseous membrane	Base of the anterior distal phalanx of the thumb	Anterior interosseous nerve (C8-T1)	Anterior interosseous artery	Flexion of the interphalangeal (IP) joint of the first digit
Pronator quadratus (layer 4)	Distal one-fourth of the ulna	Distal one-fourth of the radius	Anterior interosseous nerve (C8-T1)	Anterior interosseous artery	Forearm pro-nation

In this chapter, a thorough discussion focuses on the proximal attachment of these muscles. The muscle bellies during the palpation process are emphasized and depicted. The tendons of these forearm muscles that cross the wrist, and at times the hand, are discussed in more detail in the wrist and hand chapter.

Zone I: Anterior Aspect of the Arm

Coracobrachialis

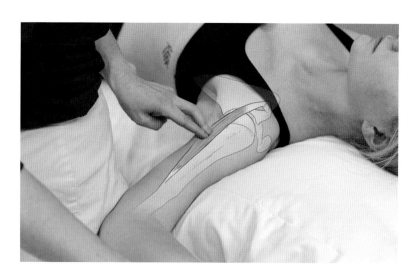

Positions

- Patient: supine
- Clinician: sitting or standing, facing the patient, on the side being palpated

Instructions

- Place the patient's shoulder into abduction and external rotation (right hand pictured).
- Using two or three fingers, palpate the lateral border of the pectoralis major.
- Move distally and palpate the medial upper arm (left hand pictured).
- To confirm palpation, have the patient gently perform resisted shoulder adduction against your thigh. You will feel a small slender muscle contraction under your fingers.

CLINICAL PEARL

The clinician should be aware that the axillary artery and the brachial plexus, specifically the lateral cord, is in this region. Pay close attention and maintain communication with the patient regarding signs of neurovascular changes in the distal aspect of the upper extremity.

Biceps Brachii

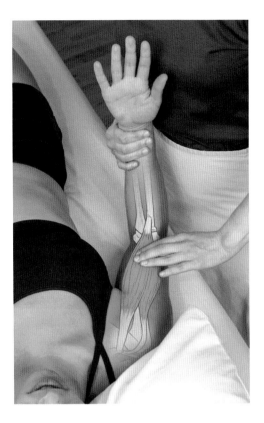

Positions
- Patient: sitting or supine
- Clinician: sitting or standing, facing the patient, on the side being palpated

Instructions
- Place the patient's forearm in supination with the elbow flexed to 90°.
- Using three fingers, palpate the entire length of the muscle belly along the anterior aspect of the upper arm (left hand pictured).
- To confirm palpation, have the patient perform resisted elbow flexion (right hand pictured). You will feel a large contraction under your fingers.

Notes
- To isolate the insertion of the biceps brachii on the radial tuberosity, refer to instructions for palpating the radial tuberosity.
- To isolate the long head of the biceps tendon, refer to the instructions for palpating the intertubercular groove in chapter 3.

Brachialis

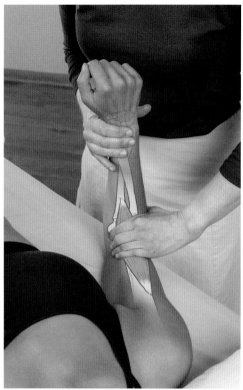

VIDEO 5.3 ▶

Positions
- Patient: supine
- Clinician: sitting or standing, facing the patient, on the side being palpated

Instructions
- Place the patient's forearm in pronation with the elbow flexed to 90°.
- Using two or three fingers, palpate the muscle's insertion near the coronoid process where it inserts (left hand pictured).
- To confirm palpation, have the patient perform resisted elbow flexion (right hand pictured). You will feel a small contraction under your fingers.

Note
The brachialis is deep to the biceps, forming the floor of the cubital fossa. It may be necessary to have the patient first contract the biceps to isolate its muscle belly and then have the patient relax so the biceps can be moved aside, allowing the deeper brachialis to be palpated.

Brachial Artery

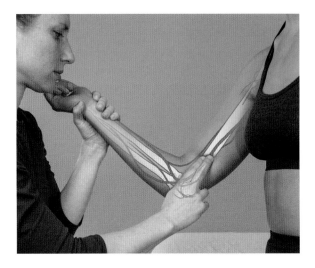

Positions

- Patient: sitting
- Clinician: sitting or standing, facing the patient, on the side being palpated

Instructions

- Place the patient's elbow in 90° of elbow flexion.
- Using the pads of your second and third digits, palpate the medial epicondyle.
- Move your fingers one-half inch (1.3 centimeters) laterally and one-half inch superiorly so they are just above the cubital fossa.
- Apply light pressure with the pads of your second and third digits to assess the brachial artery and pulse.

Note

Because this artery runs down the medial aspect of the lower two-thirds of the upper arm, this artery can be palpated anywhere along its path.

Median Nerve

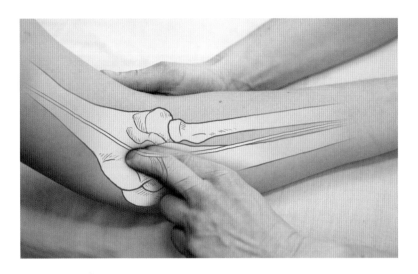

Positions

- Patient: sitting
- Clinician: sitting, facing the patient, on the side being palpated

Instructions

- Place the patient's elbow in 90° of elbow flexion.
- Palpate the brachial artery in the cubital fossa.
- Move one or two fingers slightly medially to palpate the median nerve. You will feel a small, rounded structure under your fingers.

Note

The median nerve is just medial to the brachial artery. It is a round, slender structure that should feel like a guitar string in the cubital fossa.

Zone II: Posterior Aspect of the Arm

Triceps Brachii

Positions

- Patient: supine
- Clinician: sitting or standing, behind and slightly lateral to the patient, on the side being palpated

Instructions

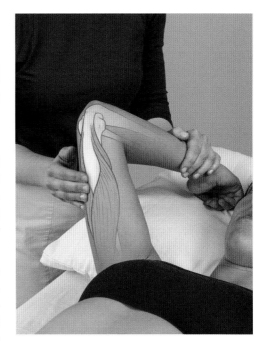

- Place the patient's forearm in supination, with the elbow flexed to approximately 110°.
- Place the patient's shoulder in approximately 90° of shoulder flexion.
- Palpate the olecranon process.
- Using the pads of three fingers, move your fingers proximally 4 to 5 inches (10 to 13 centimeters) to palpate the muscle bellies of the triceps (right hand pictured).
- To confirm palpation, have the patient perform resisted elbow extension (left hand pictured). You will feel a large contraction under your fingers to contract the muscle.

Notes

- The clinician should attempt to palpate each of the heads of the triceps.
- The medial head of the triceps is deep to the long head and may be difficult to palpate, but it can be palpated on the medial aspect of the distal end of the humerus.
- The lateral and long heads are palpated along the lateral and medial aspects of the arm, respectively.

Zone III: Posterior Aspect of the Forearm

Brachioradialis

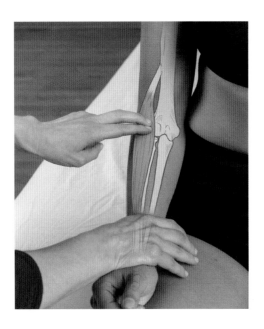

Positions

- Patient: sitting
- Clinician: sitting or standing, facing the patient, on the side being palpated

Instructions

- Place the patient's forearm in a neutral position.
- Palpate the lateral epicondyle with the pads of two or three fingers; move the fingers medially about one-half inch (1.3 centimeters) (left hand pictured).
- To confirm palpation, have the patient perform resisted elbow flexion with the forearm in neutral (right hand pictured). You will feel a large contraction under your fingers.

Extensor Carpi Radialis Longus

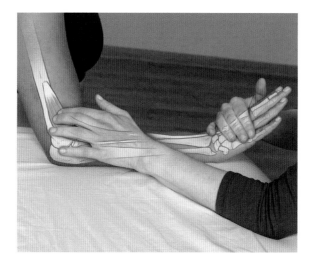

Positions

- Patient: sitting, with the forearm on a table or plinth in a pronated position
- Clinician: sitting, facing the patient, on the side being palpated

Instructions

- Palpate the lateral epicondyle.
- Using the pads of two or three fingers, move proximal to the lateral aspect of the distal humerus (lateral supracondylar ridge) (left hand pictured).
- To confirm palpation, have the patient extend and radially deviate the wrist against resistance (right hand pictured). You will feel a small contraction under your fingers.

Extensor Carpi Radialis Brevis

Common Extensor Tendon

- Extensor carpi radialis brevis (ECRB)
- Extensor digitorum (ED)
- Extensor digiti minimi (EDM)
- Extensor carpi ulnaris (ECU)

Positions

- Patient: sitting, with the forearm resting on a table or plinth in a pronated position

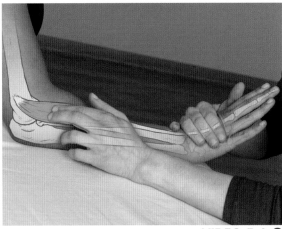

VIDEO 5.4 ▶

- Clinician: sitting, facing the patient, on the side being palpated

Instructions

- Using the pads of two fingers, palpate the lateral epicondyle.
- Move distally to palpate the radial head.
- Move your fingers slightly anteriorly to palpate the muscle belly of the ECRB (left hand pictured).
- To confirm palpation, have the patient extend the wrist against resistance (right hand pictured). You will feel the contraction under your fingers.

Note

Because the ECRB inserts on the third metacarpal, and digit 3 is the midline of the hand, the action of the ECRB from a kinesiologic perspective is predominantly wrist extension with minimal radial deviation.[1]

CLINICAL PEARL

Research has demonstrated that lateral epicondylalgia (tennis elbow) usually involves the extensor carpi radialis brevis muscle.[7]

Extensor Digitorum

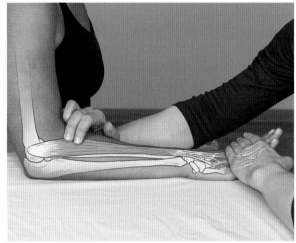

VIDEO 5.4 ▶

Positions

- Patient: sitting, with the forearm on a table or plinth in a pronated position
- Clinician: sitting, facing the patient, on the side being palpated

Instructions

- Using the pads of two fingers, palpate the ECRB.
- Move your fingers medially to palpate the muscle belly of the EDC (your fingers should be in the midline of the posterior forearm) (right hand pictured).
- To confirm palpation, have the patient extend digits 2 to 5 against resistance at the metacarpophalangeal joints (left hand pictured). You will feel the contraction under your fingers.

Extensor Digiti Minimi

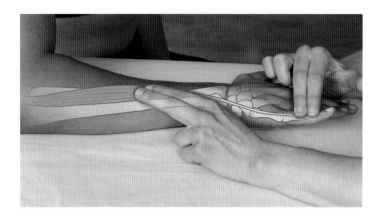

Positions
- Patient: sitting, with the forearm on a table or plinth in a pronated position
- Clinician: sitting, facing the patient, on the side being palpated

Instructions
- Using the pads of two fingers, palpate the lateral epicondyle.
- Move your fingers distally approximately two-thirds down the posterior medial forearm to palpate the muscle belly of the EDM (left hand pictured).
- To confirm palpation, have the patient extend digit 5 against resistance at the metacarpophalangeal joint (right hand pictured). You will feel a subtle contraction under your fingers.

Note
Remember that the EDM is attached to the EDC tendon and is palpable individually only at the distal one-third of the posterior medial forearm.

Extensor Carpi Ulnaris

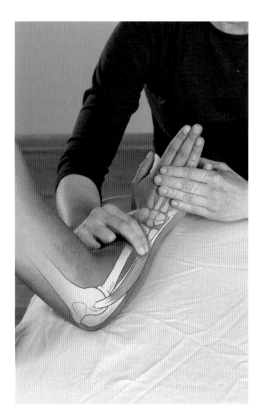

Positions
- Patient: sitting, with the forearm on a table or plinth in a pronated position
- Clinician: sitting, facing the patient, on the side being palpated

Instructions
- Using the pads of two fingers, palpate the EDC.
- Move your fingers medially approximately 1 inch (2.5 centimeters) to palpate the muscle belly of the ECU (your fingers should be on the most medial aspect of the posterior forearm) (right hand pictured).
- To confirm palpation, have the patient extend and ulnarly deviate the wrist against resistance (left hand pictured). You will feel the contraction under your fingers.

Zone IV: Anterior Aspect of the Forearm

Pronator Teres

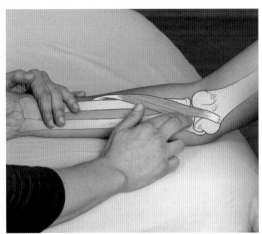

VIDEO 5.5 ▶

Common Flexor Tendon

- Pronator teres
- Flexor carpi radialis (FCR)
- Palmaris longus
- Flexor carpi ulnaris (FCU)

Positions

- Patient: sitting, with the forearm resting on a table or plinth in a supinated position
- Clinician: sitting, facing the patient, on the side being palpated

Instructions

- Using the pads of two fingers, palpate the medial epicondyle.
- Move your fingers to the medial border of the cubital fossa (pronator teres) (right hand pictured).
- To confirm palpation, have the patient pronate the forearm against resistance (left hand pictured). You will feel a subtle, small muscle contraction under your fingers.

Flexor Carpi Radialis

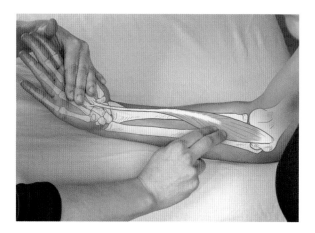

Positions

- Patient: sitting, with the forearm resting on a table or plinth in a supinated position
- Clinician: sitting, facing the patient, on the side being palpated

Instructions

- Using the pads of two fingers, palpate the pronator teres.
- Move your fingers one-half inch (1.3 centimeters) distally and medially to palpate the muscle belly of the FCR (right hand pictured).
- To confirm palpation, have the patient flex and radially deviate the wrist against resistance (left hand pictured). You will feel the contraction under your fingers.

Palmaris Longus

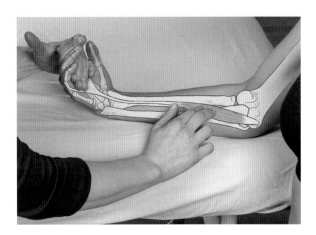

Positions
- Patient: sitting, with the forearm resting on a table or plinth in a supinated position
- Clinician: sitting, facing the patient, on the side being palpated

Instructions
- Using the pads of two fingers, palpate the FCR.
- Move your fingers one-half inch (1.3 centimeters) medially to palpate the muscle belly of the palmaris longus (right hand pictured).
- To confirm palpation, have the patient flex the wrist against resistance (left hand pictured). You will feel the contraction under your fingers.

Note
A portion of the population does not have a palmaris longus bilaterally, and some people do not have it at all.

Flexor Carpi Ulnaris

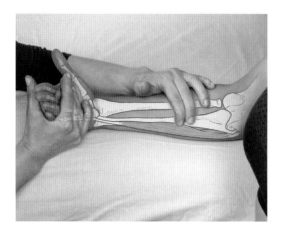

Positions
- Patient: sitting, with the forearm resting on a table or plinth in a supinated position
- Clinician: sitting, facing the patient, on the side being palpated

Instructions
- Using the pads of two fingers, palpate the palmaris longus.
- Move your fingers one-half inch (1.3 centimeters) medially to palpate the muscle belly of the flexor carpi ulnaris (left hand pictured).
- To confirm palpation, have the patient flex and ulnarly deviate the wrist against resistance (right hand pictured). You will feel the contraction under your fingers.

Note
If the patient does not have a palmaris longus, begin the palpation at the medial epicondyle and then move your fingers 1 inch (2.5 centimeters) distally to palpate the FCU.

Medial (Ulnar) Collateral Ligament

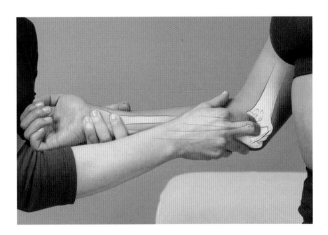

Positions
- Patient: sitting
- Clinician: sitting or standing, facing the patient, on the side being palpated

Instructions
- Place the patient's elbow in approximately 70° of flexion.
- Using the pads of the second and third digits, palpate the medial epicondyle.
- Move your fingers slightly inferior and anterior to the joint line of the elbow (humeroulnar joint).
- Apply firm pressure as you move from the medial epicondyle to the coronoid process.

Notes
- This ligament is difficult to palpate accurately on patients without elbow pathology, and it may become easier to palpate following trauma to the elbow when pain is present.
- You can apply a valgus force to the elbow joint, putting stress on the ligament, which may improve the ability to accurately palpate the medial collateral ligament of the elbow.[5] This should be done carefully and with caution in people presenting with elbow joint pathology.

Lateral (Radial) Collateral Ligament

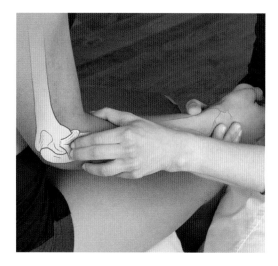

Positions

- Patient: sitting
- Clinician: sitting, facing the patient, on the side being palpated

Instructions

- Place the patient's elbow in approximately 70° of flexion.
- Using the pads of your second and third digits, palpate the lateral epicondyle.
- Move your fingers slightly inferior and anterior to the joint line of the elbow (humeroradial joint).
- Apply firm pressure as you move from the lateral epicondyle to the radius. You may not be able to feel the ligament fibers during this palpation.

Notes

- This ligament is difficult to palpate accurately on patients without elbow pathology, and it may be easier to palpate following trauma to the elbow when pain is present.
- To improve accuracy of this palpation, you can apply a varus force to the elbow joint. This will put stress through the ligament and may improve the ability to accurately palpate the lateral collateral ligament of the elbow.[8] Do this carefully and with caution in patients presenting with elbow joint pathology.

Ulnar Nerve

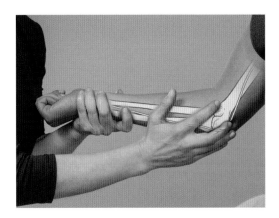

Positions

- Patient: sitting
- Clinician: sitting or standing, facing the patient, on the side being palpated

Instructions

- Place the patient's elbow in 90° of elbow flexion.
- Using the pads of the second and third digits, palpate the medial epicondyle.
- Continue to move the pad of the third digit slightly posteriorly until you palpate the cubital tunnel (groove).
- Gently palpate the ulnar nerve in the groove. You will feel a cord-like structure under your fingers.

Note

Palpation of the ulnar nerve may elicit paresthesia down the medial forearm, as far down as digits 4 and 5. If discomfort is expressed by your patient, reassess and modify your technique.

Case Study

History

A 30-year-old female presents to your clinic with reports of right elbow pain. She reports that the pain began about 2 months ago. She notes an increase in symptoms after a long day at work if she spends a lot of time typing papers on the computer and sometimes after an intense shoulder workout at the gym. She is a right hand–dominant hairdresser. She lives with a roommate and goes to school at night. She tries to go to the gym two or three times a week, where she does 30 minutes of cardio and lifts weights.

- Based on this information only, what are the three most likely diagnoses?

Examination

Past medical history	Unremarkable
Medication	Motrin
Observation	Increased right scapular winging
Active range of motion	Within normal limits, except right active wrist extension, 0° to 50° with pain
Passive range of motion	Within normal limits
Manual muscle testing	Right upper extremity 5/5, except wrist extensors 3+/5 with pain, serratus anterior 4–/5
Special tests	Pain with resisted right third-digit extension Negative cervical spine distraction test Negative quadrant test Negative median nerve upper limb tension test
Other	Sensation intact to radial nerve

- Based on the subjective and objective information together, what are the two most likely diagnoses? Give your rationale for eliminating the third diagnosis.
- What structures should you palpate on this patient based on your differential diagnoses?
- Given all the information presented, what would you expect to find upon palpation of those structures?

Case Solution and Discussion

Potential Diagnoses Based on History

- Cervical radiculopathy
- Lateral epicondylalgia
- Radial tunnel syndrome

Potential Diagnoses Based on History and Examination

- Lateral epicondylalgia
- Radial tunnel syndrome

Cervical radiculopathy: This diagnosis can be ruled out because of the negative cervical spine distraction test, negative quadrant test, and negative median nerve upper limb tension test. In addition, the lack of myotomal or dermatomal signs and symptoms makes this diagnosis highly improbable.

Structures to Be Palpated

- Lateral epicondyle
- Radial head
- Posterior forearm muscles (ECRB)

Palpation Findings

- Point tenderness at the lateral epicondyle
- Tenderness to palpation throughout posterior forearm musculature

Clinical Reasoning

- Lateral epicondylalgia: The repetitive nature of the patient's occupation places her at risk for lateral epicondylalgia. Her localized pain, point tenderness to the lateral epicondyle, tenderness throughout the posterior forearm musculature, and pain with resisted right third-digit extension and wrist extension are all indicative of this diagnosis.
- Radial tunnel syndrome: The patient's pain on the posterior–lateral aspect of the right forearm is a symptom of radial tunnel syndrome. However, the pain of radial tunnel syndrome is present more as a diffuse pain in the midposterior forearm, and there are no sensory changes, which are among the main diagnostic criteria for ruling in radial tunnel syndrome. In addition, the point tenderness to the lateral epicondyle is not present with radial tunnel syndrome.

Case Study Questions

1. What information do the palpation findings of the case give the clinician? How can this information be incorporated in the clinical decision-making process?

2. Think about how the examination findings (subjective and objective) lead to the differential diagnosis. What might you do differently?

3. What are the important considerations for the long-term management of lateral epicondylalgia?

CHAPTER REVIEW QUESTIONS

1. Name the muscles that come off the common extensor tendon.
2. Name the muscles that come off the common flexor tendon.
3. Describe blood flow to the forearm.
4. What nerve gives sensation to the lateral forearm, and where does it come from?
5. What nerve gives sensation to the medial forearm, and where does it come from?
6. What nerve gives sensation to the posterior arm, and where does it come from?

chapter 6

Wrist and Hand

CHAPTER OBJECTIVES

After completing this chapter, the reader will be able to do the following:

- Describe the key bony anatomical structures of the wrist and hand.
- Identify and describe the soft tissue anatomy of the wrist and hand, including muscles, ligaments, nerves, arteries, and veins.
- Identify the different groups of intrinsic muscles in the hand.
- Identify the structures that travel through the carpal tunnel.
- Identify on bony or skeletal models the origins and insertions of the muscles of the wrist and hand in order to aid in understanding osteokinematic action and surface palpation.
- Palpate structures of the wrist and hand.
- Integrate surface palpation findings to aid in the differential diagnosis of a patient with wrist or hand pain.

Several joints compose the anatomical complex of the wrist and hand: the distal radioulnar, radiocarpal, midcarpal, carpometacarpal, metacarpophalangeal, and interphalangeal joints. Many bones, ligaments, and muscles form and stabilize these important articulations to enable a multitude of fine-motor tasks. Several nerves and arteries cross the wrist, bringing in sensation, motor function, and arterial supply to the digits.

Functions of the Wrist and Hand

The most important function of the wrist is to maintain an ideal length–tension relationship of the long finger flexor and extensor muscles to optimize the function of the hand during its performance of tasks.[1] Any trauma, injury, disease, or immobilization to the wrist can negatively affect an individual's ability to perform activities of daily living.

In addition to the functions of the wrist, we depend on the hand for fine-motor function and manipulation of objects. For this to occur, the other joints of the upper extremity are responsible for the placement of the hand in space (gross-motor function). Proper placement of the hand allows it to perform the task required. The fine-motor and manipulation functions of the hand require highly coordinated movement with simultaneous stabilization of the many joints in the upper extremity.

The hand has the ability to perform a variety of osteokinematic movements. The digits can perform flexion, extension, abduction, and adduction, depending on the joint. In addition to the other motions, the thumb, or digit 1, has a unique structure that allows us to oppose this digit to any of the other digits on the hand. Functionally speaking, the thumb side (radial aspect) of the hand is used for dexterity, while the medial side (ulnar aspect) of the hand, especially digit 5, provides power for grip strength.[1]

Bony Anatomy

The wrist is composed of eight carpal bones, which are divided into a proximal row and a distal row (figure 6.1).

- The proximal row is formed by the scaphoid, lunate, triquetrum, and pisiform.
- The distal row is formed by the trapezium, trapezoid, capitate, and hamate.

The hamate has a large projection, called the hook of the hamate, on the anterior–lateral aspect of the bone. Of particular importance, because several soft tissue structures attach to them, are the scaphoid, lunate, hamate, and pisiform bones. The scaphoid and lunate serve as the attachment for the thenar muscles, while the hamate and pisiform bones serve as the attachment for the hypothenar muscles.[2]

The wrist is composed of two joints enclosed in the same joint capsule.

- The radiocarpal joint is a condyloid joint, formed by the distal aspect of the radius articulating with the scaphoid and lunate.
- The midcarpal joint (see figure 6.1) is also a condyloid joint, formed by the proximal scaphoid and lunate articulating with the distal capitate.

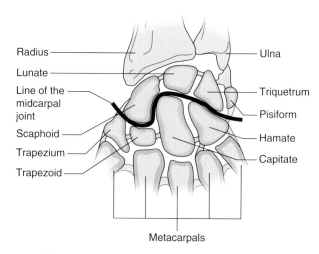

FIGURE 6.1 Bones of the wrist. See figure 6.2 for another view of the wrist bones.

Together these two joints permit wrist flexion and extension as well as radial and ulnar deviation.

Proximal to the wrist joint is another synovial joint, the distal radioulnar joint, which is formed by the ulnar head fitting into the ulnar notch of the radius. It is the movement at this joint, along with that of the proximal radioulnar joint, that permits forearm pronation and supination. In addition to the bony articulations, a thick interosseous membrane between the radius and ulna functions to transfer forces from the radius to the ulna to the humerus.[1]

The bony anatomy of the hand is quite complex because of the many bones, joints, and ligaments that not only provide stability to the hand but also promote motion in multiple planes. The hand has five digits, numbered 1 to 5, beginning with the thumb (digit 1) and ending with the pinky (digit 5) (figure 6.2).

- Distal to the carpal bones are the five metacarpal bones, which serve as attachments for many of the forearm muscles.

- Distal to the metacarpals are the phalanges, which can be divided into the proximal phalanges, middle phalanges, and distal phalanges on all digits except the thumb, which has no middle phalanx.[2] These small bones form the carpometacarpal (CMC) joints, the metacarpophalangeal (MCP) joints, the proximal interphalangeal (PIP) joints, and the distal interphalangeal (DIP) joints of the hand.

  - The first CMC joint is of particular importance to hand function because this saddle-shaped joint permits motion in both the sagittal and frontal planes, making opposition with the other four digits possible. The remaining CMC joints offer little motion except the fifth CMC joint, which works with the first CMC joint to allow cupping of the hand.

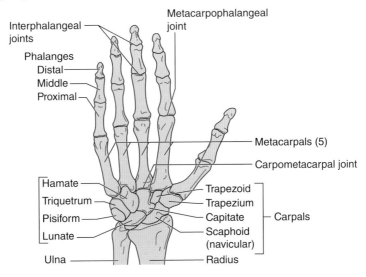

FIGURE 6.2 Bones of the wrist and hand.

- The MCP joints of the hand permit motion in both the sagittal and frontal planes, whereas the DIP and PIP joints allow only for motion in the sagittal plane.

All these joints are stabilized by a variety of soft tissues (ligaments, capsule, muscles, and fascia) to prevent unwanted motion.[1]

Soft Tissue Anatomy

Several groups of muscles cross the distal forearm, wrist, and hand. The previous chapter describes the muscles originating off the lateral and medial epicondyles and provides instructions on how to palpate their muscle bellies in the forearm. This chapter focuses on palpation of the tendons of these muscles distally as they cross the wrist and head to their insertions in the hand.

The anterior aspect of the wrist has several tendons crossing over it (figure 6.3):

- Flexor carpi radialis
- Palmaris longus
- Flexor carpi ulnaris
- Flexor digitorum superficialis
- Flexor digitorum profundus
- Flexor pollicis longus

On the anterior aspect of the wrist is the carpal tunnel, a narrow tunnel through which nine tendons and the median nerve travel to get to the hand.

- The tendons of the flexor pollicis longus, flexor digitorum superficialis, and flexor digitorum profundus all travel through the carpal tunnel, along with the median nerve and a branch of the radial artery.
- Superiorly, this tunnel is covered by the transverse carpal ligament.

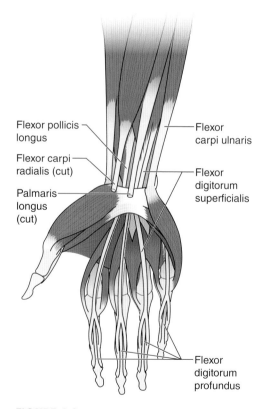

FIGURE 6.3 Anterior wrist tendons.

Superficial to the carpal tunnel and the muscles and tendons crossing the wrist is the flexor retinaculum, a thick band of fascia, which keeps the tendons from bowstringing during wrist flexion.[1]

The posterior aspect of the wrist has several tendons crossing over it (figure 6.4):

- Extensor carpi radialis longus and brevis
- Extensor digitorum communis
- Extensor digiti minimi
- Extensor carpi ulnaris

On the distal lateral aspect of the forearm is a depression called the snuff box, which is bordered by several tendons.[2]

- The abductor pollicis longus and extensor pollicis brevis tendons form the anterior border of the snuff box.
- The extensor pollicis longus forms the posterior border of the snuff box.
- The scaphoid and trapezium form the floor of the snuff box.

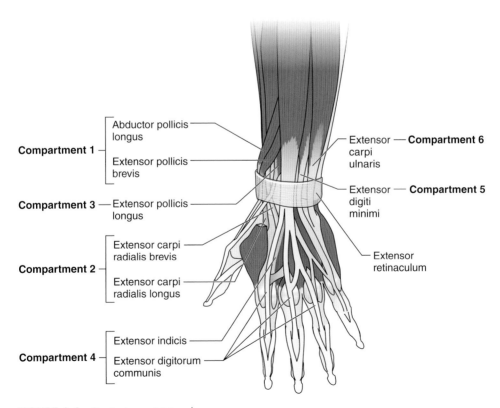

FIGURE 6.4 Posterior wrist tendons.

Superficial to these muscles and tendons is another thick band of fascia, the extensor retinaculum, which prevents the extensor tendons from bow-stringing during wrist extension.[2] The extensor retinaculum is composed of six compartments, or tunnels (see figure 6.4), through which tendons travel to insert distally on the hand.[2]

- The first compartment contains the abductor pollicis longus and extensor pollicis brevis.
- The second compartment contains the extensor carpi radialis longus and brevis.
- The third compartment contains the extensor pollicis longus.
- The fourth compartment contains the extensor digitorum communis and extensor indicis.
- The fifth compartment contains the extensor digiti minimi.
- The sixth compartment contains the extensor carpi ulnaris.

The palm of the hand consists of 20 intrinsic muscles that can be divided into several groups.

- The thenar muscle group, also known as the thenar eminence, is located on the radial aspect of the hand and includes the abductor pollicis brevis, flexor pollicis brevis, and opponens pollicis muscles (figure 6.5). In addition, to complete the muscles that are located on the radial aspect of the hand, the adductor pollicis attaches to the first digit.

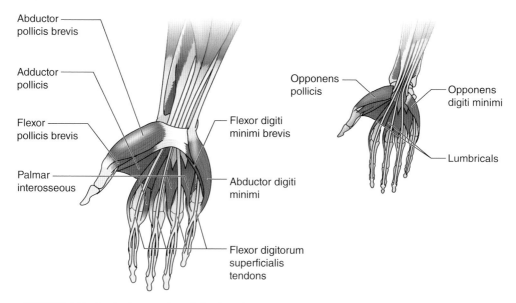

FIGURE 6.5 Intrinsic muscles of the hand.

- On the ulnar aspect of the hand is the hypothenar muscle group, also known as the hypothenar eminence. This muscle group is composed of the abductor digiti minimi, flexor digiti minimi brevis, and opponens digiti minimi muscles.

The remaining intrinsic muscles of the hand are divided into three additional groups: the lumbricals, dorsal interossei, and palmar interossei, with four muscles in each group. All of these contribute to proper biomechanical function of the hand. To complete the intrinsic muscles of the hand, the small palmaris brevis lies on the ulnar aspect of the hand and has no significant osteokinematic action, but rather functions to tighten the skin over the ulnar aspect of the hand.[2]

Surrounding the wrist and hand are important ligaments that increase the passive stability of these joints during movement. As in the elbow, passive stability of the joint is provided by the medial (ulnar) and lateral (radial) collateral ligaments, both of which are palpable (figure 6.6). There are also intrinsic wrist and hand ligaments that attach one carpal bone to another. Of particular importance is the scapholunate ligament, which runs from the scaphoid to the lunate. In cases of wrist instability or following trauma, this ligament may be torn, causing pain for patients during weight-bearing activities.[1,3,4] These smaller ligaments, however, cannot be palpated directly.

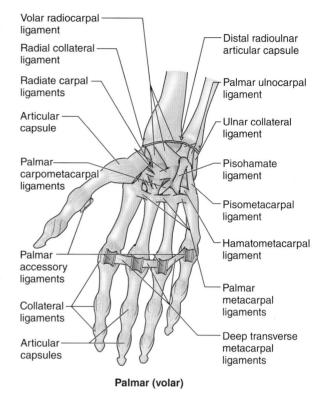

Palmar (volar)

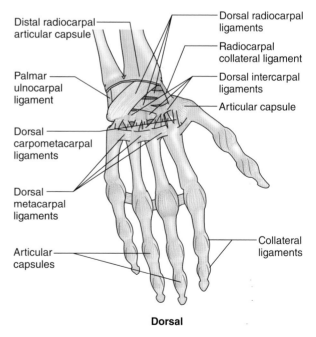

Dorsal

FIGURE 6.6 Ligaments of the wrist and hand.

Neurovascular Anatomy

Both the radial and ulnar arteries cross the anterior aspect of the wrist (figure 6.7), and they are both palpable in this location.

- The radial artery is located lateral to the tendon of the flexor carpi radialis. This artery heads into the hand and helps to form the deep palmar arterial arch.[2]
- The ulnar artery is located lateral to the flexor carpi ulnaris and subsequently heads into the hand to help form the superficial palmar arterial arch.[2]

While several nerves cross the wrist joint, the median nerve, located in the carpal tunnel, is the most commonly injured nerve in the upper extremity (figure 6.8).[5,6] This nerve enters the forearm through the heads of the pronator teres and innervates muscles in the forearm and hand. The median nerve can be compressed in the carpal tunnel, causing carpal tunnel syndrome, and also in the pronator teres, causing pronator teres syndrome. This latter condition is far less common than carpal tunnel syndrome.[2]

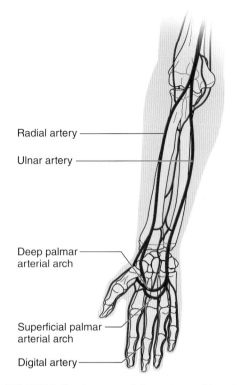

FIGURE 6.7   Arteries of the wrist and hand.

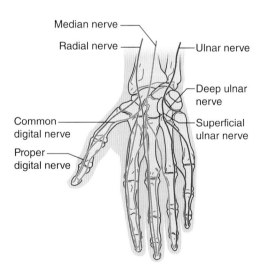

FIGURE 6.8   Nerves of the wrist and hand.

Structural Inspection

- Observation of the wrist and hand is extremely important and can provide information or clues to the clinician about multiple systems in the body.

- Because most patients with wrist and hand injuries splint their hand across the chest or abdomen for protection, the clinician should observe to see whether the patient is ambulating with reciprocal arm swing.

- Once seated, the clinician can quickly ascertain the resting position of the wrist and hand, which usually places the MCP and DIP and PIP joints in slight flexion.

- The overall gross-motor function of the wrist and hand can next be assessed by simply asking the patient to do functional activities, such as writing and eating.

- The clinician should assess for bony deformities, swelling, nodules, trophic changes, or bruising that may be indicative of trauma.

- Close inspection of the nail beds can reveal potential clubbing of the digits, which is a sign of possible vascular compromise.

- Excessive sweating can be indicative of complex regional pain syndrome and also a benign finding of hyperhidrosis.

- The clinician should use the creases of the wrist and hand palmarly to help identify the location of bony structures. These include the proximal and distal wrist creases as well as the proximal palmar crease, distal palmar crease, and creases located at the MCP, PIP, and DIP joints on digits 2 to 5.

- Dorsally, the clinician should observe the relationship between the lunate, capitate, and third metacarpal. They should form a single stable ray that is free from deviation when the patient makes a fist.

- Additionally, there should be no rotation or deviation seen along the MCP joints when the patient makes a full fist. Such deviation may be the result of a dislocation or fracture.

Radial Styloid Process (Key Reference Structure)

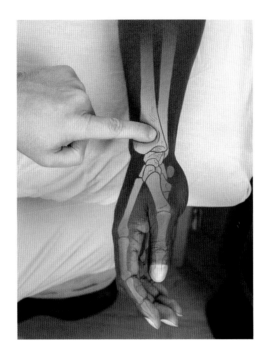

Positions
- Patient: sitting, with the forearm supported by a table or plinth in a neutral position
- Clinician: sitting, facing the patient, on the side being palpated

Instructions
- Palpate along the lateral aspect of the distal radius with one or two fingers until a bony prominence is felt proximal to the wrist.
- At the distal tip of the radial styloid process, palpate the small groove that can be felt along the lateral edge.
- Move the fingers proximally along the lateral aspect of the radius, continuing to palpate the bone until it is covered by soft tissue, approximately at the midforearm.

Ulnar Styloid Process (Key Reference Structure)

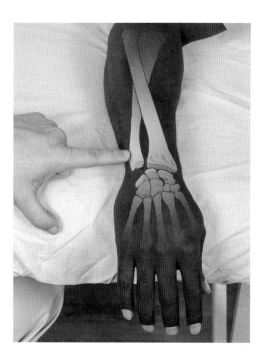

Positions

- Patient: sitting, with the forearm supported by a table or plinth in a pronated position
- Clinician: sitting, facing the patient, on the side being palpated

Instructions

- Palpate the radial styloid process.
- Move your fingers medially to the bony prominence on the other side of the wrist to palpate the ulnar styloid process with one finger.
- Keep in mind that the ulnar styloid process does not extend as far distally as the radial styloid process and is located more posteriorly than medially.
- To confirm palpation, follow digit 5 proximally to the most distal medial aspect of the forearm until a large bony prominence is felt.

Lister's Tubercle (Key Reference Structure)

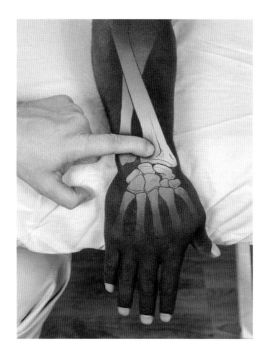

Positions

- Patient: sitting, with the forearm supported by a table or plinth in a pronated position, with the wrist passively flexed to at least 45°
- Clinician: sitting, facing the patient, on the side being palpated

Instructions

- Palpate the radial styloid process.
- Move one finger posteriorly to the radial side of the dorsum of the hand until another bony prominence is felt.

Scaphoid

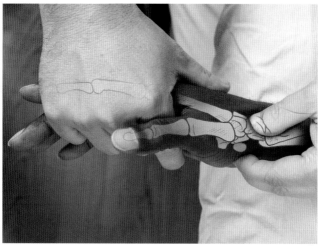

VIDEO 6.1 ▶

Positions

- Patient: sitting, with the forearm supported by a table or plinth in a neutral position
- Clinician: sitting, facing the patient, on the side being palpated

Instructions

- Palpate the radial styloid process.
- Using a pincer grasp, palpate down to the snuff box until reaching the first bony prominence located there.
- Your thumb should be on the posterior aspect of the scaphoid, with digits 2 and 3 on the anterior aspect of the scaphoid.
- To confirm palpation of the scaphoid, have the patient alternately radially and ulnarly deviate the wrist so you can feel the scaphoid move.

CLINICAL PEARL

The scaphoid is the most commonly fractured carpal bone following falls on an outstretched hand. The proximal pole of the bone has tenuous blood supply and is susceptible to developing avascular necrosis if not treated effectively. Tenderness in the anatomical snuff box is common with scaphoid fractures, which must be ruled out in a patient presenting with snuff box tenderness.[7]

Lunate

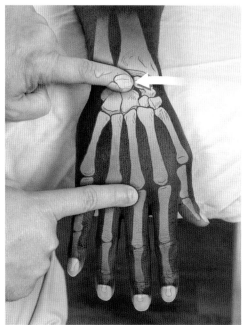

VIDEO 6.2 ▶

Positions
- Patient: sitting, with the forearm supported by a table or plinth in a pronated position
- Clinician: sitting, facing the patient, on the side being palpated

Instructions
- Palpate the scaphoid.
- Move one or two fingers medially to palpate the lunate on the dorsal aspect of the wrist just distal to the radius (left hand pictured).
- To confirm palpation, have the patient alternately flex and extend the wrist so you can feel the lunate moving. The lunate will be more prominent in flexion.

Note
The third metacarpal, capitate, and lunate form the most stable column of the wrist and hand.

Pisiform (Key Reference Structure)

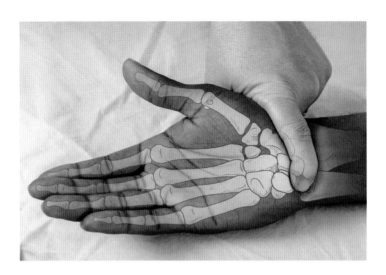

Positions
- Patient: sitting, with the forearm supported by a table or plinth in a supinated and ulnarly deviated position
- Clinician: sitting, facing the patient, on the side being palpated

Instructions
- Palpate along the anterior aspect of the distal ulna with one finger.
- A bony prominence will be felt at the distal aspect of the wrist, just proximal to the hypothenar eminence.

Triquetrum

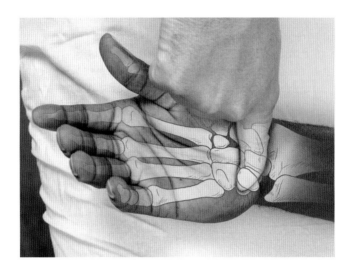

Positions

- Patient: sitting, with the forearm supported by a table or plinth in a supinated position
- Clinician: sitting, facing the patient, on the side being palpated

Instructions

- With the pad of your second digit, palpate the pisiform bone.
- Move your finger slightly laterally and apply pressure into the palm of the hand.
- You will feel a bony prominence.

Note

The pisiform bone sits on top of the triquetrum. Palpating the pisiform bone first and then sliding your finger off the pisiform will confirm the palpation of the triquetrum.

Trapezium

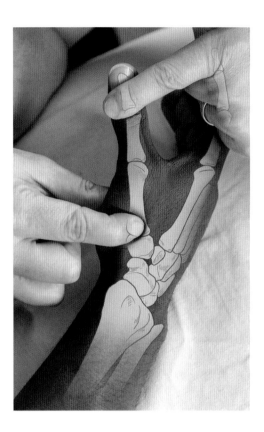

Positions
- Patient: sitting, with the forearm supported by a table or plinth in a neutral position
- Clinician: sitting, facing the patient, on the side being palpated

Instructions
- Palpate the scaphoid.
- Move distally in the snuff box with one finger to palpate the trapezium (right hand pictured).
- Confirm the palpation of the trapezium by moving slightly more distal and feeling for the joint space between the trapezium and first metacarpal.

Trapezoid

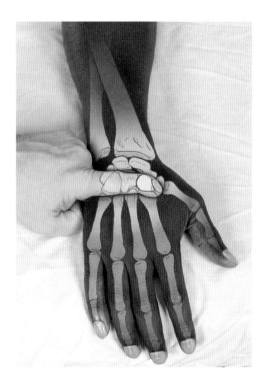

Positions

- Patient: sitting, with the forearm supported by a table or plinth in a pronated position
- Clinician: sitting, facing the patient, on the side being palpated

Instructions

- With the pad of your second digit, palpate the trapezium.
- Move your finger medially to palpate the trapezoid.

Capitate

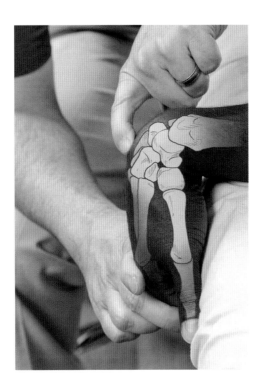

Positions
- Patient: sitting, with the forearm supported by a table or plinth in a pronated position and the wrist in a position of full passive flexion
- Clinician: sitting, facing the patient, on the side being palpated

Instructions
- Palpate the lunate.
- Move distally until a groove is felt.
- Palpate the capitate with one finger in the groove. A large bony prominence will be felt under your finger.

Hamate

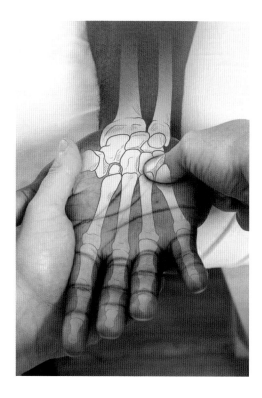

Positions

- Patient: sitting, with the forearm supported by a table or plinth in a supinated position
- Clinician: sitting, facing the patient, on the side being palpated

Instructions

- Palpate the pisiform.
- Move your thumb distally and laterally over the hypothenar eminence.
- A bony projection should be felt; this is the hook of the hamate.
- Move your fingers back medially to palpate the most medial aspect of the bone.

Metacarpals 1 to 5

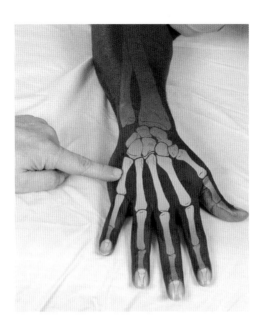

Positions

- Patient: sitting, with the forearm supported by a table or plinth in a supinated position
- Clinician: sitting, facing the patient, on the side being palpated

Instructions

- Palpate the distal row of carpal bones.
- Move one finger distally to where it articulates with the respective metacarpal.

Proximal Phalanges 1 to 5

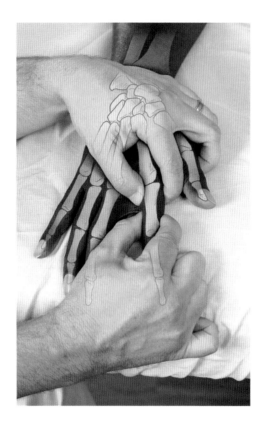

Positions

- Patient: sitting, with the forearm supported by a table or plinth in a pronated position
- Clinician: sitting, facing the patient, on the side being palpated

Instructions

- Palpate the metacarpals using the pads of digits one and two and move your fingers distally to where they articulate with the respective proximal phalanges.
- With your four fingers encircling the bone, palpate along the shaft of the bone to the distal end.

Middle Phalanges 2 to 5

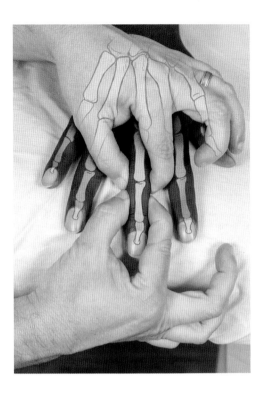

Positions

- Patient: sitting, with the forearm supported by a table or plinth in a pronated position
- Clinician: sitting, facing the patient, on the side being palpated

Instructions

- Palpate the proximal phalanges using the pads of digits one and two.
- Move your fingers distally to the point where they articulate with the respective middle phalanges.
- With your four fingers encircling the bone, palpate along the shaft of the bone to the distal end.

Distal Phalanges 1 to 5

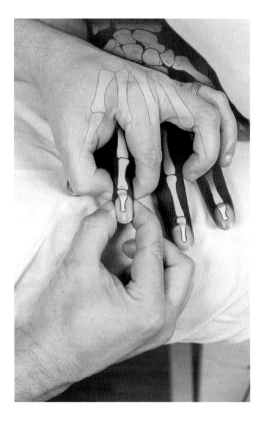

Positions

- Patient: sitting, with the forearm supported by a table or plinth in a pronated position
- Clinician: sitting, facing the patient, on the side being palpated

Instructions

- Palpate the middle phalanges using the pads of digits one and two (proximal for the first digit).
- Move your fingers distally to the point where they articulate with the respective distal phalanges.
- With your four fingers encircling the bone, palpate along the shaft of the bone to the distal end.

Intrinsic Muscles of the Hand

Name	Origin	Insertion	Innervation	Blood supply	Action
Abductor pollicis brevis	Flexor retinaculum, scaphoid, and trapezium	Lateral aspect of the proximal phalanx of digit 1 (thumb)	Recurrent branch of median nerve (C8-T1)	Superficial palmar branch of the radial artery	Abduction of digit 1 and assistance with opposition
Flexor pollicis brevis	Flexor retinaculum and trapezium	Lateral aspect of the proximal phalanx of digit 1	Recurrent branch of the median nerve (C8-T1)	Superficial palmar branch of the radial artery	Flexion of the proximal phalanx (MCP joint) of digit 1
Opponens pollicis	Flexor retinaculum and trapezium	Lateral side of metacarpal 1	Recurrent branch of the median nerve (C8-T1)	Superficial palmar branch of the radial artery	Thumb opposition
Adductor pollicis	*Oblique head:* Capitate, trapezoid, and bases of metacarpals 2 and 3	Medial aspect of the proximal phalanx of digit 1	Deep branch of the ulnar nerve (C8-T1)	Deep palmar arterial arch	Thumb adduction
Palmaris brevis	Palmar aponeurosis	Skin along the ulnar border of the palm	Superficial palmar branch of the ulnar nerve (C8)	Superficial palmar arterial arch	Deepening of the hollow of the hand
Abductor digiti minimi	Pisiform bone	Medial aspect of the proximal phalanx of digit 5	Deep branch of the ulnar nerve (C8-T1)	Deep palmar branch of the ulnar artery	Abduction of digit 5
Flexor digiti minimi	Hook of hamate	Medial aspect of the proximal phalanx of digit 5	Deep branch of ulnar nerve (C8-T1)	Deep palmar branch of ulnar artery	Flexion of the proximal phalanx (MCP joint) of digit 5
Opponens digiti minimi	Hook of hamate	Medial border of metacarpal 5	Deep branch of the ulnar nerve (C8-T1)	Deep palmar branch of the ulnar artery	Digit 5 opposition
Lumbricals (four)	Tendons of the flexor digitorum profundus	Extensor expansions of digits 2 to 5	Median nerve (lumbricals 1-2) and ulnar nerve (lumbricals 3-4) (C8-T1)	Superficial and deep palmar arterial arches	Flexion of the MCP joints and extension of the IP joints of digits 2-5
Dorsal interossei (four)	Adjacent sides of two metacarpals	Extensor expansions of digits 2 to 4	Deep branch of ulnar nerve (C8-T1)	Deep palmar arterial arch	Abduction of the digits, assistance of lumbricals in flexion of the MCP joints, and extension of the IP joints
Palmar interossei (four)	Metacarpals 1, 2, 4, 5	Extensor expansions of digits 1, 2, 4, 5	Deep branch of the ulnar nerve (C8-T1)	Deep palmar arterial arch	Adduction of the digits, assistance of lumbricals in flexion of the MCP joints, and extension of the IP joints

Please refer to chapter 5 for the anterior and posterior arm and forearm muscle chart.

Wrist Zone I: Lateral Aspect of the Wrist

Anatomical Snuff Box: Extensor Compartment I

- Abductor pollicis longus
- Extensor pollicis brevis
- Extensor pollicis longus

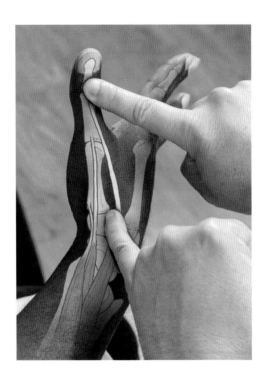

Positions
- Patient: sitting, with the forearm supported by a table or plinth in a neutral position
- Clinician: sitting, facing the patient, on the side being palpated

Instructions
- Palpate the radial styloid process (key reference structure).
- Move one finger just dorsally and distally to palpate the anatomic snuff box by having the patient extend and abduct the thumb (left hand pictured).

- Identify the visible extensor pollicis longus, which is the posterior border of the snuff box, by having the patient perform thumb extension against resistance (right hand pictured).
- Identify the visible extensor pollicis brevis, which helps form the anterior border of the snuff box, by having the patient perform thumb extension against resistance.
- Move one or two fingers slightly anteriorly to palpate the abductor pollicis longus (often not visible) by having the patient perform thumb abduction against resistance.

CLINICAL PEARL

Inflammation of the tendon sheaths of the first dorsal compartment, which contain the abductor pollicis longus and the extensor pollicis brevis, is called De Quervain's syndrome.[8]

Wrist Zone II: Dorsal Aspect of the Wrist

Extensor Compartment II

- Extensor carpi radialis longus (ECRL)
- Extensor carpi radialis brevis (ECRB)

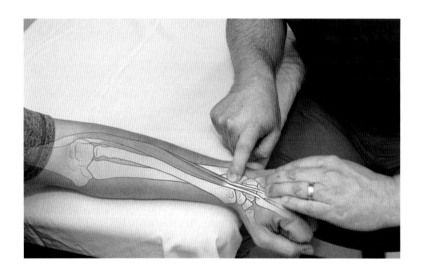

Positions

- Patient: sitting, with the forearm supported by a table or plinth in a pronated position
- Clinician: sitting, facing the patient, on the side being palpated

Instructions

- Palpate Lister's tubercle (key reference structure).
- Move your finger or fingers laterally just off the bony prominence (right hand pictured).
- To confirm palpation, have the patient make a full fist and perform wrist extension against resistance (left hand pictured). You should feel a thin tendon contract under your finger.

Extensor Compartment III

- Extensor pollicis longus

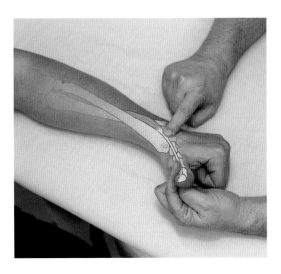

Positions
- Patient: sitting, with the forearm supported by a table or plinth in a neutral position
- Clinician: sitting, facing the patient, on the side being palpated

Instructions
- Palpate Lister's tubercle with one finger.
- Move your finger medially just off the bony prominence (right hand pictured).
- To confirm palpation, have the patient perform thumb extension against resistance (left hand pictured). You will feel a small tendon contract under your finger.

Extensor Compartment IV

- Extensor digitorum
- Extensor indicis

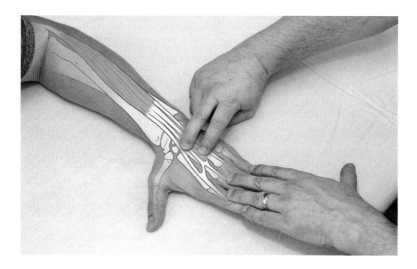

Positions
- Patient: sitting, with the forearm supported by a table or plinth in a pronated position
- Clinician: sitting, facing the patient, on the side being palpated

Instructions
- Locate the radiocarpal joint and the MCP joints of digits 2 to 5.
- Using two fingers, move distal to the radiocarpal joint to palpate extensor compartment IV (right hand pictured).
- To confirm palpation, have the patient extend the MCP joints against resistance of digits 2 to 5 (left hand pictured).

Note
The picture is demonstrating palpation of the extensor digitorum in the hand after it exits compartment number four in the posterior aspect of the wrist. The extensor digitorum tendons are not visible within the compartment as they are covered by the extensor retinaculum.

Wrist Zone III: Medial Aspect of the Wrist

Extensor Compartment V

- Extensor digiti minimi

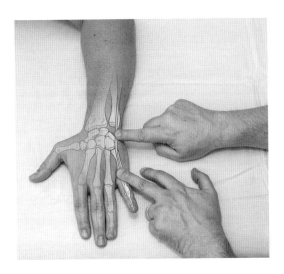

Positions

- Patient: sitting, with the forearm supported by a table or plinth in a pronated position
- Clinician: sitting, facing the patient, on the side being palpated

Instructions

- Palpate the ulnar styloid process (key reference structure).
- Move one finger just lateral to the ulnar styloid process and feel for a small groove (right hand pictured).
- To confirm palpation, have the patient extend the MCP joint of digit 5 against resistance with the hand resting on the table or plinth (left hand pictured). You will feel a subtle contraction under your finger.

Extensor Compartment VI

- Extensor carpi ulnaris

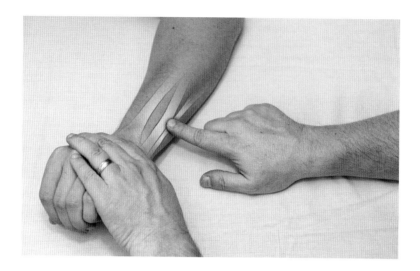

Positions

- Patient: sitting, with the forearm supported by a table or plinth in a pronated position
- Clinician: sitting, facing the patient, on the side being palpated

Instructions

- Palpate the ulnar styloid process with one or two fingers.
- Move the fingers slightly medially and distally and feel for a small groove (right hand pictured).
- To confirm palpation, have the patient extend and ulnarly deviate the wrist against resistance (left hand pictured). You will feel the tendon contract under your fingers.

Wrist Zone IV: Palmar Aspect of the Wrist

Flexor Carpi Ulnaris (FCU)

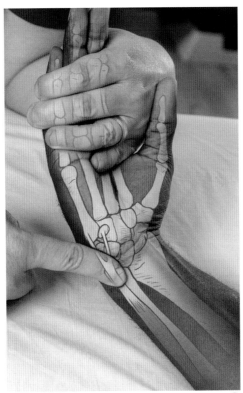

VIDEO 6.3 ▶

Positions
- Patient: sitting, with the forearm supported by a table or plinth in a supinated position
- Clinician: sitting, facing the patient, on the side being palpated

Instructions
- Using one finger, palpate the pisiform bone (key reference structure).
- Move the finger slightly proximally to palpate the FCU (right hand pictured).
- To confirm palpation, have the patient flex and ulnarly deviate the wrist against resistance (left hand pictured). You will feel the tendon contract under your finger.
- The tendon is easily visible on the ulnar side of the wrist.

Flexor Digitorum Superficialis

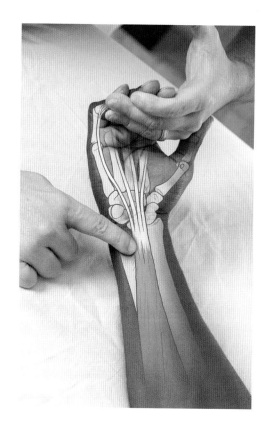

Positions

- Patient: sitting, with the forearm supported by a table or plinth in a supinated position
- Clinician: sitting, facing the patient, on the side being palpated

Instructions

- Palpate the FCU with one or two fingers.
- Move the fingers laterally toward the center of the wrist and proximal to the proximal wrist crease (right hand pictured).
- To confirm palpation, have the patient flex the PIP joints of digits 2 to 5 against resistance (left hand pictured). You will feel the tendons bulge under your fingers.
- The tendons of the flexor digitorum superficialis (FDS) will be visible between the flexor carpi ulnaris (FCU) and the palmaris longus.

Ulnar Nerve (Guyon's Canal)

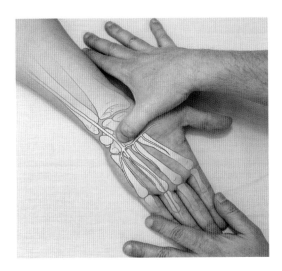

Positions

- Patient: sitting, with the forearm supported by a table or plinth in a supinated position
- Clinician: sitting, facing the patient, on the side being palpated

Instructions

- Palpate the pisiform bone.
- Palpate the hook of the hamate with one finger.
- Between the two bones is a groove, Guyon's canal (tunnel), where the ulnar nerve sits.
- Depending on the thickness of the overlying soft tissue, the ulnar nerve may be palpable in this groove. You should feel a round, narrow structure.

CLINICAL PEARL

Tenderness to palpation or reproduction of neurological symptoms in Guyon's canal can be indicative of ulnar nerve pathology.

Ulnar Artery

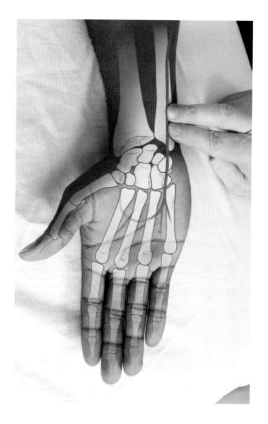

Positions

- Patient: sitting, with the forearm supported by a table or plinth in a supinated position
- Clinician: sitting, facing the patient, on the side being palpated

Instructions

- Palpate the pisiform bone.
- Palpate the FCU.
- With the pads of digits 2 and 3, palpate proximal to the pisiform bone and lateral to the FCU.
- Apply gentle pressure to assess the ulnar pulse.

Wrist Zone V: Palmaris Longus and Carpal Tunnel

Palmaris Longus

Positions

- Patient: sitting, with the forearm supported by a table or plinth in a supinated position
- Clinician: sitting, facing the patient, on the side being palpated

Instructions

- When present, the tendon lies over the midline of the wrist medial to the flexor carpi radialis (left hand pictured).
- To confirm palpation, have the patient flex the wrist against resistance (right hand pictured) while opposing the thumb with the fourth digit. You will feel a small bulge under your fingers.

Note

A portion of the population does not have a palmaris longus bilaterally, and some people do not have it at all. In the second photo, note the lack of a clearly defined tendon, which would be the palmaris longus. The tendon in this photo is the flexor carpi radialis, which is less defined than the palmaris longus.

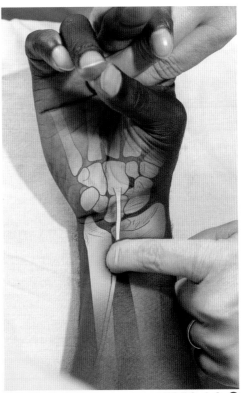

VIDEO 6.3 ▶

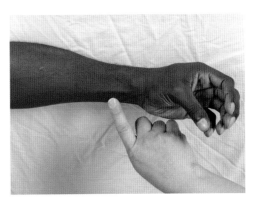

Carpal Tunnel

Positions

- Patient: sitting, with the fore-arm supported by a table or plinth in a supinated position
- Clinician: sitting, facing the patient, on the side being palpated

Instructions

- Palpate the palmaris longus.
- Palpate the four bony promi-nences that define the carpal tunnel.
  - Proximally, the pisiform medially and the scaphoid laterally
  - Distally, the hook of the hamate medially and the trapezium laterally.
- Palpate deep to the palmaris longus through the FDS and flexor digitorum profundus (FDP) muscles, assessing for tenderness while palpating.

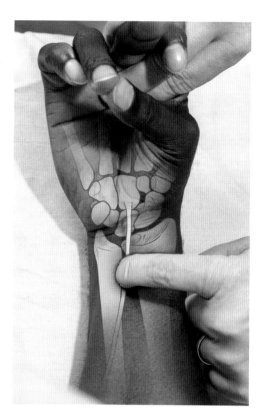

CLINICAL PEARL

The median nerve runs through the carpal tunnel. Compression of this nerve results in carpal tunnel syndrome, the most common compression neuropathy of the upper extremity. This presents as pain and paresthesia along the first three digits, which is usually worse during sleeping.[5]

Flexor Carpi Radialis

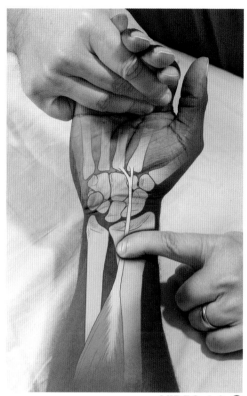

VIDEO 6.3 ▶

Positions

- Patient: sitting, with the forearm supported by a table or plinth in a supinated position
- Clinician: sitting, facing the patient, on the side being palpated

Instructions

- Palpate the palmaris longus if present with one finger.
- Move the finger laterally to palpate the flexor carpi radialis (FCR) (left hand pictured).
- To confirm palpation, have the patient perform flexion and radial deviation against resistance (right hand pictured). You will feel a small bulge under your finger.

Radial Artery

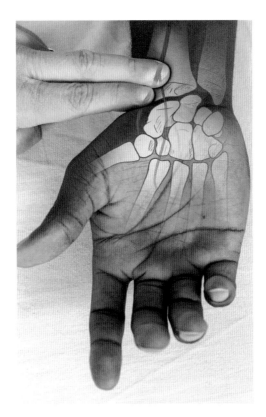

Positions

- Patient: sitting, with the forearm supported by a table or plinth in a supinated position
- Clinician: sitting, facing the patient, on the side being palpated

Instructions

- Palpate the flexor carpi radialis (FCR).
- With the pads of digits 2 and 3, palpate between the FCR and the radial styloid process.
- Apply gentle pressure to assess the radial pulse.

Hand Zone I: Thenar Eminence

- Abductor pollicis brevis
- Flexor pollicis brevis
- Opponens pollicis

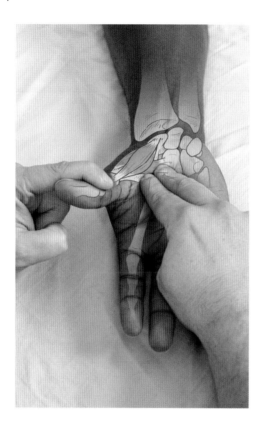

Positions
- Patient: sitting, with the forearm supported by a table or plinth in a supinated position
- Clinician: sitting, facing the patient, on the side being palpated

Instructions
- Using the pads of digits 2 and 3, identify the first MCP joint.
- Move your fingers medially and palpate along the anterior aspect of the thumb to identify the thenar muscle group (right hand pictured).
- To confirm palpation, have the patient perform various thumb movements (abduction, flexion, opposition) against resistance (left hand pictured). You should feel a firm contraction under your fingers.

Adductor Pollicis

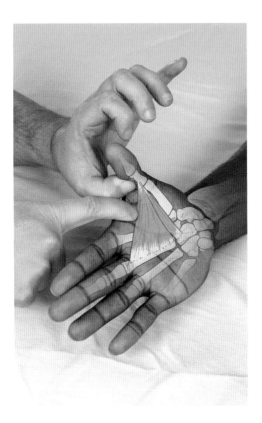

Positions
- Patient: sitting, with the forearm supported by a table or plinth in a supinated position
- Clinician: sitting, facing the patient, on the side being palpated

Instructions
- Using the pads of digit 2, identify the first MCP joint.
- Move your finger medially into the web space and palpate between the first and second digits (right hand pictured).
- To confirm palpation, have the patient perform thumb adduction against resistance (left hand pictured). You should feel a firm contraction under your finger.

Hand Zone II: Hypothenar Eminence

- Abductor digiti minimi
- Flexor digiti minimi
- Opponens digiti minimi

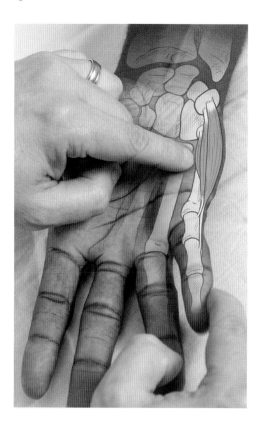

Positions
- Patient: sitting, with the forearm supported by a table or plinth in a supinated position
- Clinician: sitting, facing the patient, on the side being palpated

Instructions
- Palpate the pisiform bone.
- Using the pads of digit 2, move your finger distally to palpate along the anterior aspect of the hand near the fifth digit (left hand pictured).
- To confirm palpation, have the patient perform various movements with the fifth digit (abduction, flexion, opposition) against resistance (right hand pictured). You will feel a firm contraction under your finger.

Hand Zone III: Palm

Palmar Aponeurosis

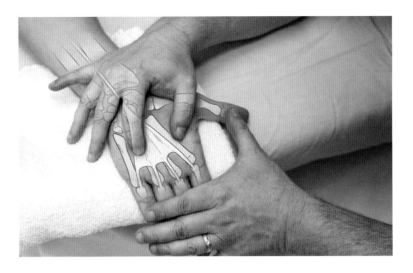

Positions
- Patient: sitting, with the forearm supported by a table or plinth in a supinated position
- Clinician: sitting, facing the patient, on the side being palpated

Instructions
- Gently, passively extend the MCP joints to place the palmar aponeurosis on stretch (left hand pictured).
- Using digits 1 and 2, palpate along the palmar aponeurosis to assess for nodules along the fascia (right hand pictured).

CLINICAL PEARL
Prolonged nodules that develop along the palmar aponeurosis can develop into a condition called Dupuytren's contracture, which is a flexion deformity of digits 4 and 5 most commonly.[9]

Finger Flexor Tendons

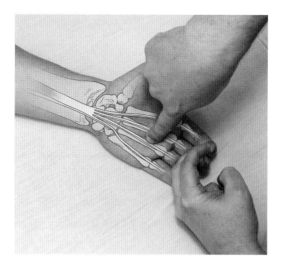

Positions

- Patient: sitting, with the forearm supported by a table or plinth in a supinated position
- Clinician: sitting, facing the patient, on the side being palpated

Instructions

- Palpate the palmar aspect of the MCP joints of digits 2 to 5.
- Move your finger or fingers proximally into the palm of the hand to assess for the long finger flexors (right hand pictured). Of note, the FDP is deep to the FDS.
- To confirm palpation, have the patient flex the fingers against resistance at the MCP joints or the PIP joints (left hand pictured). You should feel the tendon bulge under your fingers.

CLINICAL PEARL

Trigger finger is experienced when the flexor tendon does not glide smoothly in the sheath because of tenosynovitis. This results in a palpable and audible snapping during finger flexion and extension, which is indicative of a trigger finger.[10]

Hand Zone IV: Dorsum

Extensor Tendons

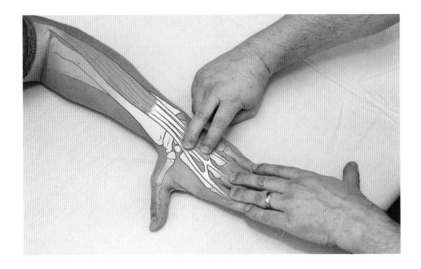

Positions
- Patient: sitting, with the forearm supported by a table or plinth in a pronated position
- Clinician: sitting, facing the patient, on the side being palpated

Instructions
- Palpate the dorsal aspect of the MCP joints of digits 2 to 5.
- Move two fingers proximally on the dorsum of the hand to palpate the extensor tendons.
- To confirm palpation, have the patient extend the fingers against resistance at the MCP joints (left hand pictured). You should feel the tendons bulge under your fingers.

Dorsal Interossei

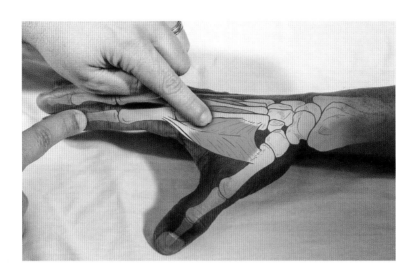

Positions
- Patient: sitting, with the forearm supported by a table or plinth in a pronated position
- Clinician: sitting, facing the patient, on the side being palpated

Instructions
- Palpate the dorsal aspect of the first MCP joint.
- Move your finger posteriorly and medially into the posterior web space between the first and second digits (left hand pictured).
- To confirm palpation of the first dorsal interossei, have the patient abduct the second digit against resistance (right hand pictured). You should feel a firm contraction under your finger.

Case Study

History

A mother brings her 12-year-old daughter, who has been complaining of left wrist pain, into your office. The mother reports that her daughter fell while ice skating 1 week ago. She reports having taken her daughter to the emergency room that day. Radiographs were taken, and she was told that her daughter did not have a fracture but had sprained her wrist. Her daughter was given a splint to wear. The mother reports being concerned because her daughter is still complaining of significant wrist pain on the radial side of the wrist and hand and having difficulty completing daily activities.

- Based on this information only, what are the three most likely diagnoses?

Examination

Past medical history	Asthma
Medication	Albuterol as necessary
Observation	Edema and ecchymosis over posterior, lateral aspect of the wrist Patient presents in splint After splint is removed, patient is reluctant to move her wrist
Active range of motion	Wrist flexion and extension limited to 0° to 20° due to pain Pronation and supination within normal limits Radial and ulnar deviation 0° to 10° with significant pain
Passive range of motion	Same as for active
Manual muscle testing	Not assessed because of mechanism of injury and extreme pain
Special tests	Negative triangular fibrocartilaginous complex load test Negative piano key test
Other	Sensation intact to median, radial, and ulnar nerves Radial and ulnar pulses 2+

- Based on the subjective and objective information together, what are the two most likely diagnoses? Give your rationale for eliminating the third diagnosis.
- What structures should you palpate on this patient based on your differential diagnoses?
- Given all the information presented, what would you expect to find on palpation of those structures?

Case Solution and Discussion

Potential Diagnoses Based on History

- Colles' fracture
- Scaphoid fracture
- Triangular fibrocartilage complex tear

Potential Diagnoses Based on History and Examination

- Colles' fracture
- Scaphoid fracture

Triangular fibrocartilage complex (TFCC) tear: This diagnosis can be eliminated because of the negative triangular fibrocartilaginous complex load test and negative piano key test. Additionally, the subjective report of pain on the radial aspect of the wrist is inconsistent with the pain pattern associated with a TFCC tear.

Structures to Be Palpated

- Scaphoid
- Trapezium
- Distal radius
- Distal ulna

Palpation Findings

- Exquisite tenderness to palpation within the anatomical snuff box

Clinical Reasoning

- Colles' fracture: The patient's mechanism of injury, reports of pain, and bruising and swelling of her wrist in addition to pain and limitations to her active range of motion in the wrist are all consistent with a Colles' fracture. However, this would have been detected immediately after injury on the radiographs. Furthermore, her active range of motion pronation and supination are within normal limits but would be limited if a Colles' fracture were present.

- Scaphoid fracture: The patient's mechanism of injury and reports of pain are consistent with a scaphoid fracture. This is often not immediately detected on radiographs. Other imaging studies are more reliable at detecting this type of fracture, specifically bone scans, computed tomography scans, and magnetic resonance imaging. Clinically, there is exquisite tenderness to palpation of the anatomical snuff box, which is a potential red flag for scaphoid fracture. This, the pain and limitations of wrist active range of motion, and the bruising and swelling of her wrist are all indicative of a scaphoid fracture.

For this diagnosis, the patient *must* be referred to a physician for further diagnostic imaging and proper diagnosis before treatment is administered.

Case Study Questions

1. What information do the palpation findings of the case give the clinician? How can this information be incorporated in the clinical decision-making process?

2. Think about how the examination findings (subjective and objective) lead to the differential diagnosis. What might you do differently?

3. If initial radiographs were negative, what should the clinician recommend to the patient?

CHAPTER REVIEW QUESTIONS

1. List the carpal bones from lateral to medial.
2. Name the tendons that travel through the carpal tunnel.
3. List and group the intrinsic muscles of the hand.
4. Describe the blood supply to the wrist and hand.
5. Describe the nerve supply to the muscles of the hand.
6. What is the most commonly fractured carpal bone?

chapter 7

Cervical Spine and Thorax

After completing this chapter, the reader will be able to do the following:

- Identify the key bony anatomical structures of, and functional relationship between, the cervical spine, thoracic spine, and rib cage.
- Identify and describe the soft tissue anatomy of the cervical spine, thoracic spine, and rib cage, including muscles, ligaments, nerves, arteries, and veins.
- Differentiate the layers of muscles in the cervical and thoracic spine.
- Identify on bony or skeletal models the origins and insertions of the muscles of the cervical and thoracic spine in order to aid in understanding osteokinematic action and surface palpation.
- Describe blood supply to the cervical spine, including the circle of Willis.
- Palpate structures of the cervical spine, thoracic spine, and rib cage.
- Integrate surface palpation findings to aid in the differential diagnosis of a patient with neck or thoracic spine.

The cervical spine, thoracic spine, and rib cage compose an intricate system encompassing many bones, soft tissues, and joints. Neck pain is a prevalent condition in society, with approximately 20% of people in the United Kingdom experiencing neck pain at some point.[1] Evidence has emphasized the importance of regional interdependence between the cervical spine, thoracic spine, and upper quadrant.[2,3] The function of any of these joints can easily affect the function of any other joint in the area. It is important to be mindful of these relationships while studying these joint functions and throughout the clinical examination and management of patients with neck pain.

Functions of the Cervical Spine, Thoracic Spine, and Rib Cage

The cervical spine is the most mobile region of the spine and performs many important functions. One function is to support the head, and another is to protect the spinal cord. The cervical spine is dependent on muscles and ligaments to provide the intersegmental stability that is required to protect the spinal cord from serious injury.[4,5] However, the bony architecture of the cervical spine protects the vital vertebral artery as it passes up to the brainstem. The cervical spine has a more complex function as part of a proprioceptive system to keep the eyes level with the horizon in addition to helping maintain balance.[6]

Unlike the highly mobile cervical spine, the thoracic spine predominantly permits motion in the frontal plane. It functions to maintain an erect posture, which is accomplished by the orientation of the facet joints, as well as its articulations with the rib cage. The thoracic spine functions mainly as a stable base on which the thoracic cage can move. Despite the strong bony articulation between the sternum and rib cage, movement in this anatomical region does occur and is extremely important. The thoracic cage moves to accommodate changes in the diaphragm and lungs throughout inhalation and exhalation. Any trauma to the thoracic spine, rib cage, or sternum can be quite painful for the patient and can potentially interfere with normal breathing patterns.[4,5]

Bony Anatomy

The cervical spine consists of seven vertebrae, which are divided into an upper cervical spine (C0-C2) and a lower cervical spine (C3-C6).

- The first two cervical vertebrae, the atlas and axis (figure 7.1), are considered *atypical*, with C3 to C6 referred to as *typical* cervical vertebrae.[4] The axis has a large projection called the dens, which articulates with the anterior arch of the atlas.

- The skull and atlas form the atlanto-occipital (AO) joint, and the atlas and axis form the atlantoaxial (AA) joint. These joints provide motion so the upper cervical spine can be placed in a multitude of positions.

The third through sixth cervical vertebrae all have small bodies with bifid spinous and transverse processes (figure 7.2). In addition, there is a transverse foramen, through which the vertebral artery passes on its way to the brainstem.[4] Of particular importance is the orientation of the facet joints in the cervical spine, which permits motion in all three cardinal planes.[5]

With respect to the cervical and thoracic spine, the seventh cervical vertebra is a transitional vertebra with some features of cervical and thoracic vertebrae. Thoracic vertebrae have the following features (figure 7.3):

- These heart-shaped bodies have larger spinous and transverse processes.

- In the thoracic spine, the spinous processes project in an inferior direction, making the level of the spinous and transverse processes somewhat controversial during palpation.

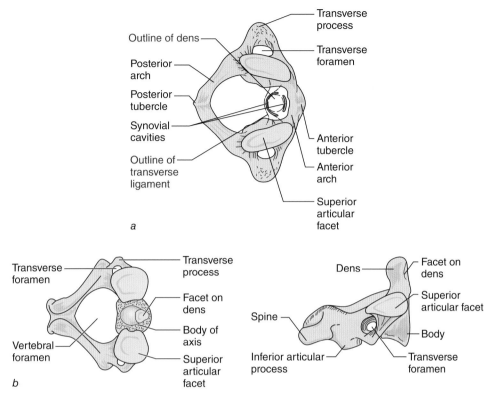

FIGURE 7.1 *(a)* Superior aspect of the atlas. *(b)* Superior and right lateral aspects of the axis.

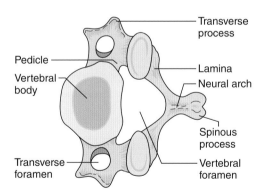

FIGURE 7.2 Superior view of a typical cervical vertebra.

- The hallmark features of the thoracic vertebrae are their costal facets. These facets allow the ribs to articulate with each vertebra at both the transverse processes (costotransverse joint) and the vertebral body (costovertebral joint).

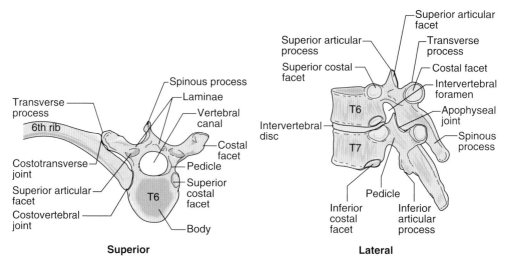

FIGURE 7.3 Typical thoracic vertebrae.

These joints function like other synovial joints in the body and can be a source of pain, degeneration, or both. Of particular importance in this region is the rib angle, which is found just lateral to the transverse processes. At times, this angle can be exquisitely tender to palpation, indicating dysfunction in the thoracic spine or rib cage (or both).[4,5]

Soft Tissue Anatomy

The numerous muscles that surround the cervicothoracic spine and rib cage can all provide dynamic stability. These muscles can be divided into local stabilizing muscles, which increase segmental stability, and global muscles, which produce gross motion.[7] While a thorough discussion of these muscles is beyond the scope of this book, a brief review of the various layers of muscles crossing the cervicothoracic spine and rib cage is necessary here.

The trapezius, levator scapulae, latissimus dorsi, and rhomboids have all been previously discussed (see chapter 3). Deep to the trapezius muscle in the posterior aspect of the neck are the following muscles, running from superficial to deep: splenius capitis and cervicis, semispinalis capitis and cervicis, longissimus capitis, and the suboccipital muscles (figure 7.4). While some of these muscles cannot be palpated individually, understanding their function as a group can help facilitate surface palpation. These muscles collectively perform extension of the upper and lower cervical spine, side-bending, and rotation.[4]

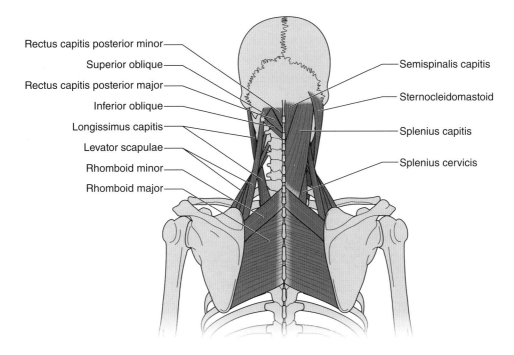

Rectus capitis posterior minor
Superior oblique
Rectus capitis posterior major
Inferior oblique
Longissimus capitis
Levator scapulae
Rhomboid minor
Rhomboid major

Semispinalis capitis
Sternocleidomastoid
Splenius capitis
Splenius cervicis

FIGURE 7.4 Muscles of the posterior cervical spine.

Attached to the upper cervical spine are the superior oblique, inferior oblique, rectus capitis posterior major, and rectus capitis posterior minor muscles, collectively known as the suboccipital muscles (figure 7.5). These muscles function to produce head and neck movement in the upper cervical spine.[4] Often these muscles can become shortened by prolonged forward head posture and can be a source of chronic pain and disability.[8,9]

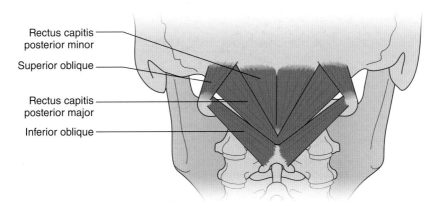

Rectus capitis posterior minor
Superior oblique
Rectus capitis posterior major
Inferior oblique

FIGURE 7.5 Suboccipital muscles.

Anteriorly in the cervical spine are two other important muscles that control the craniocervical region. These are the longus capitis and longus colli muscles (figure 7.6). The longus capitis and colli function to counteract the action of the suboccipital muscles by producing craniocervical flexion.[4] Often these muscles have poor neuromuscular endurance following injury to the cervical spine.[10]

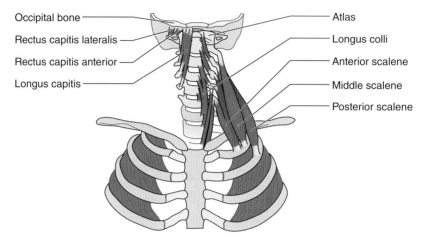

FIGURE 7.6   Muscles of the anterior craniocervical region.

On the anterior–lateral aspect of the neck is the sternocleidomastoid (SCM) (figure 7.7). This muscle is an important landmark that separates the anterior cervical triangle from the posterior cervical triangle.

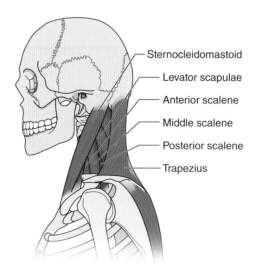

FIGURE 7.7   Muscles of the posterior cervical triangle.

- The anterior cervical triangle is bordered anteriorly by the midline of the neck, posteriorly by the SCM, and superiorly by the mandible.
  - This triangle is further subdivided by the omohyoid and digastric muscles into the carotid, submandibular, submental, and muscular triangles.
  - The suprahyoid and infrahyoid muscles are located in the anterior cervical triangle.[4]
- The posterior cervical triangle is bordered anteriorly by the SCM, posteriorly by the trapezius, and inferiorly by the clavicle.
  - This triangle is further subdivided into the occipital and supraclavicular triangles by the inferior belly of the omohyoid. There are five muscles in the posterior cervical triangle: the anterior, middle, and posterior scalenes, the levator scapulae, and the splenius capitis.[4]
  - The scalene muscles assist in respiration and are referred to as the lateral stabilizers of the cervical spine.
  - Running behind the posterior scalene is the levator scapulae (see chapter 3), which is then followed by the splenius muscle.[4]

Clinically, the muscles of the thoracic spine are collectively known as the erector spinae (thoracic paraspinals). The erector spinae consist of three groups: the iliocostalis, longissimus, and spinalis (figure 7.8). When the erector spinae contract bilaterally, they perform spinal extension; when they contract unilaterally, the result is lateral flexion to the ipsilateral side.[4]

Several ligaments attach to the cervical spine to increase stability in the region. These include the posterior longitudinal ligament (tectorial membrane), the alar ligaments, and the transverse ligament of the atlas (figure 7.9).

- The posterior longitudinal ligament is a broad ligament that runs from the sacrum to the occiput, posterior to the vertebral bodies.
  - In the cervical spine this ligament spans out, widens, and subsequently changes its name to the tectorial membrane.
  - It functions to prevent excessive cervical spine flexion.[4,5]
- The alar ligaments run from the C2 vertebra to the occipital bone. These ligaments function primarily to prevent excessive cervical spine rotation, but also to limit the extremes of all motion.[4,5]
- The transverse ligament of the atlas is a thick band that runs across the atlas and stabilizes the odontoid process of C2 against the anterior arch of the atlas. It functions to prevent the odontoid process of C2 from impinging on the spinal cord.[4,5]

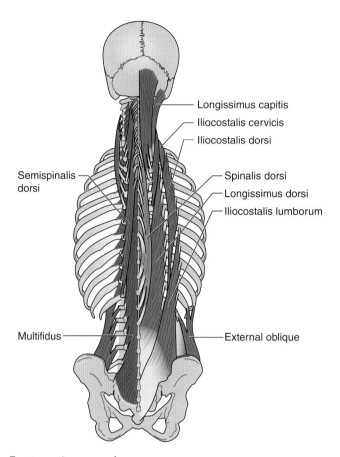

FIGURE 7.8 Erector spinae muscles.

Longissimus capitis

Iliocostalis cervicis

Iliocostalis dorsi

Semispinalis dorsi

Spinalis dorsi

Longissimus dorsi

Iliocostalis lumborum

Multifidus

External oblique

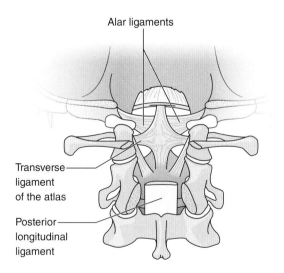

FIGURE 7.9 Ligaments of the cervical spine.

Alar ligaments

Transverse ligament of the atlas

Posterior longitudinal ligament

Neurovascular Anatomy

During the examination and treatment of patients with cervical spine pathology, you should be mindful of important neurovascular structures in the anterior lateral neck region. As mentioned in chapter 2, the common carotid artery travels up through the anterior cervical triangle, and this is where you palpate for the carotid pulse.[4] As with the brachial artery, this should be done carefully with light pressure to avoid occluding the artery.

Blood supply to the cervical spine comes from branches of the vertebral and cervical arteries as they ascend up the neck. The vertebral artery ascends up through the transverse foramen of the cervical spine on its way to help form the circle of Willis (figure 7.10). This artery is located in the suboccipital triangle formed between the inferior and superior oblique muscles. While this artery is not palpable, it is important to be mindful of its path when placing the cervical spine in extreme positions of rotation and extension, which may occlude the vessel and thus cut off blood supply to the brain.[4] We advocate avoiding end-range positions of cervical spine extension and rotation throughout your examination and treatment techniques. As always, maintain good communication with your patient throughout this process to monitor for signs of neurovascular compromise.

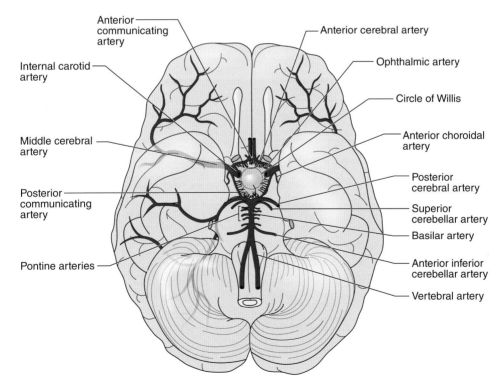

FIGURE 7.10 Circle of Willis.

Directly anterior to the SCM is the carotid sheath. This sheath contains the common carotid artery, internal jugular vein, and vagus nerve. Care must be taken to avoid stimulating the vagus nerve when performing soft tissue mobilization or palpation of the area because this may cause an unwanted drop in heart rate and may lead to the patient losing consciousness.[4]

Posterior to the SCM, between the anterior and middle scalene muscles, are the trunks of the brachial plexus.[4] Aggressive soft tissue mobilization in this area may cause neurological symptoms, which can radiate down the ipsilateral upper extremity. It is important to maintain continuous communication with your patient throughout your examination and treatment session so you can ascertain whether any of these symptoms occur. The presence of symptoms requires immediate modification of that particular examination or treatment technique.

In the cervical spine, there are eight cervical nerves but only seven cervical vertebrae. This is the case because the first cervical nerve exits above C1, with the remaining cervical nerves exiting below the corresponding vertebrae (figure 7.11), similar to the 12 thoracic nerves, as well as the nerves of the lumbosacral spine. The spinal cord starts at the medulla oblongata and runs inferiorly to the L1 to L2 interspace, at which point it is known as the cauda equina, a collection of spinal nerve roots that look like a horse's tail.[4] In the cervical region there is an enlargement of the nerve roots between C5 and T1, which contribute to forming the brachial plexus. Each spinal nerve contains an anterior root and a posterior root.

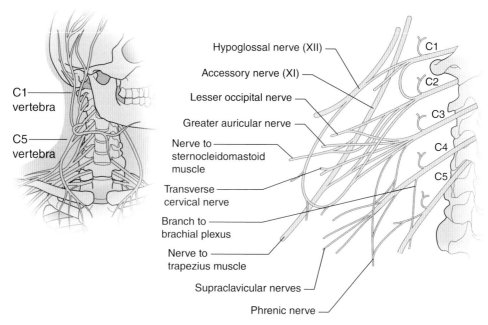

FIGURE 7.11   The cervical plexus, from C1 through C5 nerve roots.

The anterior roots of spinal nerves contain the motor (efferent) fibers innervating skeletal muscles, while the posterior roots contain the sensory (afferent) fibers from the skin and other subcutaneous tissues. The anterior and posterior nerve roots unite to form a spinal nerve that exits the intervertebral foramen.[4]

Structural Inspection

- The structural inspection begins once the patient is comfortably in the examining room in the appropriate attire.
- The clinician should start by noticing the overall movement and attitude of the patient.
- If appropriate, observe for guarded or unnatural movement as the patient disrobes, which can alert the clinician to the possibility of pathology or increased muscle tone or both.
- The head and neck should be in a neutral position, free from side-bending or rotation.
- The clinician should next observe for normal muscle tone and skin color and make sure the region is free from blisters, scars, or abnormal skin markings.
- The clinician should observe the normal curves of the spine (cervical and lumbar lordosis, thoracic and sacral kyphosis) from the anterior, lateral, and posterior views.
- The relationship between the spine and scapula should also be documented and assessed for symmetry.

Thyroid Cartilage

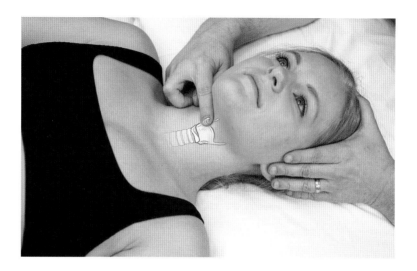

Positions

- Patient: supine, with a pillow under the knees and the head and neck in a neutral position
- Clinician: sitting at the head of the table or standing to the side of the patient

Instructions

- Palpate the hyoid bone using one finger.
- Move inferiorly, staying in midline until your finger palpates the superior aspect (notch) of the thyroid cartilage.
- Continue to move your fingers slightly inferiorly and palpate the prominent upper portion of the thyroid cartilage (Adam's apple). You should feel a small projection under your finger.

Note

The superior aspect of the thyroid cartilage is located at the C4 vertebral level, while the inferior aspect marks the C5 vertebral level.

First Cricoid Ring

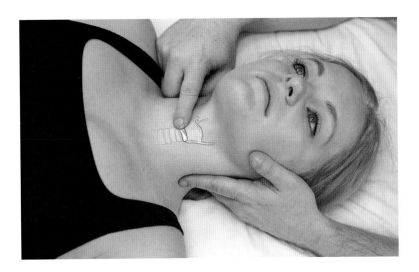

Positions

- Patient: supine, with a pillow under the knees and the head and neck in a neutral position
- Clinician: sitting at the head of the table or standing to the side of the patient

Instructions

- Palpate the inferior border of the thyroid cartilage.
- Move your finger just inferiorly, staying in midline until you palpate the first cricoid ring. You will feel a small circular structure under your finger.

Notes

- The clinician should palpate this structure gently because too much pressure may cause the patient to gag.
- The first cricoid ring is usually at the C6 vertebral level.
- It is the only complete cricoid ring, which is an important part of the trachea. It provides attachments for muscles, cartilages, and ligaments involved in opening and closing the airway and in speech production.

CLINICAL PEARL

This structure is important clinically because it is immediately above the site for emergency tracheostomy.

Carotid Tubercle

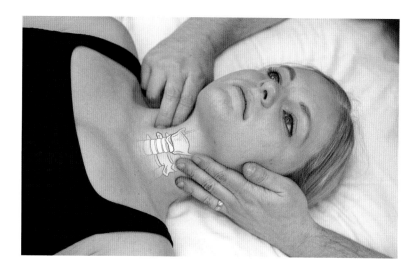

Positions

- Patient: supine, with a pillow under the knees and the head and neck in a neutral position
- Clinician: sitting at the head of the table or standing to the side of the patient

Instructions

- Palpate the first cricoid ring.
- Move two fingers just laterally (approximately 1 inch [2.5 centimeters]) until you palpate the carotid tubercle, which is the anterior tubercle of the C6 transverse process (right hand pictured).
- The remainder of the anterior tubercles of the transverse processes can then be palpated by moving the fingers in a superior direction.

Notes

- The carotid tubercle may be small, but it can be palpated if you use care.
- Carefully palpate each carotid tubercle separately so you do not occlude the carotid arteries, which run along the tubercle, simultaneously.

Spinous Process of C2

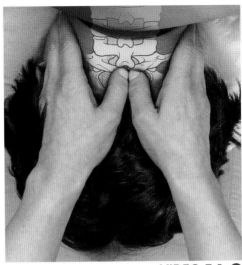

VIDEO 7.1 ▶

Positions
- Patient: prone, with the upper cervical spine in slight flexion
- Clinician: standing or sitting at the head of the table

Instructions
- Palpate the external occipital protuberance, a large bony prominence on the back of the head (see chapter 2).
- Palpate with the first digit of both hands down the midline of the spine, moving inferiorly along the suboccipital tissues.
- Continue inferiorly until a large midline projection is palpated; this is the spinous process of C2.

Note
This is an important palpation because the spinous process of C2 will serve as the anatomical landmark for palpation of the remainder of the cervical spinous processes.

CLINICAL PEARL
Once you are comfortable palpating the spinous process of C2 prone (simpler method), you should learn how to palpate the spinous process of C2 supine. This is because the facet joints can subsequently be palpated by moving just lateral to the spinous processes in the cervical spine. This is an important landmark for the application of manual therapy techniques.

Spinous Processes of C3 to C7

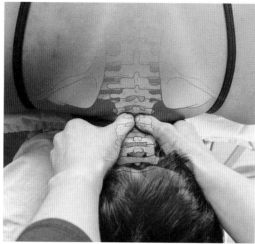

VIDEO 7.2 ▶

Positions

- Patient: prone, with the lower cervical spine in slight flexion
- Clinician: standing or sitting at the head of the table

Instructions

- Palpate the spinous process of C2 with the first digit of both hands.
- Keeping your thumbs in midline, move slightly inferior to palpate the C3, C4, C5, C6, and C7 spinous processes.
- To confirm palpation of the C6 spinous process, have the patient flex and extend the neck; the spinous process of C6 will be more prominent with neck flexion.

Notes

- If assessment of cervical spine motion is difficult in a prone position, it can also be assessed with the patient in a seated position.
- Rotation of the cervical spine can be used in addition to flexion and extension to verify palpation of the spinous processes of C6 and C7. Rotation of the cervical spine will cause much greater movement of the C6 and C7 spinous processes compared to the T1 spinous process.

Transverse Processes of C1

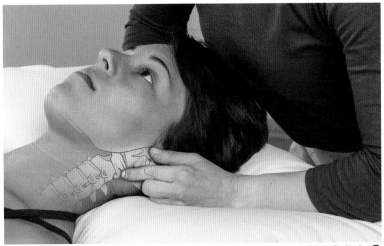

VIDEO 7.3 ▶

Positions
- Patient: supine, with the cervical spine in a neutral position
- Clinician: standing or sitting at the head of the table

Instructions
- Palpate the mastoid process (a bony prominence posterior to the external auditory meatus; see chapter 2) bilaterally with the second digit of both hands.
- Move the pads of both index fingers slightly inferiorly, making sure you are posterior to the insertion of the SCM.
- Abduct both of your shoulders to 45° to orient your second digits directly toward the transverse processes of C1.
- Firmly, but gently, apply force in a medial direction to palpate the transverse processes of C1 bilaterally.
- To confirm palpation, have the patient gently rotate the head side to side. You should feel a small bony projection through the soft tissue on both sides.

Note
The transverse processes of C1 are the largest and easiest to palpate with some practice. They are important landmarks for the palpation of other transverse processes and serve as a bony landmark for the application of manual therapy techniques.

Transverse Processes of C2 to C7

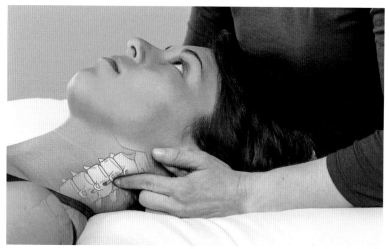

VIDEO 7.4 ▶

Positions

- Patient: supine, with the cervical spine in a neutral position
- Clinician: standing or sitting at the head of the table

Instructions

- Palpate the transverse processes of C1 bilaterally using the pads of both second digits.
- While maintaining firm pressure, begin to move your fingers inferiorly approximately one fingerwidth to palpate the transverse processes of C2.
- Continue to move your fingers in an inferior direction to assess and palpate the remaining transverse processes. You should feel a small bony projection under your fingers.

CLINICAL PEARL

These structures are extremely important during the examination of a patient with cervical or thoracic spine pain. Accurate palpation of these anatomical landmarks is imperative for joint mobility assessment. During palpation of the spinous and transverse processes, you can assess both the amount of movement available at each segment and the presence or absence of pain.

Spinous Processes of T1 to T12

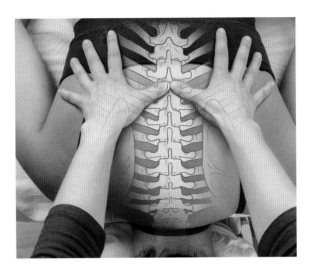

Positions
- Patient: prone, with a pillow under the abdomen
- Clinician: standing to the side of the patient or at the head of the table

Instructions
- Palpate the spinous process of C7.
- Place the third digit (of the hand that is closer to the patient's head) on the spinous process of C7 and the second digit in the space between C7 and T1 (not shown).
- Now place your second digit on the spinous process of T1 and your middle finger in the space between T1 and T2 (not shown).
- Continue to follow these steps until all spinous processes of the thoracic spine have been palpated.
- Finish the palpation by having one or two thumbs on the specific spinous process. You should feel a prominent bony projection under your fingers.

Note
Due to the size of the spinous processes of the thoracic vertebrae, the clinician may use two fingers (or thumbs) to palpate the spinous processes.

Transverse Processes of T1 to T12

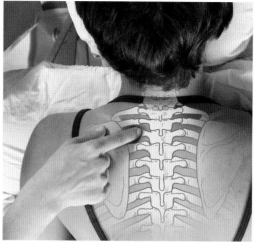

VIDEO 7.5 ▶

Positions

- Patient: prone, with a pillow under the abdomen
- Clinician: standing to the side of the patient

Instructions

- Palpate the spinous process of T1 using one finger.
- Move your finger approximately 1 inch (2.5 centimeters) laterally to identify the transverse processes of the thoracic vertebra.
- Continue to follow these steps as you move down the spine until all transverse processes of the thoracic spine have been palpated. You should feel a subtle bony projection through the soft tissue under your fingers.

Note

Identification of the transverse process of a particular vertebral level can be somewhat difficult because the transverse processes are not at the same level as the spinous processes in the thoracic spine. To palpate a specific transverse process, follow these steps:

- Palpate the spinous process at the desired level with the first digit (thumb) of one hand.
- Place the thumb of your other hand 1 inch (2.5 centimeters) lateral to the spinous process being palpated.
- Using a posterior-to-anterior force, push on the transverse process felt under your thumb.
- Repeat these steps on the next few levels above and below until motion is felt under the thumb palpating the spinous process.

Rib Angles of Thoracic Vertebrae

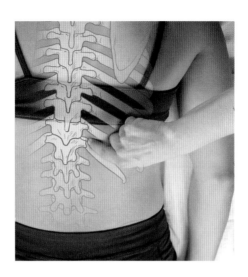

Positions
- Patient: prone, with a pillow under the abdomen
- Clinician: standing to the side of the patient

Instructions

Method 1
- Palpate the transverse process at the desired level with one finger.
- Move your finger about half a fingerwidth laterally.
- Apply firm pressure using a posterior–anterior force.
- A bony prominence should be palpable under your finger.

Method 2
- Palpate the shaft of the desired rib.
- Continue palpating along the shaft of the rib, moving in a medial direction, until a bony prominence is felt, approximately 1.25 inches (3 centimeters) from the spinous process.

Muscles of the Cervical and Thoracic Spine

Muscle	Origin	Insertion	Innervation	Blood supply	Action
Sternocleidomastoid	*Sternal head:* Anterior aspect of the manubrium of the sternum *Clavicular head:* Superior surface of the medial aspect of the clavicle	Mastoid process and the lateral half of the superior nuchal line	Accessory nerve (cranial nerve XI)	Branch of the superior thyroid artery and occipital arteries and muscular branch of the suprascapular artery	*Acting bilaterally:* upper cervical spine (head) extension, lower cervical spine (neck) flexion *Acting unilaterally:* ipsilateral side-bending and contralateral rotation
Anterior scalene	Anterior tubercles of the transverse processes of C3 to C6	Superior aspect of rib 1	Ventral rami of C5 to C8	Ascending cervical branch of the inferior thyroid artery	*Acting bilaterally:* neck flexion *Acting unilaterally:* ipsilateral side-bending, contralateral rotation, and elevation of the first rib
Middle scalene	Posterior tubercles of the transverse processes of C2 to C7	Superior aspect of rib 1	Ventral rami of C3 to C7	Muscular branches of ascending cervical arteries	*Acting bilaterally:* neck flexion *Acting unilaterally:* ipsilateral side-bending, contralateral rotation, and elevation of the first rib
Posterior scalene	Posterior tubercles of the transverse processes of C4 to C6	Lateral aspect of rib 2	Ventral rami of C5 to C8	Muscular branches of ascending cervical division of inferior thyroid artery and superficial branch of transverse cervical artery	*Acting bilaterally:* neck extension *Acting unilaterally:* ipsilateral side-bending, contralateral rotation Assistance with respiration

Muscle	Origin	Insertion	Innervation	Blood supply	Action
Splenius capitis	Ligamentum nuchae and spinous processes C7 to T4	Mastoid process and superior nuchal line	Dorsal rami of C7 to C8	Occipital and transverse cervical arteries	*Acting bilaterally:* head and neck extension *Acting unilaterally:* ipsilateral side-bending and rotation of head and neck
Semispinalis capitis	Transverse processes of C7 to T6	Occipital bone between the superior and inferior nuchal lines	Dorsal rami C1 to C6	Posterior intercostal arteries, occipital artery, and costocervical trunk	Extension of the head and ipsilateral side-bending
Superior oblique	Transverse process of C1	Occiput	Suboccipital nerve	Vertebral artery and descending branch of occipital artery	Extension of the head and ipsilateral side-bending
Inferior oblique	Spinous process of C2	Transverse process of C1	Suboccipital nerve	Vertebral artery, descending branch of occipital artery	*Acting bilaterally:* head extension *Acting unilaterally:* ipsilateral rotation
Rectus capitis posterior major	Spinous process of C2	Inferior nuchal line	Suboccipital nerve	Vertebral artery and descending branch of occipital artery	Extension of the head and ipsilateral rotation
Rectus capitis posterior minor	Posterior arch of the atlas (C1)	Inferior nuchal line	Suboccipital nerve	Vertebral artery and descending branch of the occipital artery	Extension of the head
Longus capitis	Anterior tubercles of the transverse processes of C3 to C6	Inferior aspect of the occipital bone	Ventral rami C1 to C3	Ascending cervical branch of inferior thyroid artery and muscular branches of vertebral artery	Flexion of the head (upper cervical spine)

> continued

MUSCLES OF THE CERVICAL AND THORACIC SPINE   > *continued*

Muscle	Origin	Insertion	Innervation	Blood supply	Action
Longus colli	Anterior tubercles of the transverse processes of C5 to T3	Atlas (C1)	Ventral rami C2 to C8	Muscular branches of ascending cervical and vertebral arteries	Flexion of the head and neck and ipsilateral rotation
Iliocostalis thoracis and lumborum	Iliac crest	Ribs	Posterior branches of spinal nerves	Intercostal and lumbar arteries	*Acting bilaterally:* extension of the spine *Acting unilaterally:* ipsilateral side-bending of the spine
Longissimus thoracis	Lower ribs	Higher ribs	Posterior branches of spinal nerves	Lateral sacral artery	*Acting bilaterally:* extension of the spine *Acting unilaterally:* ipsilateral side-bending of the spine
Spinalis thoracis	Sides of lower spinous processes	Sides of higher spinous processes	Posterior branches of spinal nerves	Lateral sacral artery and posterior intercostal arteries	*Acting bilaterally:* extension of the spine *Acting unilaterally:* ipsilateral side-bending of the spine

Zone I: Anterior Lateral Aspect

Sternocleidomastoid

Positions

- Patient: supine, with a pillow under the knees, or sitting in a chair
- Clinician: sitting at the head of the table or standing to the side of the patient

Instructions

- Palpate the sternoclavicular joint.
- Move your fingers just superior to the sternoclavicular joint.
- Using two fingers, follow the muscle from origin to insertion, palpating both heads distally.
- To confirm palpation, have the patient rotate the head and neck contralaterally.
- For additional confirmation, have the patient lift the head and neck off the table. You should feel a prominent contraction under your finger.

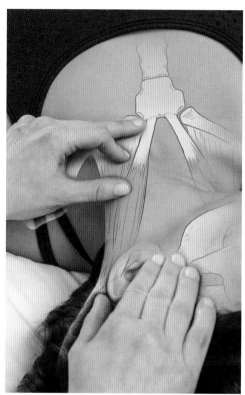

VIDEO 7.6 ◉

Note

In certain cases it may be painful for the patient to lift the head off the table. In these instances, palpate the SCM using only cervical spine rotation.

Longus Capitis and Colli

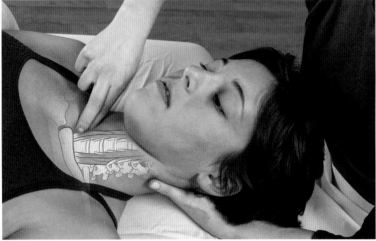

VIDEO 7.7 ▶

Positions
- Patient: supine, with a pillow under the knees
- Clinician: sitting at the head of the table

Instructions
- Palpate the SCM.
- With the pads of digits 2 and 3, slide anteriorly until you roll off the anterior, inferior border of the muscle belly.
- With the pads of your fingers, pull the SCM laterally.
- Begin to apply gentle but firm pressure in an anterior-to-posterior direction toward the transverse processes.
- To confirm palpation of these muscles, ask the patient to perform flexion of the upper cervical spine (craniocervical flexion, or nodding). You will feel a slight contraction under your finger.

Note
During this palpation, you may feel a pulse. This is the common carotid artery, and deeper palpation should not be performed directly over this structure. Move your fingers slightly anterior or posterior to assess the deep longus capitis and colli muscles.

CLINICAL PEARL
These muscles are antagonistic to the suboccipital muscles and often become chronically lengthened secondary to forward head posture. Motor retraining of these muscles can have a beneficial effect in people with chronic neck pain and people with whiplash-associated disorders.[6-9]

Scalenes

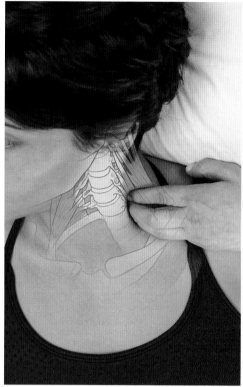

VIDEO 7.6 ▶

Positions

- Patient: supine, with a pillow under the knees, or sitting in a chair
- Clinician: sitting at the head of the table or standing to the side of the patient

Instructions

- Palpate the SCM.
- Using two or three fingers, move your fingers just posterior to the SCM.
- To confirm palpation, have the patient side-bend the head and neck toward, and rotate away from, the side being palpated. You should feel a small contraction under your fingers.
- Try to identify the anterior, middle, and posterior scalenes by moving your fingers from anterior to posterior.

Note

To further confirm palpation of the scalenes, have the patient take quick breaths in through the nose. This will cause the scalenes to contract under your fingers.

Lymph Node Chain

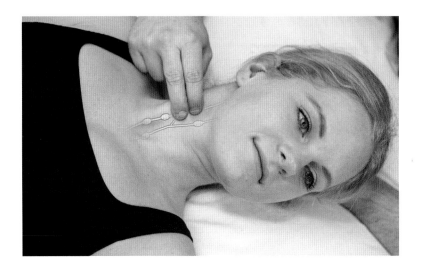

Positions

- Patient: supine, with a pillow under the knees and the head and neck rotated slightly in the contralateral direction
- Clinician: sitting at the head of the table or standing to the side of the patient

Instructions

- Palpate the medial aspect of the SCM, moving two fingers from superior to inferior.
- The lymph node chain is normally not palpable, but when it is enlarged, it will be felt as small lumps that are tender to palpation.

CLINICAL PEARL

Tenderness to palpation of the lymph nodes medial to the SCM is usually a sign of an upper respiratory infection.

Thyroid Gland

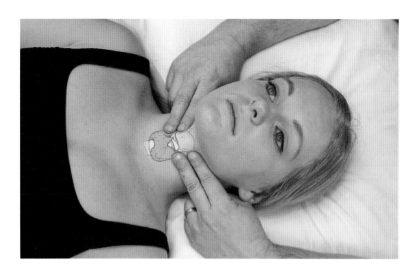

Positions

- Patient: supine, with a pillow under the knees and the head and neck in a neutral position
- Clinician: sitting at the head of the table or standing to the side of the patient

Instructions

- Palpate the thyroid cartilage anteriorly along the C4 to C5 vertebral levels.
- Using the pads of digits 2 and 3 of both hands, move your fingers laterally on both sides to palpate the thyroid gland, which may be indistinguishable and not palpable.

Note

When enlarged, clinicians will be able to palpate and identify the thyroid gland more distinctly.

Parotid Gland

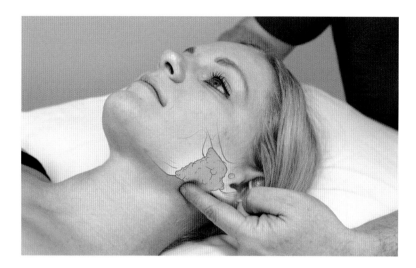

Positions

- Patient: supine, with a pillow under the knees and the head and neck in a neutral position
- Clinician: sitting at the head of the table or standing to the side of the patient

Instructions

- Palpate the angle of the mandible using one finger.
- The parotid gland is superficial to the angle of the mandible.
- When normal, the gland is not palpable, but it can become palpable when it is swollen and inflamed.

Carotid Pulse

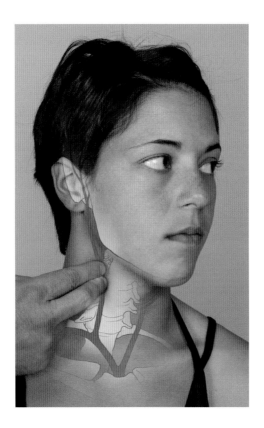

Positions

- Patient: sitting
- Clinician: sitting at the head of the table or standing to the side of the patient

Instructions

- Have the patient rotate the head and face away from the side being palpated.
- Identify the large SCM in the anterior–lateral aspect of the neck with the pads of the first two digits.
- Using mild pressure, move your fingers anteriorly and superiorly.
- A firm pulse should be felt under your fingers, around the level of the C3 to C4 vertebrae.

Note

This palpation should not be carried out bilaterally simultaneously. If you want to assess both carotid arteries, you should do so one at a time.

Zone II: Posterior Aspect

Splenius Capitis

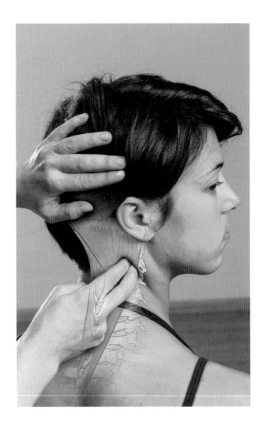

Positions
- Patient: sitting
- Clinician: standing behind and to the side of the patient

Instructions
- Using two fingers, palpate just posterior to the insertion of the SCM and just below the occipital bone.
- To make this muscle more palpable, inhibit the upper trapezius muscle by having the patient rotate the head and neck toward the side being palpated (right hand pictured).
- To confirm palpation, simultaneously resist head and neck extension (left hand pictured). You should feel a slight contraction under your fingers.

Semispinalis Capitis

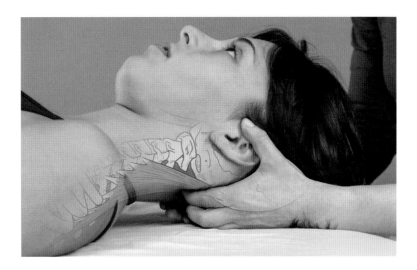

Positions
- Patient: supine, with a pillow under the knees
- Clinician: sitting at the head of the table

Instructions
- Palpate the external occipital protuberance.
- Using three fingers from both hands, move your fingers inferior to the occiput and lateral to the spinous processes.
- Have the patient rotate the head and neck ipsilaterally.
- To confirm palpation, palpate deep to the trapezius and have the patient extend the head and neck into your fingers. You should feel a small, subtle contraction under your fingers.

Notes
- Having the patient place the hand behind the back downwardly rotates the scapula, thus inhibiting the trapezius muscle.
- Having the patient rotate the head to the same side further inhibits the trapezius muscle.

Suboccipital Muscles

Positions

- Patient: supine, with a pillow under the knees
- Clinician: sitting at the head of the table

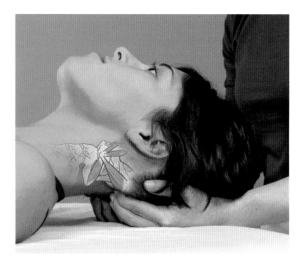

Instructions

- Palpate the external occipital protuberance.
- Palpate the spinous process of C2.
- Using three fingers from both hands, place the fingers between the external occipital protuberance and C2.
- Attempt to identify each of the following muscles by following the fibers from origin to insertion.
  - Superior oblique: transverse process of C1 to the occipital bone
  - Inferior oblique: spinous process of C2 to the transverse process of C1
  - Rectus capitis posterior major: spinous process of C2 to the occipital bone
  - Rectus capitis posterior minor: transverse process of C1 to the occipital bone
- To confirm palpation of the superior oblique and the rectus capitis posterior major and minor, have the patient perform extension of the upper cervical spine.
- To confirm palpation of the inferior oblique, have the patient perform ipsilateral rotation of the upper cervical spine. You should feel a small, subtle contraction under your fingers.

CLINICAL PEARL

The suboccipital muscles often become chronically shortened secondary to forward head posture. These muscles may develop spasm and associated trigger points, which may cause headaches as well as orofacial pain. In addition to these symptoms, the overexcited nerve roots traveling through these muscles may cause disturbances in balance and proprioception.[6-9]

Erector Spinae

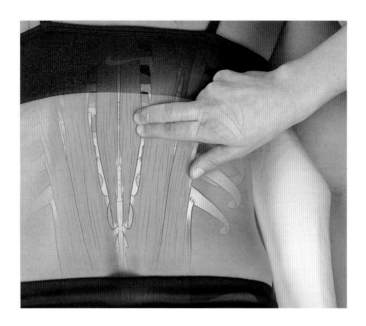

Positions
- Patient: prone
- Clinician: standing to the side of the patient, on the side being palpated

Instructions
- Place the pads of two or three fingers lateral to the midline of the spine.
- Apply your force in a posterior-to-anterior direction.
- To confirm palpation, have the patient slightly extend the spine. You will feel a large contraction under your fingers.

Note
Depending on the area of the spine you are palpating, the degree to which the patient extends the spine to confirm the palpation will vary. When you are addressing the cervical and upper thoracic spines, lifting the head off the table should suffice. If you are addressing the midthoracic spine, the shoulders and even possibly the chest may need to be lifted off the table. For the lower thoracic and lumbar spines, more extension of the spine is needed, and the chest may need to be lifted farther off the table.

Case Study

History

A 45-year-old female presents to your clinic reporting right-sided cervical spine pain that runs down the right arm. She reports that the symptoms began about 2 months ago while she was at work. She reports an increase in symptoms over the past month, with symptoms moving farther down her right arm and into her thumb. She states this is worse at the end of the day, after having been at work and on the phone and computer. She reports minimal relief after a hot shower. She says she thought the problem would get better on its own, but it has not, and she is now seeking help. She is married with two children, ages 6 and 8 years. She works as an administrative assistant (part time) and is right-hand dominant. She walks the family dog (40 pounds, or 18 kilograms) two times a day, takes a spinning class two times a week, and plays tennis once a week.

- Based on this information only, what are the three most likely diagnoses?

Examination

Past medical history	Unremarkable
Medication	Denies taking any medications, vitamins, or supplements
Observation	No acute distress, no bruising, no gross deformity noted Decreased cervical lordosis Mild left cervical spine side-bending
Active range of motion	Within normal limits, except right side-bending = 0° to 10°
Passive range of motion	Same as for active
Manual muscle testing	Right upper extremity 4/5 throughout
Special tests	Positive Spurling's test Positive distraction test Positive quadrant test—extension, right side-bending, and rotation Positive median nerve upper limb tension test Negative cervical flexion lateral rotation test Negative Roos test
Other	Decreased biceps and triceps reflexes Diminished light-touch sensation to anterior aspects of digits 1 and 2 Limited cervical spine right → left side-gliding Elevated first rib with limited mobility

- Based on the subjective and objective information together, what are the two most likely diagnoses? Give your rationale for eliminating the third diagnosis.
- What structures should you palpate on this patient based on your differential diagnoses?
- Given all the information presented, what would you expect to find on palpation of those structures?

Case Solution and Discussion

Potential Diagnoses Based on History
- Cervical radiculopathy
- Mechanical neck pain
- Thoracic outlet syndrome

Potential Diagnoses Based on History and Examination
- Cervical radiculopathy
- Thoracic outlet syndrome

Mechanical neck pain: The positive Spurling's test, positive distraction test, positive quadrant test, and positive median nerve upper limb tension test, as well as decreased biceps and triceps reflexes and decreased sensation in digits 1 and 2 (C6-C7 dermatomal distribution) are all indicative of neurological involvement. Therefore, by definition, this diagnosis, which is purely mechanical in nature, can be ruled out.

Structures to Be Palpated
- Radial pulse
- First rib
- Spinous and transverse processes C1 to C7
- Upper trapezius
- Levator scapulae
- SCM
- Scalenes
- Pectoralis minor

Palpation Findings
- Muscle spasm right upper trapezius, levator scapulae, SCM
- Tenderness to palpation C3 to C7 spinous processes
- Tenderness to palpation right first rib

Clinical Reasoning

- Cervical radiculopathy: The patient's report of pain down the right upper extremity in a dermatomal pattern and in addition the positive tests (Spurling's, distraction, and quadrant tests), the limited side-gliding of the vertebrae, and tenderness to palpation of C3 to C7 are more indicative of a C6 to C7 radiculopathy.

- Thoracic outlet syndrome: The patient's report of pain down the right upper extremity, diminished sensation, and an elevated first rib are signs and symptoms of thoracic outlet syndrome. However, because of the negative Roos and cervical rotation lateral flexion tests, as well as positive nerve root signs, thoracic outlet syndrome is less likely.

Case Study Questions

1. What information do the palpation findings of the case give the clinician? How can this information be incorporated in the clinical decision-making process?

2. Think about how the subjective and objective examination findings lead to the differential diagnosis. What might you do differently?

3. What important patient education is critical in a case like this?

CHAPTER REVIEW QUESTIONS

1. Which region of the spine has the most amount of movement?
2. Which plane of movement does the thoracic spine predominantly move in?
3. Name the suboccipital muscles located posteriorly.
4. List the insertion of the scalene muscles.
5. What are the borders of the anterior and posterior cervical triangles?
6. What major arteries give blood supply to the cervical spine?

chapter 8

Lumbosacral Spine

CHAPTER OBJECTIVES

After completing this chapter, the reader will be able to do the following:

- Identify the key bony anatomical structures and the functional relationships of the lumbopelvic region.
- Identify and describe the soft tissue anatomy of the lumbopelvic region, including muscles, ligaments, nerves, arteries, and veins.
- Differentiate the layers of muscles in the lumbosacral spine.
- Identify on bony or skeletal models the origins and insertions of the muscles of the lumbosacral spine in order to aid in understanding osteokinematic action and surface palpation.
- Draw and discuss the lumbar and sacrococcygeal plexi.
- Palpate structures of the lumbosacral spine.
- Integrate surface palpation findings into the differential diagnosis of a patient with back pain.

The lumbosacral spine comprises an intricate system encompassing many bones, soft tissues, and joints. Low back pain is a common and costly condition worldwide, with lifetime prevalence between 11% and 84%.[1-3] Evidence has emphasized the importance of regional interdependence between the lumbar spine, sacral spine, and lower quadrant.[4-6] Dysfunction of the proximal segments in the kinetic chain (lumbar spine) can manifest as impairments of distal segments in the kinetic chain (hip, knee, and ankle.) It is important to be mindful of these relationships while studying these joint functions and throughout the clinical examination.

Functions of the Lumbosacral Spine

The most important function of the lumbosacral region is to support the weight of the body. Proper stability of this region is important for successful transfer of forces from the trunk to the lower extremities and vice versa. While the lumbar spine needs stability to perform many functional activities, movement is also available in this region, especially in the sagittal plane. As a result of the vertical orientation of the facet joints in the lumbar spine, flexion and extension are the primary osteokinematic motions. This orientation does allow some side-bending and a minimal amount of rotation.[7] Similar to the cervical and thoracic spine, the lumbar spine is dependent on muscles and ligaments to provide the intersegmental stability that is necessary during performance of functional tasks.

Compared to the cervical, thoracic, and lumbar sections of the spine, the sacral region does not permit a great deal of motion. While there is controversy regarding the actual function of the sacrum and sacroiliac joints, most agree that slight, subtle movement is available at the sacroiliac joints, which serves to fine-tune and coordinate overall movement between the pelvis and lower extremities.[7-10] The sacrum functions as a link between the trunk and lower extremities, and the distribution of forces must occur evenly in this region to prevent unnecessary imbalance of forces.[7-10]

Bony Anatomy

The lumbar spine consists of five vertebrae (L1-L5), which all possess similar features and can be broken into two main parts: a large vertebral body and a neural arch (figure 8.1). The primary function of the lumbar vertebral bodies is to support over 80% of body weight.[7,11] The vertebral body is connected to the neural arch by the pedicle. Located on the neural arch is the lamina, which contains several processes.[11]

- One large spinous process
- Two transverse processes
- The superior and inferior articular processes, or facets
- The mammillary process, which is located on the superior articular facet and serves as the attachment for the multifidus muscle

The sacral region consists of four segments (S1-S4) that usually fuse into one piece called the sacrum (figure 8.2). This large, broad bone is much wider than any of the other vertebrae. The sacrum has a base, which is the superior portion of the bone, and an apex, which is the inferior aspect of the bone. Distally, the sacrum articulates with the coccyx, forming the

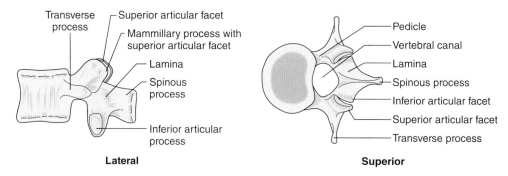

Lateral

Superior

FIGURE 8.1   Aspects of the lumbar vertebra.

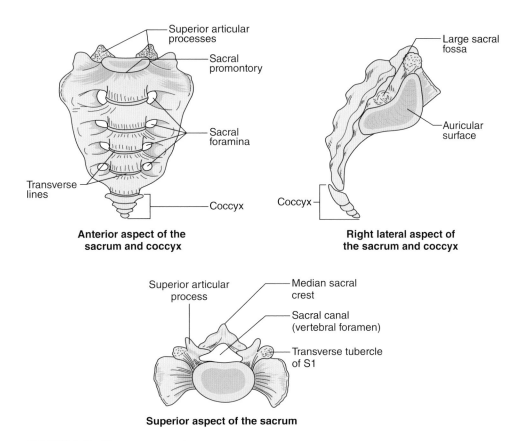

FIGURE 8.2 The sacrum and coccyx.

sacrococcygeal joint.[11] Movement of the sacrum in the sagittal plane is known as nutation (flexion) and counter-nutation (extension).[7] The sacrum also articulates laterally with both ilia to form the sacroiliac joints (SIJ). These joints may be considered synovial joints, but unlike other synovial joints, the amount of movement available is limited to a small amount of gliding and rotation, which many would consider an amphiarthrotic articulation.[7-11]

Soft Tissue Anatomy

The muscles that surround the lumbosacral spine all provide dynamic stability. These muscles are divided into two groups[12-17] (figure 8.3):

- The local stabilizing muscles (multifidus, internal oblique, and transversus abdominis), which are designed to increase segmental stability
- The global muscles (latissimus dorsi, rectus abdominis, and external oblique), which produce gross motion

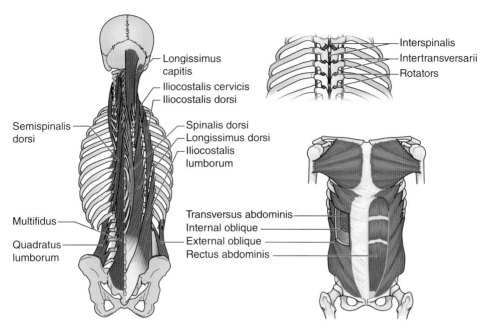

FIGURE 8.3 Muscles of the anterior and posterior trunk.

The latissimus dorsi is the most superficial muscle that crosses the lumbosacral spine and has an attachment into the thoracolumbar fascia. This muscle is discussed in chapter 3. The thoracolumbar fascia, which covers the deep muscles of the trunk, is a fascial sheet composed of three layers and serves as an attachment for both local and global muscles that contribute to increased lumbosacral stability.[11]

- The quadratus lumborum muscle lies between the anterior and middle layers.
- The erector spinae muscles lie between the middle and posterior layers.
- The thoracolumbar fascia contains both longitudinal and transverse fibers, and its deepest fibers have attachments to the lumbar vertebrae.

Like the erector spinae in the thoracic spine, the lumbar erector spinae (lumbar paraspinals) are composed of three groups of muscles: the iliocostalis, longissimus, and spinalis (see figure 8.3). When the erector spinae contract bilaterally, they perform spinal extension; when the erector spinae contract unilaterally, the result is lateral flexion to the ipsilateral side.[11] These muscles are discussed in detail in chapter 7.

The transversospinalis muscle group lies deep to the erector spinae. This group of muscles is composed of the multifidus, semispinalis, and rotator muscles (see figure 8.3). Collectively, these muscles function to produce contralateral rotation of the trunk.[11] The multifidus is the only palpable muscle of this group. It is a broad muscle that has received much attention in the literature for its control of local segmental spinal stability.[11,13-15,17] The multifidus is often broken into superficial and deep layers.

- The superficial fibers of the multifidus insert along the posterior-medial aspect of the iliac crest. These fibers are often hypertonic and tender to palpation with lumbosacral pathology.

- The deeper fibers of the multifidus are located just lateral to the spinous processes in the lumbar spine or just lateral to the median sacral crest. These fibers are more involved with local segmental stabilization and often become inhibited in the presence of low back pain.[18]

Muscles of the anterior–lateral abdominal wall act on the lumbar spine. The abdominal muscles consist of the rectus abdominis, external abdominal oblique, internal abdominal oblique, and transversus abdominis. In addition, on the posterior–lateral abdominal wall are the psoas major and quadratus lumborum muscles. Collectively, these muscles (see figure 8.3) function to produce either gross spinal movements (i.e., rectus abdominis, external oblique, quadratus lumborum) or increase segmental stability (i.e., internal oblique, multifidus, transversus abdominis).[11,13-15,17] Further detail regarding the abdominal muscles will be discussed in chapter 9.

In addition to the muscles adding stability to the lumbosacral spine, several ligaments, as well as the intervertebral discs, add important passive stability to the spine. Each intervertebral disc sits between two vertebrae and provides a strong attachment for the vertebral bodies. The intervertebral disc is composed of an outer portion called the annulus fibrosus and an inner portion called the nucleus pulposus (figure 8.4). Its main function is to absorb and dissipate forces over a large surface area.[11]

The annulus fibrosus is a fibrocartilaginous ring that forms the outer surface of the intervertebral disc. It has layers that run at right angles to each other to increase stability of the disc. The annulus fibrosus attaches to the vertebral endplates, which are the rims of the vertebral bodies. Both the annulus and vertebral endplates have good blood supply, which is carried to the nucleus pulposus by movement.[11] The inner portion of the disc, the nucleus pulposus, receives nutrients through compression and decompression during movement. It is made up predominantly of water and has the ability to broaden with compressive forces and thin with tensile forces.[11]

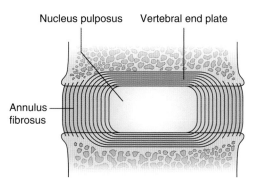

FIGURE 8.4 Intervertebral disc.

Spanning the entire anterior and posterior aspects of the vertebrae are the anterior longitudinal and posterior longitudinal ligaments, respectively (figure 8.5). These ligaments provide resistance to excessive flexion or extension during movement.

- The anterior longitudinal ligament becomes taut with lumbar extension, while the posterior longitudinal ligament becomes taut with lumbar flexion. These ligaments increase stability of the anterior and posterior aspects of the spinal column.[7,11]

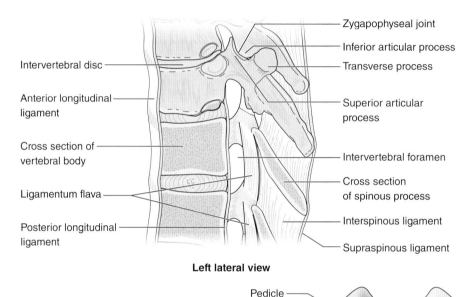

Left lateral view

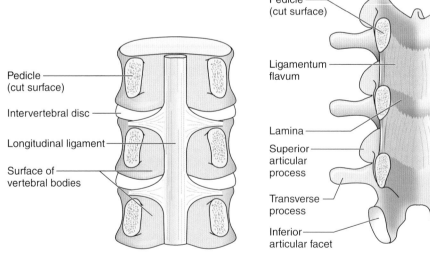

Anterior vertebral segments, posterior view

Posterior vertebral segments, anterior view

FIGURE 8.5 Vertebral ligaments.

- Running along the laminae of successive vertebrae is the ligamentum flavum. This ligament functions to form the posterior wall of the vertebral canal and prevents excessive flexion of the vertebral column, thereby protecting the intervertebral disc from injury.[7,11]

Neurovascular Anatomy

Blood supply to the lumbar spine comes from the subcostal and lumbar arteries in the abdomen. Traveling directly anterior to the lumbar vertebral bodies is the abdominal aorta. This is a large artery that bifurcates into the right and left common iliac arteries at the level of L2. This artery further divides into the internal iliac artery and the external iliac artery. It is the external iliac artery that becomes the femoral artery as it passes under the inguinal ligament (figure 8.6).[11]

In the lumbosacral region are five lumbar and five sacral nerves. These nerves exit below the corresponding vertebrae. The spinal cord runs from the medulla oblongata (brainstem) to the L1 to L2 interspace, at which point it becomes known as the cauda equina, which is a collection of spinal nerve roots.[11]

- In the lumbosacral region there is an enlargement of the nerve roots between L1 and S3, which contribute to the lumbar plexus (L1-L4) and the sacrococcygeal plexus (L4-S3) (figure 8.7).

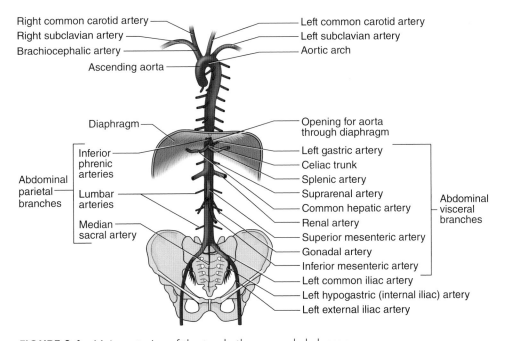

FIGURE 8.6 Major arteries of the trunk, thorax, and abdomen.

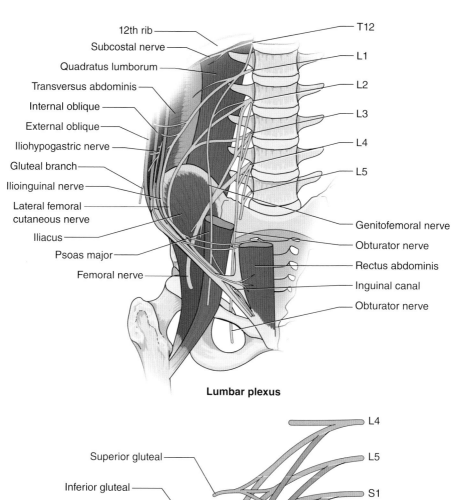

Lumbar plexus

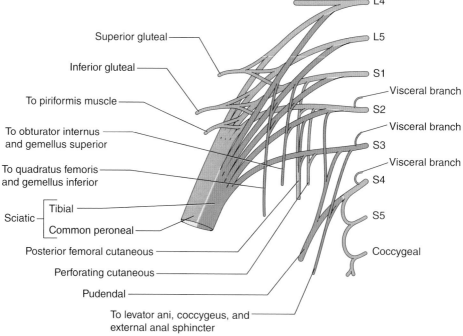

Sacral plexus

FIGURE 8.7   Lumbar and sacrococcygeal plexi.

- Each spinal nerve has both an anterior and a posterior root.
  - The anterior roots of spinal nerves contain motor (efferent) fibers innervating skeletal muscles.
  - The posterior roots of spinal nerves contain sensory (afferent) fibers from the skin and other subcutaneous tissues.
  - The anterior and posterior nerve roots unite to form a spinal nerve that exits through the intervertebral foramen (figure 8.7).[11]

Structural Inspection

- Begin the inspection by initially observing the patient walking into the examining room. This will provide a gross assessment of motion throughout the lumbar spine so the clinician can observe for painful or guarded movements that may help guide the examination process.
- Once in the examination room, the clinician should assess the skin for unusual moles, markings, or areas of redness.
- The clinician should now perform a thorough postural assessment by observing the patient from the anterior, posterior, and lateral views.
  - The clinician should assess for the lordosis present in the lumbar spine when observing from the lateral view. Muscle spasm or increased tone of the paraspinals may present with a decreased lumbar lordosis in standing. Conversely, an exacerbated or increased lordosis could be a sign of hip flexor shortness and weakening of the abdominal muscles.
  - From the posterior view, the clinician should carefully observe the relationship between the shoulders and pelvis for signs of a lateral shift or true spinal scoliosis.

Spinous Processes of L1 to L5

Positions
- Patient: prone, with two pillows under the abdomen
- Clinician: standing to the side of the patient

Method 1

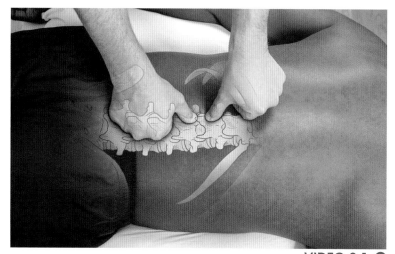

VIDEO 8.1 ▸

Instructions
- Palpate the spinous process of T12 with the first digit (thumb) of both hands.
- Keeping one thumb over the spinous process of T12, move the other thumb inferiorly along the midline of the spine.
- Continue inferiorly until a large midline projection is palpated; this is the spinous process of L1.
- Continue to move your thumb inferiorly to palpate the remaining spinous processes. You will feel a prominent bony projection under your finger.

Method 2

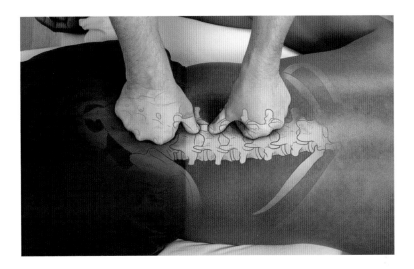

Instructions

- Palpate the iliac crests with both hands (which are at the level of the L4 to L5 interspace).
- Keeping both hands on the trunk, move your thumbs to the midline of the back until they meet.
- Move your thumbs superiorly to identify the L4 spinous process.

Notes

- Always maintain contact with the previously palpated spinous process before moving inferiorly.
- Because the lumbar spine has a natural lordosis, palpation of individual spinous processes can be difficult because they may be in close proximity to one another. For this reason, placement of two or more pillows under the abdomen will put the lumbar spine in relative flexion, thus increasing the space between spinous processes.
- Recent evidence has suggested that palpation of the spinous process in the lumbar spine may yield different results based on anatomical variation and clinician experience.[19-22] It is for this reason that we present a couple of ways to identify the levels of the spinous processes in the lumbar spine.
- A third method that clinicians use to identify the spinous processes of the lumbar spine involves palpating S2 first and then counting up.

Transverse Processes of L1 to L5

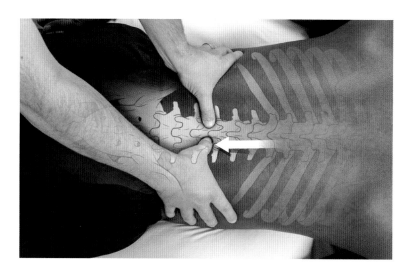

Positions
- Patient: prone, with two pillows under the abdomen
- Clinician: standing to the side of the patient

Instructions
- Palpate the spinous process of L1 with the first digit of both hands.
- Keep one first digit on the spinous process of L1 and move the other first digit in a lateral direction approximately 1 inch (2.5 centimeters).
- To confirm palpation of the L1 transverse process, apply firm posterior-to-anterior pressure (right hand pictured). You will feel a small bony projection through the soft tissue under your finger.
- Repeat these steps to palpate the other lumbar transverse processes.

Notes
- The spinous process under your thumb should move if you are applying pressure to the transverse process.
- Palpation of the transverse processes in the lumbar spine is extremely difficult, if not impossible, at times because of the large erector spinae muscle mass that completely covers these anatomical landmarks. Careful assessment and practice are necessary to palpate these structures effectively.

Sacral Base

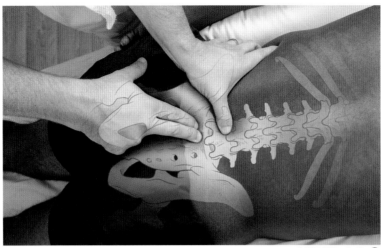

VIDEO 8.2 ▶

Positions

- Patient: prone, with two pillows under the abdomen
- Clinician: standing to the side of the patient

Instructions

- Palpate the spinous process of L5 with your thumb (left hand pictured).
- While keeping your thumb on the spinous process of L5, move the pads of digits 2 and 3 in an inferior direction (right hand pictured).
- You should feel a bony ridge that is a few inches wide; this is the sacral base (S1).

Sacral Apex

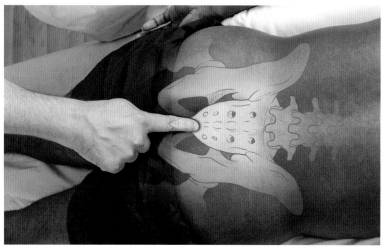

VIDEO 8.2 ▶

Positions

- Patient: prone, with two pillows under the abdomen
- Clinician: standing to the side of the patient

Instructions

- Palpate the sacral base (S1) with digit 2.
- Continue to move your second digit in an inferior direction until you get to the inferior-most aspect of the sacrum (S4).

Inferior Lateral Angle of the Sacrum

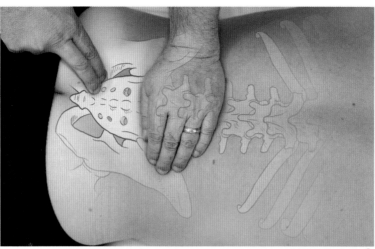

VIDEO 8.3 ▶

Positions
- Patient: prone with two pillows under the abdomen
- Clinician: standing to the side of the patient

Instructions
- Palpate the spinous process of S1.
- Using two fingers, move inferiorly and palpate S2, using the posterior superior iliac spine as a reference (see chapter 10).
- Continue inferiorly to S3 and S4.
- Move your fingers laterally from S4, palpating for a small ridge on the posterior lateral aspect of the sacrum (right hand pictured).

CLINICAL PEARL
Palpation of the inferior lateral angle is often used as a reference point to assess for sacral rotations. The clinician should keep in mind that this can be difficult and has been met with diagnostic challenges in the literature. It should also be mentioned that the majority of anatomy books do not identify the inferior lateral angle of the sacrum as a specific bony landmark on the posterior sacrum, thus raising the question of whether the structure exists in all people.

Coccyx

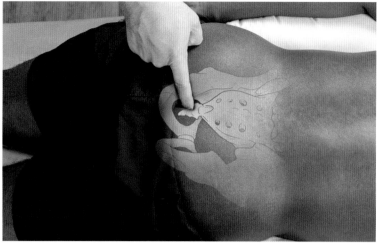

VIDEO 8.2 ▶

Positions

- Patient: prone, with two pillows under the abdomen
- Clinician: standing to the side of the patient

Instructions

- Palpate the sacral apex (S4) with the pad of digit 1 (not shown).
- While maintaining this palpation, place another finger inferiorly to palpate the coccyx (right hand pictured).

Note

Many people are uncomfortable with palpation of this area. Before palpating this structure, explain to the patient what you are doing and why it is necessary.

Muscles of the Lumbar Spine and Abdominal Region

Muscle	Origin	Insertion	Innervation	Blood supply	Action
Multifidus	Posterior surface of the sacrum, ilium, and transverse processes of T1 to T12 and lumbar vertebrae	Spinous processes of the lumbar vertebrae (L2-L5)	Dorsal rami of spinal nerves	Lumbar arteries and the dorsal branches of the lateral sacral arteries	*Acting bilaterally:* spinal extension *Acting unilaterally:* rotation to the opposite side
Pyramidalis	Body of pubis, anterior to rectus abdominis	Linea alba	Iliohypogastric nerve	Inferior epigastric artery	Tension of the linea alba
Rectus abdominis	Costal cartilages and ribs 5 to 7 and xiphoid process	Pubic tubercle	Anterior rami of the inferior 6 thoracic nerves	Superior and inferior epigastric arteries	Flexion of the trunk and support of the abdominal viscera
External oblique	External surfaces of ribs 5 to 12	Linea alba, pubic tubercle, anterior half of the iliac crest, and inguinal ligament	Anterior rami of the inferior 6 thoracic nerves	Superior and inferior epigastric arteries	Flexion of the trunk, rotation of the trunk to the opposite side, and support of abdominal viscera
Internal oblique	Inferior border of ribs 8 to 12, linea alba, pubis via conjoint tendon	Anterior two-thirds of the iliac crest, lateral half of the inguinal ligament, and the thoracolumbar fascia	Anterior rami of the inferior 6 thoracic and first lumbar nerves	Superior and inferior epigastric and deep circumflex iliac arteries	Flexion of the trunk, rotation of the trunk to the same side, and support of the abdominal viscera
Transversus abdominis	Internal surfaces of costal cartilages 7 to 12, thoracolumbar fascia, iliac crest, and lateral third of the inguinal ligament	Linea alba, aponeurosis of the internal oblique, pubic crest, and conjoint tendon	Anterior rami of the inferior 6 thoracic and first lumbar nerves	Deep circumflex iliac and inferior epigastric arteries	Increase in intersegmental stability

Zone I: Posterior Aspect

Supraspinous Ligaments

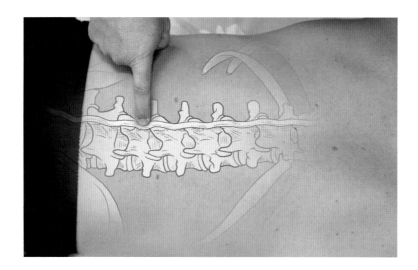

Positions
- Patient: prone, with one or two pillows under the abdomen
- Clinician: standing to the side of the patient

Instructions
- Palpate the spinous processes beginning with L1 using one finger.
- Move your finger inferiorly between each spinous process to palpate the supraspinous ligaments. You may feel a broad band of tissue under your finger.

Note
The supraspinous ligaments are broad, thick structures in the lumbar spine, and the clinician can palpate them lying superficial to the spinous processes.

> **CLINICAL PEARL**
>
> Tenderness to palpation directly over the spinous processes in the lumbar spine is often associated with a ligamentous injury, in which the supraspinous ligaments may have been sprained or ruptured, often leading to pain and guarded motion.

Multifidus

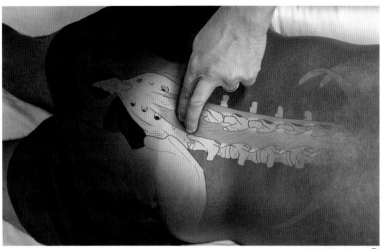

VIDEO 8.4 ▶

Positions
- Patient: prone, with one or two pillows under the abdomen
- Clinician: standing to the side of the patient

Instructions
- Palpate the spinous process of L4 to S1.
- Move laterally to the spinous processes using two fingers and follow the superficial fibers of the multifidus inferiorly to the medial aspect of the iliac crest.
- Palpate the deep fibers of the multifidus just lateral to the spinous processes of the lumbar spine, or just lateral to the median sacral crest.
- To confirm palpation, have the patient visualize bringing their posterior superior iliac spines (PSIS) together. If this is not possible, have the patient gently begin to lift the thigh off the table (hip extension).

CLINICAL PEARL
This muscle is extremely important in stabilizing the lumbar spine during functional activities.[13,15-18] Certain people have the ability to isolate contraction of the multifidus by attempting to pull their posterior superior iliac spines together. This is extremely difficult, and it usually takes practice for someone to successfully accomplish this task.

Zone II: Anterior–Lateral Aspect

Rectus Abdominis

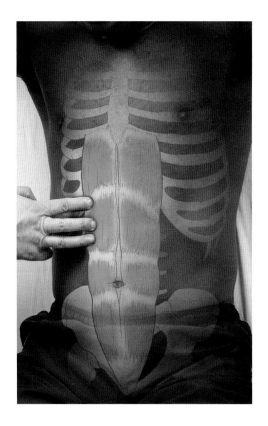

Positions
- Patient: supine, with the hips at about 45° of flexion and the knees at about 110° of flexion
- Clinician: standing to the side of the patient

Instructions
- Identify the umbilicus.
- Using three fingers, palpate the anterior aspect of the abdomen just lateral to the midline, bilaterally.
- To verify palpation, have the patient perform a crunch. You should feel a strong contraction under your fingers.

Notes
Superficial to the rectus abdominis is the pyramidalis. This muscle runs from the pubic bone to the linea alba. When present (in 80% of people), it increases the size of the lower end of the rectus abdominis.

External Oblique

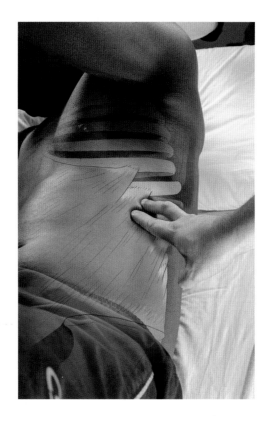

Positions
- Patient: supine, with the hips at about 45° of flexion and the knees at about 110° of flexion
- Clinician: standing next to the patient, on the side being palpated

Instructions
- Palpate the anterior–lateral aspect of the abdomen.
- Using two fingers, palpate perpendicular to the fibers from origin to insertion.
- To verify palpation of the external oblique, have the patient flex and rotate the trunk to the opposite side. You should feel a small contraction under your fingers.

Note
The fibers of the external oblique run in an anterior–medial direction (like putting your hands in your pockets).

Internal Oblique

Positions

- Patient: supine, with the hips at about 45° of flexion and the knees at about 110° of flexion
- Clinician: standing next to the patient, on the side being palpated

Instructions

- Palpate the anterior–lateral aspect of the abdomen.
- Using two fingers, palpate perpendicular to the fibers of the internal oblique from origin to insertion.
- To verify palpation of the internal oblique, have the patient flex and rotate the trunk to the same side. You should feel a small contraction under your finger.

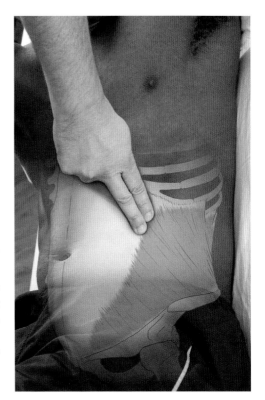

Notes

- The fibers of the internal oblique run in a posterior–lateral direction.
- When asking the patient to rotate the trunk to isolate the external or internal oblique muscle, watch for excessive trunk flexion; this will cause both obliques to contract at the same time.
- Differentiating the fibers of the external and internal obliques can be difficult.

Transversus Abdominis

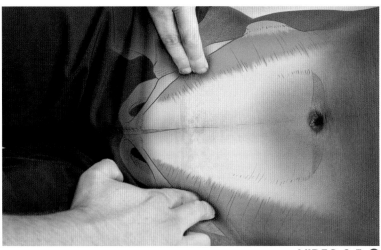

VIDEO 8.5 ▶

Positions
- Patient: supine, with the hips at about 45° of flexion and the knees at about 110° of flexion
- Clinician: standing to the side of the patient

Instructions
- Palpate the anterior superior iliac spine (ASIS), which is a bony prominence just below the waistline on the anterior aspect of the hip bone.
- Using digits 2 and 3 from both hands, move your fingers 2.5 inches (6.3 centimeters) medially and inferiorly to the ASIS.
- To verify palpation, ask the patient to bring the belly button to the spine; you should feel a contraction under your fingers. The patient can also contract the pelvic floor muscles (see clinical pearl about layered palpation of abdominal muscles).

Note
If a large bulge is felt during contraction, this is the internal oblique, and the patient is contracting too aggressively. Have the patient relax and try again.

CLINICAL PEARL

Palpation of the abdominal muscles can also be performed in a layered approach (see the following photo) so the clinician does not misinterpret one of the three key muscles: external oblique, internal oblique, or transversus abdominis.[18]

- Palpate the fascia from just below the umbilicus down to the pubic tubercle and assess its mobility.
- With both thumbs, palpate 2.5 inches (6.3 centimeters) medial and slightly inferior to the anterior superior iliac spine and press into the fascia of the external oblique.
- Palpate through the external oblique and assess whether it is easy to move into the fascia above the internal oblique muscle.
- The internal oblique is very muscular at this level.
- Assess both sides of the internal oblique.
- Palpate deeper to the fascia of the transversus abdominis.
- Apply tension to the transversus abdominis by adducting your thumbs, making a shallow V parallel to the line of the inguinal ligament.
- At this point, you can assess the contraction of the transversus abdominis, which should cocontract with the pelvic floor. Clinician can use the following cues:
  - Slowly and gently, squeeze the muscles around your urethra as if to stop your urine flow.
  - Slowly and gently, draw your vagina (or testicles) up into your body.
  - Imagine there is a wire connecting your anus to the back of your pubic bone and slowly connect this line.

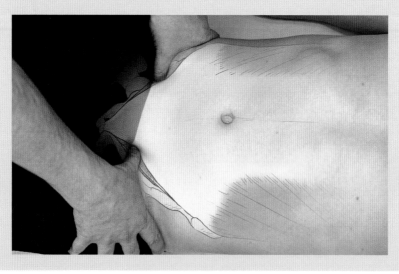

Case Study

History

A 35-year-old woman presents to your office complaining of lower back and buttock pain. She reports that the pain is not constant and that when it occurs, it is in her left lower back and pelvic and buttock area, and it is worse with standing. She gave birth to her second child 5 months ago. She reports that the pain began toward the end of her pregnancy. She is married and lives in a three-story house with her husband and 3-year-old and 5-month-old children. She recently returned to running and is training for a marathon later this year.

- Based on the subjective information alone, what are the three most likely diagnoses?

Examination

Past medical history	Two vaginal deliveries
Medication	Denies taking medications, vitamins, or supplements
Observation	Increased lumbar spine lordosis Difficulty with bed mobility: rolling over and supine to sitting
Active range of motion	Within normal limits throughout lumbar spine
Passive range of motion	Same as for active
Manual muscle testing	Left gluteus maximus and medius 4–/5 with pain Left hamstring 4–/5
Special tests	Positive sacral thrust test Positive sacroiliac distraction test Positive sacroiliac compression test Positive left Gaenslen's test Positive left active straight-leg raise test Negative quadrant test Negative straight-leg raise and crossed straight-leg raise tests bilaterally
Other	Anterior rotation of left innominate Decreased left stance phase Shortened right stride length Pain with grade II left sacral rotation No pain with posterior-to-anterior glides throughout the lumbar spine No change in pain pattern with repeated directional movement testing

- Based on the subjective and objective information together, what are the two most likely diagnoses? Give your rationale for eliminating the third diagnosis.
- What structures should you palpate on this patient based on your differential diagnoses?
- Given all the information presented, what would you expect to find upon palpation of those structures?

Case Solution and Discussion

Potential Diagnoses Based on History
- Hip (femoral) stress fracture
- Low back pain
- Sacroiliac joint dysfunction

Potential Diagnoses Based on History and Examination
- Low back pain
- Sacroiliac joint dysfunction

Hip (femoral) stress fracture: The location of pain, specifically the lack of groin pain, as well the timing of the onset of symptoms (at the end of pregnancy, *before* returning to running), makes this diagnosis unlikely. In addition, the multiple positive special tests are more indicative of a sacroiliac joint dysfunction.

Structures to Be Palpated
- Anterior superior iliac spine
- Posterior superior iliac spine
- Sacrum
- Psoas (see chapter 9)
- Adductors
- Gluteal muscles
- Superficial multifidi
- Lumbosacral paraspinals

Palpation Findings
- Tenderness to palpation immediately below the posterior superior iliac spine and gluteal region
- Left anterior superior iliac spine lower than right, left posterior superior iliac spine higher than right
- Tenderness to palpation left greater than right psoas
- Tenderness to palpation left greater than right adductors

Clinical Reasoning

- Low back pain: The patient's report of diffuse pain in her left lumbosacral and gluteal region, the gait deviations she presents with, and the musculature that is tender to palpation are all consistent with the diagnosis of low back pain. However, the lack of pain with posterior-to-anterior glides in the lumbar spine, the negative low back pain special tests, and the positive sacroiliac joint provocation tests all indicate a sacroiliac joint dysfunction and not low back pain.

- Sacroiliac joint dysfunction: The patient's history of the pain beginning toward the end of her pregnancy and two vaginal births, her pain pattern, anterior rotation of her left innominate (left half of the pelvis), gait deviations, positive sacroiliac joint provocation tests, and the musculature that is tender to palpation all indicate a left sacroiliac joint dysfunction.

Case Study Questions

1. What information do the palpation findings of the case give the clinician? How can this information be incorporated in the clinical decision-making process?

2. Think about how the examination findings (subjective and objective) lead to the differential diagnosis. What might you do differently?

3. What important patient education is critical in a case like this?

CHAPTER REVIEW QUESTIONS

1. Which plane of movement does the lumbar spine predominantly move in?

2. List all of the muscles attaching to the thoracolumbar fascia.

3. List the muscles that form the erector spinae group.

4. List the muscles that form the transversospinalis group.

5. Which major arteries give blood supply to the lumbar spine?

6. What is the function of the ligamentum flavum?

chapter 9

Abdomen and Pelvis

The authors recognize the contributions of Dean Hazama
and Gregory Scott Johnson to this chapter.

CHAPTER OBJECTIVES

After completing this chapter, the reader will be able to do the following:

- Understand the structural and functional relationships of the abdominal and pelvic regions.
- Identify and describe the soft tissue anatomy of the abdominal and pelvic regions, including muscles, ligaments, nerves, arteries, and veins.
- Identify and describe the muscle layers in the abdominal and pelvic regions.
- Identify on bony or skeletal models the origins and insertions of the muscles of the abdominal and pelvic regions in order to aid in understanding osteokinematic action and surface palpation.
- Describe the various visceral organs and their functions.
- Palpate structures of the abdominal and pelvic regions.
- Integrate surface palpation findings to aid in the differential diagnosis of a patient with abdominal or pelvic girdle pain.

It is becoming more and more common for multiple health care professionals to be part of the management team for people with abdominal and pelvic girdle dysfunction. This requires an understanding of the functional anatomy of the abdominal and pelvic regions. The visceral structures, specifically, can have a profound effect on the neuromusculoskeletal system, and accurately identifying them is important in aiding in the diagnosis and management of these patients. This understanding of anatomical structure leading to potential dysfunction must also be placed in the context of the biopsychosocial management of patients.[1]

Functions of the Abdomen and Pelvis

While the abdominal and pelvic cavities are continuous and interrelated with many similarities, they also represent unique anatomical regions of the body that have different functions. The abdomen is situated between the thorax and pelvis. This area is different from other regions of the body because the visceral contents of the abdominal cavity do not have direct bony protection as do the brain, spinal cord, heart, lungs, and pelvic viscera. This places the vital contents of the abdominal cavity, which primarily function in digestion and reabsorption of important nutrients, at a higher risk for trauma.[2] The pelvis, however, and its contents are offered bony protection through the pelvic ring that is formed by both innominate bones. The contents of the pelvis function to aid in proper elimination of waste following digestion of food and in proper sexual function and reproduction. While certain organs are anatomically placed in the abdominal cavity and others in the pelvic cavity, some organs and structures bridge the two cavities and are technically located in both the abdominal and pelvic cavities. On occasion, the position of some organs in the pelvic cavity can change. For example, the uterus and bladder can move into the abdominal cavity when distended.

Bony Anatomy

The only bony anatomy relevant to the abdominal region is the sternum and lower ribs, which were discussed in chapter 4. The clinician should remember that while there is no direct bony protection to the midportion of the abdominal region, the upper abdominal viscera, which lie under the diaphragm, are protected by the thoracic skeleton. Much of the lower abdominal viscera are protected by the pelvic girdle. Therefore, the contents of the abdominal cavity are provided support and stability through their fascial and ligamentous attachments to the ribs, lumbar vertebrae, and pelvic girdle.[2]

The pelvic ring, or girdle, is formed by the fusion of both innominate bones, with the sacrum and coccyx serving as the bridge between the two innominate bones (figure 9.1).

- The inside of the pelvic girdle, which is often referred to as the pelvic inlet, is anatomically defined by a line that extends from the promontory of the sacrum, along the arcuate line of the ilium, to the superior border of the pubic symphysis, where both pubic tubercles join to form an amphiarthrotic joint.[2]

- The pelvic outlet is a ring that is formed by a line connecting the coccyx, sacrotuberous ligaments, ischial tuberosities, ischiopubic rami, and the inferior border of the pubic symphysis.[2]

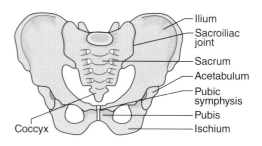

FIGURE 9.1 Pelvic bony anatomy, anterior view.

The pelvic ring is an important functional unit of the body. It is responsible for the proper transmission of forces throughout the lower kinetic chain during weight-bearing activities, such as gait. Each innominate is formed by the fusion of the ilium, ischium, and pubis, which come together to form the acetabulum. The bony anatomy for the hip and groin region are discussed in detail in chapter 10.

Soft Tissue Anatomy

Several layers of soft tissue cover the anterior and lateral aspects of the abdomen. From superficial to deep, these are the skin, subcutaneous tissue, fascia, muscles, extraperitoneal tissue, and the peritoneum. Collectively, they provide protection to the underlying viscera in addition to supporting the deeper organs of the abdominal cavity. The muscles of the abdominal region can be divided into the following (figure 9.2):

- Anterior abdominal wall (pyramidalis, rectus abdominis)
- Anterior–lateral abdominal wall (external oblique, internal oblique, and transversus abdominis)
- Posterior–lateral abdominal wall (psoas major and quadratus lumborum).

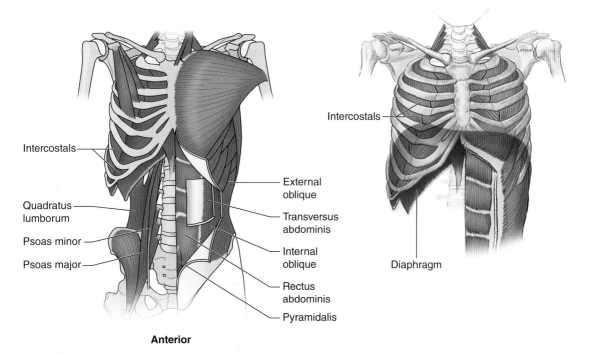

Anterior

FIGURE 9.2 Muscles of the anterior, lateral, and posterior abdominal wall. The second image shows the location of the diaphragm.

Collectively, these muscles work with the muscles of the posterior trunk (latissimus dorsi, erector spinae, and the transversospinales) either to produce gross spinal movements or to increase intersegmental stability of the spine during functional movement patterns. The superficial, global muscles (rectus abdominis, external oblique, quadratus lumborum, psoas major) are responsible for producing gross spinal movements, while the deeper, local muscles (internal oblique, transversus abdominis, multifidus, and parts of the psoas) are responsible for intersegmental stability.[3-7]

The muscles of the anterior–lateral abdominal wall act like sheets. The anterior portions are extremely aponeurotic (fascia-like) and fuse to form a thick sheath around the rectus abdominis muscle. In addition to flexing and rotating the trunk, these muscles aid in respiration, coughing, vomiting, and defecation.[8] In addition, the fascia of the anterior–lateral abdominal wall blends with the thoracolumbar fascia on the posterior–lateral aspect of the trunk.

The muscles of the pelvic girdle support the trunk and pelvic viscera and move the lower extremities. They are best described by their location.

- The lateral pelvic wall consists of the obturator internus, which arises from the internal surface of the obturator membrane, travels through the lesser sciatic foramen, and inserts on the greater trochanter.

- The posterior pelvic wall is formed by the piriformis muscle. It originates on the anterior sacrum, travels through the greater sciatic foramen, and also inserts on the greater trochanter.

It is important to remember that the nerves of the sacral plexus lie directly anterior and medial to the origin of the piriformis and, therefore, may become compressed with hypertonicity in the muscle.[8]

The pelvic floor (pelvic diaphragm; figure 9.3) is composed of the levator ani and coccygeus muscles:

- The three muscles (puborectalis, pubococcygeus, and iliococcygeus) that comprise the levator ani occupy the space between the body of the pubis, ischial spine, and coccyx.

- The coccygeus muscle is superior and lateral to the levator ani.

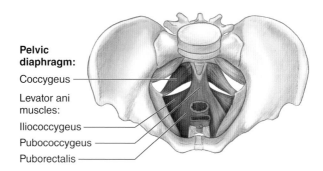

FIGURE 9.3 Muscles of the pelvic diaphragm.

These muscles collectively function to support the pelvic viscera during functional activities, urination, and defecation.

When discussing the muscles of the abdomen and pelvis, it is important to consider the trunk as a large canister. The top portion of the canister is the diaphragm as it functions to separate the thoracic cavity from the abdominal cavity. In addition to being the primary muscle of respiration, the diaphragm is the most superior aspect of the trunk. Along with the abdominal and pelvic floor muscles, it is designed to increase intrathoracic and intra-abdominal pressure. The diaphragm, abdominal muscles, lumbar muscles, and pelvic floor muscles work synergistically to increase stability to the thoracolumbar and pelvic regions during functional activities.

In addition to the muscles of the abdominal wall and pelvic girdle, strong ligaments increase the passive stability to the lower lumbar spine and pelvic regions (figure 9.4). The ligaments of the pelvic girdle are some of the strongest ligaments in the body.

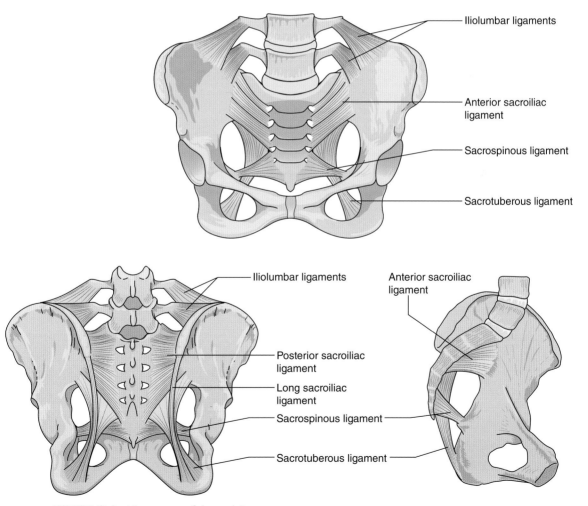

FIGURE 9.4 Ligaments of the pelvis.

- The iliolumbar ligament spans from the transverse processes of L5 to the ilium. It adds stability to the L5 to S1 vertebral levels during functional movements.
- The sacrotuberous and sacrospinous ligaments each have an attachment on the sacrum and then traverse posteriorly and laterally to attach to the ischial tuberosity and ischial spine, respectively. These ligaments resist sacral nutation.
- The long and short posterior sacroiliac ligaments run from the posterior aspect of the ilium, just inferior to the posterior superior iliac spine and attach to the posterior–lateral aspect of the sacrum. Clinically, these ligaments can be a source of pain in people with pelvic girdle dysfunction.[9-11]

Neurovascular Anatomy

The abdominal aorta is the main artery that supplies the posterior abdominal wall (figure 9.5). It is responsible for giving off branches to both the viscera and the abdominal wall itself. At the L4 level, the artery bifurcates into the right and left common iliac arteries. Subsequently, each common iliac artery divides into the internal and external iliac arteries.

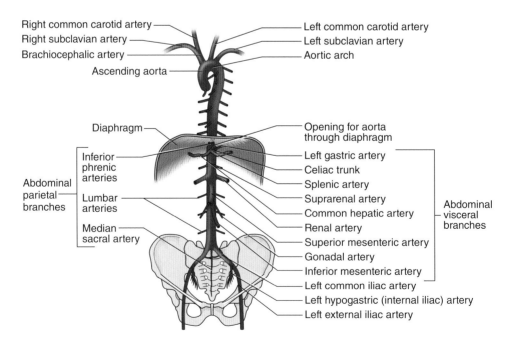

FIGURE 9.5   Major arteries of the abdominal and pelvic regions.

The internal iliac artery supplies blood to the structures in the pelvic girdle, the gluteal region, and the genitalia. It has anterior and posterior divisions that divide near the sacroiliac joints (figure 9.6).

- The anterior divisions branch into the umbilical, obturator, inferior vesical, middle rectal, vaginal, uterine, internal pudendal, and inferior gluteal arteries, which collectively supply the pelvic reproductive organs, the bladder, and the rectum.

- The posterior division of the internal iliac artery branches into the superior gluteal, iliolumbar, lateral sacral, and ovarian arteries, which supply the gluteal muscles, the muscles of the posterior abdominal wall, the sacrum and cauda equina, and the ovaries, respectively.

The external iliac artery is the main blood supply of the lower limb as it travels under the inguinal ligament where it becomes the femoral artery.[8] A further discussion of lower extremity blood supply is covered in chapters 10 through 12.

The nerve supply to the abdominal and pelvic regions is also quite extensive (figure 9.7). The anterior rami of the L1 to L4 nerves form the lumbar plexus within the psoas major muscle and is responsible for providing

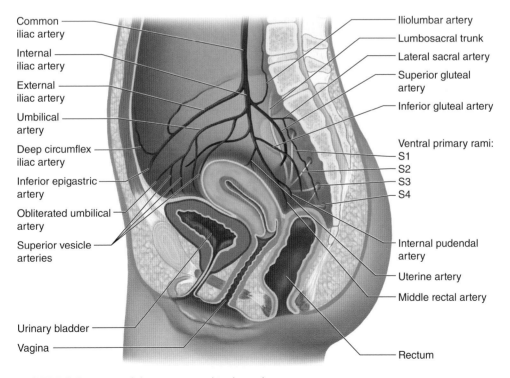

FIGURE 9.6 Internal iliac artery and its branches.

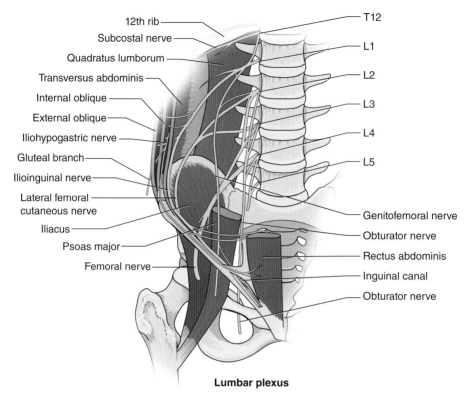

12th rib
Subcostal nerve
Quadratus lumborum
Transversus abdominis
Internal oblique
External oblique
Iliohypogastric nerve
Gluteal branch
Ilioinguinal nerve
Lateral femoral cutaneous nerve
Iliacus
Psoas major
Femoral nerve

T12
L1
L2
L3
L4
L5
Genitofemoral nerve
Obturator nerve
Rectus abdominis
Inguinal canal
Obturator nerve

Lumbar plexus

FIGURE 9.7   Lumbar plexus.

both sensory and motor innervation to the lower abdomen, pelvis, and lower extremity.

The upper part of the lumbar plexus has three branches: the iliohypogastric (L1), ilioinguinal (L1), and genitofemoral (L1-L2) nerves.[8]

- The iliohypogastric nerve is responsible for innervating the skin above the inguinal ligament and the muscles on the anterior abdominal wall.
- The ilioinguinal nerve is responsible for innervating the skin of the external genitalia and the muscles of the anterior abdominal wall.
- The genitofemoral nerve is responsible for innervating the fascia of the scrotum, the skin of the genital region, and the skin on the most medial aspect of the thigh.

The lower lumbar plexus has three additional nerves that branch off of it.[8]

- The lateral femoral cutaneous nerve (L2-L3) crosses over the iliacus and enters the thigh under the inguinal ligament.
- The femoral nerve (L2-L4) crosses lateral and deep to the psoas major. After innervating the iliacus and psoas major, it enters the thigh under

the inguinal ligament and is responsible for innervating the skin and muscles of the anterior thigh.

- The obturator nerve (L2-L4) crosses medial and deep to the psoas major and enters the thigh through the obturator foramen, innervating the skin and muscles along the medial aspect of the thigh.

The nerve supply to the pelvis is a combination of somatic and autonomic innervation. The autonomic innervation is beyond the scope of this book, and therefore readers are encouraged to consult other sources for detailed information.[2] The somatic innervation comes from the sacral plexus (L4-L5, S1-S3; figure 9.8). Several nerves arise off this plexus, which some refer to as the lumbosacral plexus.[2]

- The superior gluteal nerve (L4-S1) exits the pelvis through the greater sciatic foramen, entering the gluteal region and innervating the gluteus medius and minimus and tensor fasciae latae.
- The inferior gluteal nerve (L5-S2) also exits the pelvis through the greater sciatic foramen, entering the gluteal region and innervating the gluteus maximus.

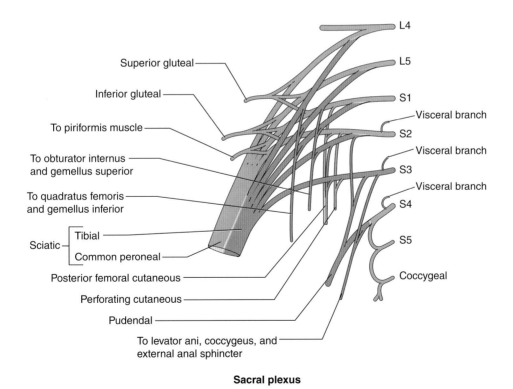

Sacral plexus

FIGURE 9.8 Sacrococcygeal plexus.

- The nerve to the quadratus femoris, which is small, also innervates the inferior gemellus.

- The nerve to the obturator internus, which is small, also innervates the superior gemellus

- The sciatic nerve (L4-S3), the largest nerve in the body, leaves the pelvis through the greater sciatic foramen and is responsible for innervating the structures of the posterior thigh and leg and the ankle and foot.

- The pudendal nerve (S2-S4) exits the pelvis through the greater sciatic foramen, medial to the posterior femoral cutaneous nerve, where it then travels through the lesser sciatic foramen to innervate structures of the perineum and ischiorectal fossa.

Abdominal Visceral Anatomy

The organs of the abdominal cavity are divided into two groups: the abdominal organs that compose the gastrointestinal tract (esophagus, stomach, small intestine, and large intestine) and the accessory abdominal organs (liver, gall bladder, pancreas, and kidneys) (figure 9.9). Each of these organs can be found in one of four quadrants of the abdominal cavity: upper right (UR), upper left (UL), lower right (LR), or lower left (LL).

The esophagus is the first part of the gastrointestinal tract and where the bolus of food first enters as it descends into the stomach. The esophagus is approximately 10 inches (25 centimeters) long, lies posterior to the trachea, and is slightly off-center to the left of the vertebral bodies. This long tube enters the abdomen through a hiatus in the diaphragm, the diaphragmatic constrictor, at the level of the T10 vertebra. It joins the stomach at the gastroesophageal sphincter, also known as the cardiac sphincter.

The stomach is situated in the upper left quadrant. Once food is in the stomach, the gastroesophageal sphincter prevents the backflow of food from the stomach back into the esophagus. The stomach breaks down large food particles into smaller ones that can better be processed for digestion. The stomach has three parts: the fundus, body, and pyloric regions. The entire stomach is covered with the peritoneum (greater omentum) and has both greater and lesser curvatures that help maintain the stomach's shape inside the gastrointestinal canal. The majority of digestion occurs in the body of the stomach, which is the longest part.

The pyloric sphincter is the opening at the end of the pyloric region of the stomach and is where the food bolus passes through on its way into the small intestine. The small intestine is the longest part of the gastrointestinal tract (over 16 feet, or about 5 meters, long) and is composed of the duodenum, jejunum, and ileum.

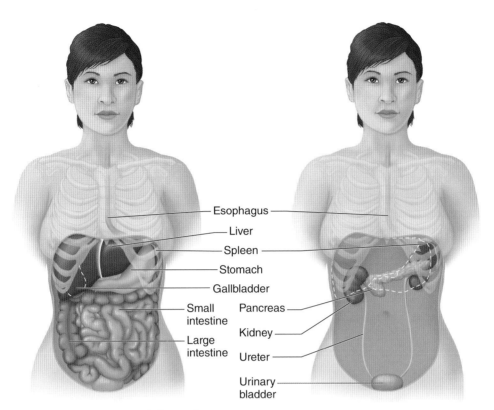

Esophagus
Liver
Spleen
Stomach
Gallbladder
Small
intestine
Large
intestine
Pancreas
Kidney
Ureter
Urinary
bladder

FIGURE 9.9 Accessory abdominal organs.

- The duodenum (7.8 to 10 inches [20 to 25 centimeters] long) is the first part of the small intestine. It has four parts: superior, descending, inferior, and ascending. The majority of the duodenum is retroperitoneal with the exception of the superior part.[8]
  - The superior part wraps around the head of the pancreas and is situated in the epigastric and umbilical regions of the abdomen at the L1 to L3 levels of the spine, just anterior to the inferior vena cava, aorta, and right kidney.
  - The descending (second part) portion of the duodenum is the most important part because this is where liver and pancreatic secretions that are vital for digestion are introduced via the hepatopancreatic sphincter (sphincter of Oddi).
- The jejunum (6.5 feet, or 2 meters, long) is the second part of the small intestine and is located in the left hypochondrium of the abdomen. The jejunum is the site for lipid and protein digestion, whereas most starch digestion occurs in the stomach.

- The ileum (10 feet, or 3 meters, long) is the last part of the small intestine and is where most digested nutrients are absorbed. It is situated in the lower right quadrant of the abdomen.

The last part of the gastrointestinal tract is the large intestine and is approximately 5 feet (1.5 meters) long. The ileocecal valve is the direct connection between the ileum and the large intestine. The large intestine is made up of the cecum, appendix, colon (ascending, transverse, descending, and sigmoid), rectum, and anal canal, which formally complete the gastrointestinal tract within the pelvis. The function of the large intestine is primarily water reabsorption before the remaining waste is eliminated from the body.

While a thorough discussion of the accessory abdominal organs is beyond the scope of this book, a brief review is appropriate to provide pertinent anatomical facts that will aid in palpation of these structures and comprehension of the contents and function of the abdominal cavity. The liver is the largest organ (glandular) in the body and is somewhat protected by the lower aspect of the rib cage. It is situated in both upper quadrants of the abdominal cavity, with most of it being in the upper right quadrant, with a small segment (left lobe) found in the upper left quadrant. The organ receives blood supply from the hepatic portal vein, which brings nutrients to the liver from the gastrointestinal tract. The main function of the liver is to clean and filter the blood coming from the gastrointestinal tract before it passes on to the remainder of the body. On the undersurface of the right lobe (upper right quadrant) is the gallbladder, a small pea-shaped organ. The gallbladder is responsible for storing approximately 1 to 1.7 ounces (30 to 50 milliliters) of bile, which is secreted into the small intestine to aid in the digestion of fat.[8]

The pancreas and kidneys (whose palpation will not be discussed) are the remaining accessory abdominal organs. They are retroperitoneal, lying behind the peritoneal lining of the abdominal cavity. The pancreas functions as both an endocrine gland and an exocrine gland. In its endocrine function, it is largely responsible for controlling blood glucose levels, while its exocrine function is the release of enzymes to aid in the digestive process. The pancreas has a head, body, and tail. The kidneys are inferior to the pancreas and are located at about the T11 to L1 or L2 vertebral levels. The kidneys function as the body's main filtration center and are responsible for the removal of urea and waste. In addition, the kidneys regulate blood pressure and overall blood volume.[8]

Pelvic Visceral Anatomy

The pelvic viscera includes the urinary bladder, distal end of the ureters, rectum, and reproductive organs (see figure 9.9). The ureters are muscular tubes that transport urine from the kidney to the bladder. They are unique in that they are actually part of both the abdominal and pelvic cavities. The ureters become pelvic structures at approximately the bifurcation of the common iliac arteries. They receive blood supply from branches of the common and internal iliac arteries, while receiving nerve supply from a collection of autonomic plexi in the abdominal and pelvic cavities.[8]

The urinary bladder is a saclike structure with strong muscular support within its walls. The apex of the bladder is situated at the superior aspect of the pubic symphysis, while the base (fundus) of the bladder is attached to the seminal vesicles and rectum in males and is attached to the uterus and vagina in females. When it starts to fill with urine, the parasympathetic nerve innervation causes the detrusor muscle to contract and the urethral sphincter to relax. This permits the flow of urine into the urethra and subsequently eliminates it from the body through the external urethral orifice. In men, the urethra is 7 to 8 inches (18 to 20 centimeters) long; in women it is only 1.6 inches (4 centimeters) long.

Male Pelvic Viscera

The prostate gland, two seminal glands, bladder, and rectum are part of the male pelvic viscera (figure 9.10), which function in sexual activity, reproduction, urination, and defecation.[8]

- The prostate is a gland, about 1.2 inches (3 centimeters) long, through which the first part of the urethra passes. It produces secretions that are added to the ejaculation fluid during sexual intercourse and orgasm.[8]

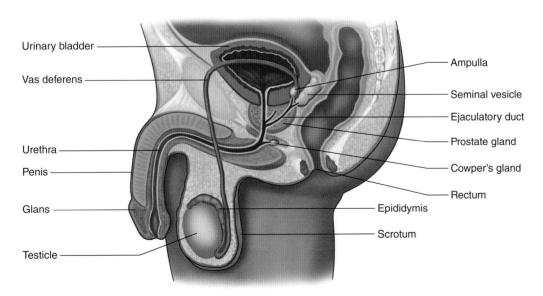

FIGURE 9.10 Male pelvic viscera.

- The prostate gland is inferior to the urinary bladder at the base of the penis, between the bladder and rectum.
  - From a bony landmark perspective, it is just posterior and inferior to the pubic symphysis. This positioning allows the palpation of the posterior segment by way of digital rectal examination (not covered in this text).
- The two seminal glands are located between the rectum and bladder. They produce a thick seminal fluid that will pass into the ejaculatory duct.[8]

Female Pelvic Viscera

The female pelvic viscera include the vagina, uterus, uterine (fallopian) tubes, and ovaries (figure 9.11).

- The uterus is a thick muscular organ that is located just superior to the bladder. It has a body, fundus, isthmus, and cervix.
  - The body of the uterus, which forms the superior two-thirds, is the largest portion, and this is where the uterine tubes enter the uterus.
  - The middle one-third of the uterus is the fundus, which narrows and becomes the isthmus of the uterus before joining with the cervix, which enters the vaginal canal.

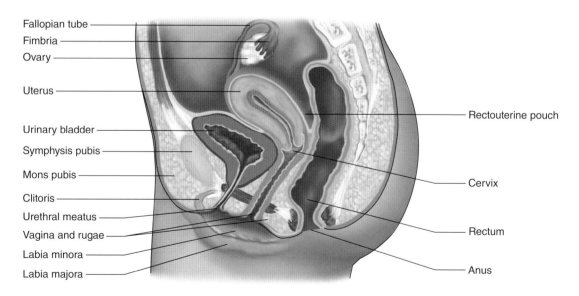

FIGURE 9.11 Female pelvic viscera.

- Two important ligaments support the uterus.[8]
  - The round ligament of the uterus attaches to the posterior aspect of the body of the uterus and traverses laterally to attach to the deep inguinal ring.
  - The broad ligament of the uterus is a fold in the peritoneum that descends from the uterine tubes to the cervix and lateral pelvic wall.
- The ovaries are small pea-shaped organs that are suspended in the pelvis by ligaments.
  - The ovaries are connected to the uterus by the ligament of the ovary, which runs from the medial aspect of the ovary to the uterus.
  - The suspensory ligament of the ovary connects the lateral aspect of the ovary to the lateral pelvic wall.
- The vagina is a fibromuscular tube that is situated between the uterus and perineum, and is the opening to the female pelvic viscera. It is anterior to the rectum and rectouterine pouch and posterior to the urethra and bladder. The vagina has two sets of skin folds.[8]
  - The outer labia majora, which contain sweat and sebaceous glands, are longitudinal skin folds that meet superiorly at the mons pubis, which is a collection of fatty tissue anterior to the pubic symphysis.
  - Medial to the labia majora are the labia minora, which are hairless skin folds that surround the vestibule of the vagina.

Structural Inspection

- The clinician should observe and look for deviations or asymmetries in the abdominal and pelvic regions such as anterior or posterior pelvic tilt or pelvic obliquities.
- Have the patient stand in a normal resting stance. For complete observation, the clinician should observe from the anterior, posterior, and lateral views.
- Pay particular attention to holding patterns (increased muscle tone), especially if it is asymmetrical.
- Observation of skin changes such as increased or decreased color, abrasions, moles, or rashes should be noted and discussed with the patient.
- Perform a careful assessment to identify areas of ecchymosis.
- Postsurgical incisions and scars should be cleared for signs of infection or delayed healing.

Muscles of the Abdomen and Pelvis

Muscle	Origin	Insertion	Innervation	Blood supply	Action
Diaphragm	Xiphoid process, lower 6 costal cartilages, and lateral and medial arcuate ligaments	Central	Phrenic nerve C3 to C5	Pericardiacophrenic, musculophrenic, and superior and inferior phrenic arteries	Primary muscle of respiration
Psoas major	T12 to L5 lumbar vertebrae	Lesser trochanter	Ventral rami L2 to L4	Iliolumbar artery	Hip flexion and lumbar stabilization
Iliacus	Iliac fossa	Blends into the psoas major	Femoral nerve L2 to L4	Iliolumbar artery	Hip flexion
Quadratus lumborum	Rib 12 and upper lumbar (L1-L3) transverse processes	Iliac crest	Ventral rami T12 to L3	Iliolumbar artery	Hip hiking and ipsilateral side-bending of the spine
Piriformis	Anterior aspect of the sacrum	Greater trochanter	Ventral rami S1 to S2	Superior and inferior gluteal arteries and internal pudendal artery	Hip abduction and external rotation
Obturator internus	Obturator membrane and fossa	Greater trochanter	Nerve to obturator internus	Internal pudendal artery and obturator artery	Hip external rotation
Levator ani	Body of pubis, obturator fascia, and ischial spine	Perineal body, coccyx, prostate or vagina, rectum, and anal canal	S4 nerve root	Inferior gluteal artery and internal pudendal artery (inferior rectal and perineal branches)	Support of pelvic viscera
Coccygeus or ischiococcygeus	Sacrum	Ischial spine	S4 to S5 nerve roots	Inferior gluteal artery	Flexion of coccyx

Zone I: Diaphragm and Posterior Abdominal Wall

Diaphragm (Indirect)

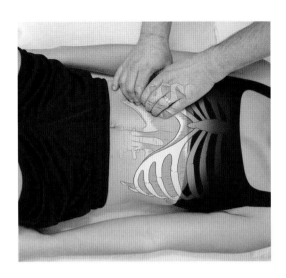

Positions
- Patient: supine, with the hips and the knee flexed to about 45°
- Clinician: Sitting or standing, facing the patient, on the side being palpated

Instructions
- Palpate the lower end of the rib cage using the pads of three to four fingers with both hands.
- To confirm palpation, have the patient breathe and note the timing and amount of movement of the diaphragm's ability to expand the lower thorax (rib cage).

Notes
- Dysfunction of the diaphragm can affect both the movement and forces through the lumbopelvic hip complex and the thorax.
- If there is hypertonicity in the abdominal muscles or the erector spinae, the lower rib cage will expand minimally during inspiration, and most movement will come from the chest (apical breathing).
- The clinician can also palpate the rib cage while the patient is in other positions, such as sitting, standing, or child's pose, to assess the movement of the diaphragm.

Psoas Major

Positions

- Patient: supine, with the hips at about 45° of flexion and the knees at 90° of flexion
- Clinician: standing, facing the patient, on the side being palpated

Instructions

- Palpate the anterior superior iliac spine (ASIS) and slide your hand medial onto the inner surface of the iliacus.
- Using three fingers, slide this hand medially and deep to the viscera and palpate the lateral aspect of the psoas. Place the opposite hand (left hand pictured) over the right hand to continue to add gentle, but firm pressure.
- To confirm palpation, have the patient perform hip flexion against resistance. You should feel a firm contraction under your fingers.

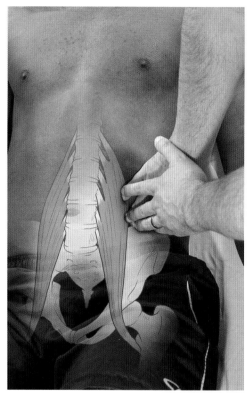

VIDEO 9.1 ▶

CLINICAL PEARL

The psoas is important for segmental control of the lumbar spine and hip and for its role as a hip flexor. Timing delays in people with primary hip pathology (femoracetabular impingement) often result in clicking, which is often the result of hypertonicity of the superficial hip flexors.

Iliacus

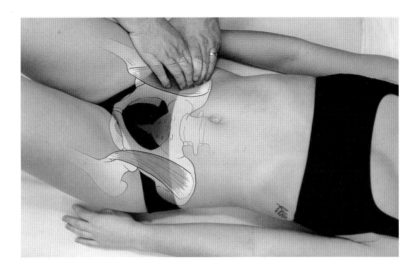

Positions

- Patient: supine, with the hips at about 45° of flexion and the knees at 90° of flexion
- Clinician: standing, facing the patient, on the side being palpated

Instructions

- Palpate the medial aspect of the iliac crest.
- Hook four fingers from both hands around the ASIS and follow along the medial aspect of the ilium as if you were scooping along the sides of a bowl.
- To confirm palpation, have the patient perform hip flexion against resistance. You will feel a firm contraction under your fingers.

Quadratus Lumborum

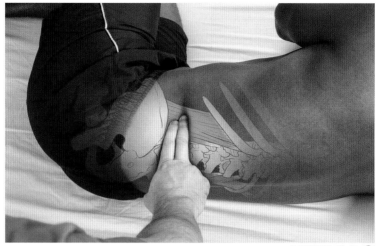

VIDEO 9.2 ▶

Positions

- Patient: side-lying, with the hips at about 45° of flexion and the knees at about 90° of flexion
- Clinician: standing, facing the patient, on the side being palpated

Instructions

- Palpate rib 12 posteriorly.
- Using two fingers, move just inferior to the rib until soft tissue is felt.
- To confirm palpation, have the patient hike the hip or side-bend the spine until a contraction is felt. You should feel a small contraction under your fingers.

Notes

- This muscle is deep and should not be confused with the posterior fibers of the external oblique.
- It is important to differentiate between the quadratus lumborum and the posterior fibers of the external oblique by isolating the function of the quadratus lumborum.

Zone II: Pelvic Wall and Floor

Piriformis

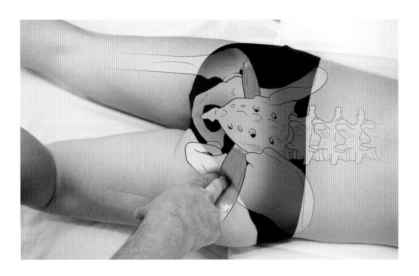

Positions
- Patient: prone, with the lumbar spine in a neutral position and a pillow under the abdomen with the knee flexed to 90°
- Clinician: standing, facing the patient, on the side being palpated

Instructions
- Palpate the sacrum along S2 to S4 with one finger.
- Using two fingers, move lateral from the sacrum.
- Continue to follow the fibers laterally to the insertion on the greater trochanter.
- To confirm palpation, have the patient perform gentle external rotation of the hip against resistance. You should feel a small contraction as the patient slowly increases the force of contraction.

Notes
- If the patient performs rapid external rotation of the hip, the gluteus maximus will contract as opposed to the piriformis.
- This muscle can compress all aspects of the sacroiliac joint, making it difficult to assess motion.
- Be careful about passively stretching this muscle in people with radicular symptoms, and consider using a more active flossing technique (the nerve gliding back and forth along its path as opposed to passive stretching).

Coccygeus, or Ischiococcygeus

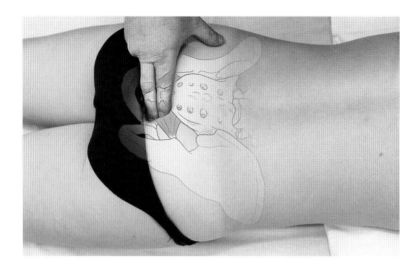

Positions

- Patient: prone, with the lumbar spine in a neutral position and a pillow under the abdomen
- Clinician: standing, facing the patient, on the side not being palpated

Instructions

- Palpate the piriformis muscle.
- Move your fingers directly inferior, keeping them along the lateral border of the sacrum.
- Here you should be able to palpate the coccygeus muscle using two fingers, which is deep to the sacrotuberous and sacrospinous ligaments.
- To confirm palpation, have the patient perform a contraction of the pelvic floor as if to stop the flow of urine. You should feel a subtle muscle contraction.

Notes

- This can be performed either prone or supine, depending on patient comfort.
- This muscle can compress the inferior aspect of the sacroiliac joint.
- Hypertonicity of this muscle can cause aberrant movements of the pelvis.

Levator Ani

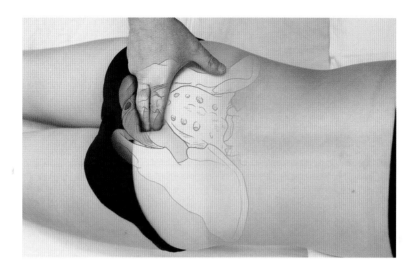

Positions

- Patient: prone, with the lumbar spine in a neutral position and a pillow under the abdomen
- Clinician: standing, facing the patient, on the side not being palpated

Instructions

- Palpate the coccygeus muscle.
- Move two fingers directly inferior, keeping them along the lateral border of the coccyx.
- The levator ani is relatively superficial but is usually under subcutaneous fascia and fat.
- To confirm palpation, have the patient perform a contraction of the pelvic floor as if to stop the flow of urine. You should feel a subtle muscle contraction.

Note

Palpation of the coccygeus, or ischiococcygeus, and levator ani are easier if the clinician is standing on the opposite side being palpated. This allows the clinician to work from medial to lateral, which is more comfortable and less intrusive for the patient.

Obturator Internus

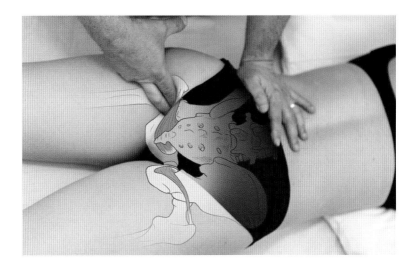

Positions

- Patient: prone, with a pillow under the abdomen.
- Clinician: standing, facing the patient, on the side being palpated

Instructions

- Palpate the ischial tuberosity using the pads of two or three fingers, making sure your proximal interphalangeal and distal interphalangeal joints are flexed.
- Move your fingers directly medial to the ischial tuberosity.
- To confirm palpation, have the patient perform external rotation of the hip against resistance. You should feel a subtle contraction under your finger.

Note

It is difficult to isolate this muscle externally from the other small external rotators of the hip (superior and inferior gemelli, quadratus femoris).

Visceral Palpation

Before discussing the specific visceral structures, a connection between the role of visceral palpation and treatment of regional dysfunction will be described. Clinicians can easily see the relationship and connection between palpation of certain structures such as muscles or ligaments and their subsequent treatment during manual therapy interventions. Oftentimes, however, visceral structures are not assessed during the examination and management of patients with neuromusculoskeletal dysfunction because this vital skill is not included in many entry-level health care professional programs.[12,13]

We encourage you to consider this information to be as important as learning, for example, to palpate the pectoralis minor or psoas to perform soft tissue mobilization. The visceral organs have fascial attachments to various bones and muscles, and increased tension in these organs or decreased mobility can lead to added stress on other joints or musculoskeletal tissues. While comprehensive treatment of these visceral structures is not the goal of this book, information useful during the structure identification and assessment is discussed in the clinical pearls. One suggestion is to palpate the viscera and assess for changes in the tissue's ability to lengthen and fold and its overall excursion of mobility during movement patterns, such as trunk flexion, extension, and rotation.[13] While visceral structures cannot be palpated and confirmed as clearly as musculoskeletal tissues, palpation of the viscera is a skill that will continue to help clinicians develop the art and science of palpation.

Zone III: Gastrointestinal Tract and Accessory Abdominal Organs

Esophagus

Positions

- Patient: supine, with a pillow under the knees
- Clinician: standing or sitting depending on the part of the esophagus being palpated

Instructions

- For the superior part of the esophagus, palpate posterior to the cricoid cartilage using two or three fingers.

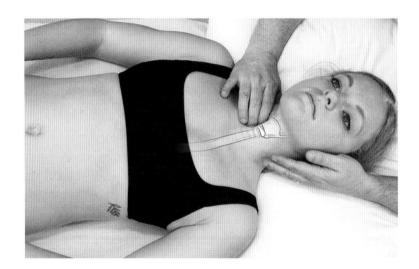

- For the inferior part of the esophagus (gastroesophageal junction), sink two fingers approximately 1 to 2 inches (2.5 to 5 centimeters) deep near the seventh sternochondral junction.

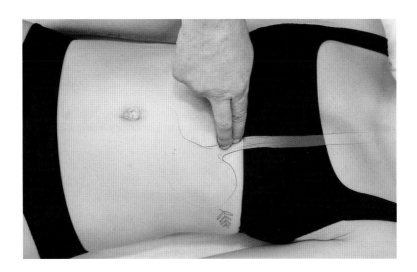

- Have the patient swallow to confirm palpation of both of these segments. You should feel a subtle movement under your fingers at the superior aspect of the esophagus. For the inferior portion of the esophagus, you may feel a small wavelike movement under your fingers.

Notes

- When palpating the superior aspect of the esophagus, be careful and don't irritate the trachea.
- The esophagus is directly anterior to the spine, so this can be used as a guide during palpation.

CLINICAL PEARL

Restrictions in the esophagus can lead to limitations in cervical extension as well as dysfunction in rotation at C7 to T1.

Stomach

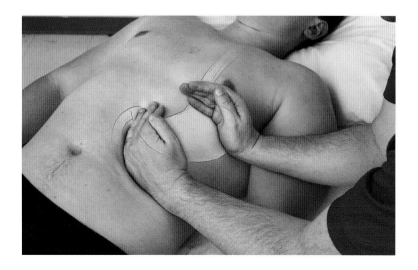

Positions

- Patient: supine, with a pillow under the knees
- Clinician: standing, on the left side of the patient, facing the head of the table

Instructions

- With the left hand, identify the medial aspect of the stomach (along the lesser curvature) just below the xiphoid process.
- Use the right hand to identify the lateral aspect (along the greater curvature) along the left lateral abdominal region.
- You should feel a broad firm structure through the rib cage.

Note

A radiographic classification has been developed to assess the shape of the stomach.[14]

- Hypertonic stomach: shaped like a steer's horn, increased tone, empties in 2 to 3 hours
- Orthotonic stomach: shaped like the letter J, normal tone, empties in 3 to 4 hours
- Hypotonic stomach: shaped like the letter U, decreased tone, empties in 4 to 5 hours
- Atonic stomach: shaped like the letter U, no tone, empties in 5 to 6 hours

CLINICAL PEARL

Clinicians can assess changes in symptoms by checking the mobility of the stomach in a medial-to-lateral and a superior-to-inferior direction.

Pyloric Sphincter

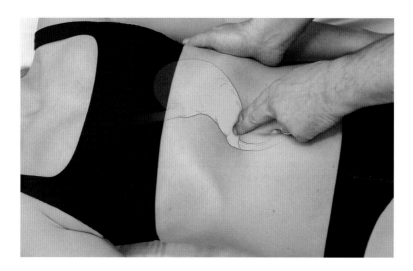

Positions

- Patient: supine, with a pillow under the knees
- Clinician: standing, on the right side of the patient, facing the head of the table

Instructions

- Use one hand to palpate about 2.5 inches (6 to 7 centimeters) above the umbilicus.
- The pyloric sphincter (approximately 2 centimeters in diameter) is vertically oriented and may be found immediately to the right or left of midline.
- Use two fingers (left hand pictured) to palpate deep through the soft tissue to the level of the sphincter. You should feel a density under your fingers.

Note

The pylorus, a strong ring of smooth muscle, connects the stomach to the duodenum.

CLINICAL PEARL

Clinicians can assess the mobility of the sphincter by checking the end feel in the clockwise and counterclockwise directions.

Duodenum (Superior Part)

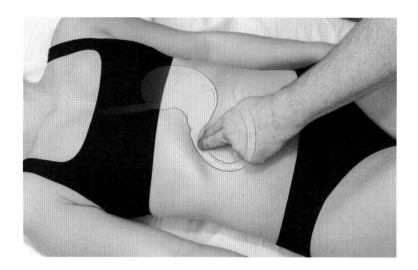

Positions

- Patient: supine, with a pillow under the knees
- Clinician: standing, on the right side of the patient, facing the head of the table

Instructions

- Palpate the pyloric sphincter using two or three fingers of the right hand (not shown).
- Palpate the superior part of the duodenum with the left hand by placing two fingers slightly to the right and superior to the pylorus (left hand pictured). You should feel a fibrous structure under your fingers.

Note

Most of the duodenum is retroperitoneal and therefore only the superior part is palpable.

CLINICAL PEARL

- Restrictions in the duodenum can lead to limited range of motion in the thoracic and lumbar spine and to pain along the right T12 to L1 segment and sixth costovertebral joint.
- Clinicians can use movements of the hip and pelvis to perform visceral mobilization with movement of this structure.

Small Intestine and Greater Omentum

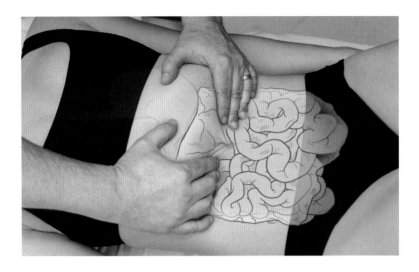

Positions
- Patient: supine, with the knees bent
- Clinician: standing, on one side, facing either the head or foot of the table

Instructions
- Using digits 2 to 5 of both hands, palpate immediately above the umbilicus.
- Gently but firmly sink in deeply and from inferior to superior, hook your fingers under as if scooping up the small intestine and greater omentum.

Notes
- The small intestine is attached to the posterior abdominal wall by the mesentery.
- Because of its attachment and vascularity, the small intestine is extremely mobile.

CLINICAL PEARL
- Restrictions in the small intestine and greater omentum can lead to low back or thoracic spine pain.
- Clinicians should assess the mobility of the small intestine and greater omentum from a superior-to-inferior and posterior-to-anterior direction.

Cecum

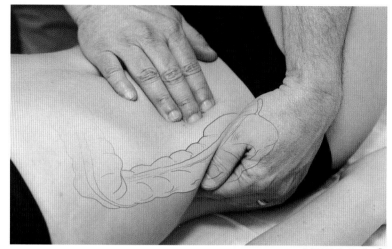

VIDEO 9.3 ▶

Positions

- Patient: supine, with a pillow under the knees
- Clinician: standing on the left side, reaching across to palpate the cecum

Instructions

- With both hands, palpate along the medial aspect of the right ilium, with fingers angled slightly medially.
- Palpate the iliacus.
- Move your fingers medially and apply more pressure until palpating the lateral border of the cecum. The texture of the tissue is softer than the iliacus, and the structure is about 2.75 inches (7 centimeters) wide.

CLINICAL PEARL

- Restrictions in the cecum can lead to right innominate dysfunction and to limitations in all planes of lumbar spine motion.
- The cecum can also adhere to the iliacus muscle, causing restrictions during functional movements such as the terminal stance phase of gait.

Ileocecal Valve

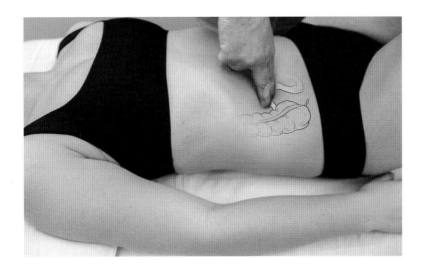

Positions

- Patient: supine, with the knees bent
- Clinician: standing on the left side of the patient

Instructions

- Palpate the right anterior superior iliac spine.
- Palpate the umbilicus.
- The ileocecal valve is palpated one-third of the way between these two structures by using two fingers and a fair amount of anterior-to-posterior force. You should feel a firm density under your fingers.

Notes

- The valve is vertically oriented and approximately 1.75 centimeters in diameter.
- The ileocecal valve connects the ileum, which is the last part of the small intestine, and the cecum, which is the first part of the large intestine.

Ascending Colon

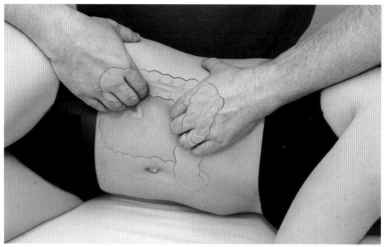

VIDEO 9.4 ▶

Positions

- Patient: left side-lying, with the knees flexed and a pillow between the knees
- Clinician: standing on the right side of the patient

Instructions

- Palpate the right ninth rib by starting at rib 12 and moving superiorly.
- The ascending colon stops at approximately this level.
- Palpate the ascending colon with two hands, using all fingers and gently, but firmly, assess medial-to-lateral mobility.

Notes

- The ascending colon is considered retroperitoneal and is about 10 inches (25 centimeters) long.
- The ascending colon can also be palpated with the patient sitting, with his or her feet on the ground and the clinician standing behind the patient.

CLINICAL PEARL

To assess the ability of the ascending colon and other structures to fold and lengthen, have the patient perform trunk side bending. Restrictions in the ascending colon can cause shortness (tightness) in the right quadratus lumborum and right psoas major. Limited left side bending and right lateral and posterior thoracolumbar pain may also be seen in these patients.

Transverse Colon

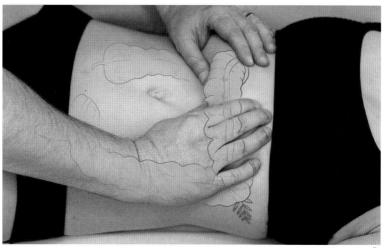

VIDEO 9.5 ▶

Positions
- Patient: supine, with the knees bent
- Clinician: standing at the bottom of the table, facing the patient

Instructions
- Palpate the umbilicus.
- Move your hands approximately 1.75 inches (4 to 5 centimeters) above the umbilicus.
- Using the thumbs of both hands, palpate the transverse colon and assess the mobility superiorly and inferiorly.

Notes
- The transverse colon is intraperitoneal and is the longest (18 inches or 45 centimeters) and most mobile part of the large intestine.
- This structure can also be palpated with the patient sitting with slight trunk flexion and feet on the ground.

CLINICAL PEARL
The clinician may consider using a half-round foam roller under the sacrum to perform visceral mobilization with movement.

Descending Colon

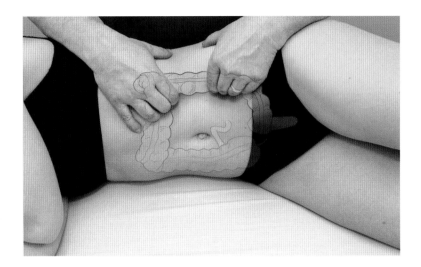

Positions

- Patient: right side-lying, with the knees bent and a pillow between the knees
- Clinician: standing behind the patient on the right side

Instructions

- Palpate the left ninth rib by starting at rib 12 and moving superiorly.
- The descending colon ends at approximately this level.
- Palpate the descending colon with two hands, using all fingers and gently, but firmly, assess medial-to-lateral mobility.

Note

The descending colon is retroperitoneal and is approximately 6 inches (15 centimeters) long.

CLINICAL PEARL

- Restrictions in the descending colon can cause shortness and tightness in the left quadratus lumborum and left psoas major.
- Limited right side bending and left lateral and posterior thoracolumbar pain may also be seen in these patients.

Liver

Positions

- Patient: supine, with a pillow under the knees
- Clinician: standing or sitting on the right side of the patient, facing the foot of the table

Instructions

- Palpate the right 10th rib, which is at the level of the lower border of the right lobe of the liver.

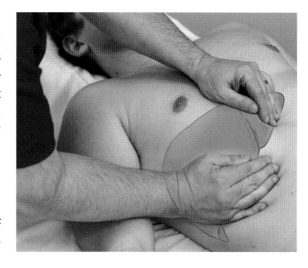

- Palpate the right fourth and fifth intercostal spaces, which is at the level of the superior border of the right lobe of the liver.
- With both hands, apply gentle inward pressure on the ribs, visualizing the borders of the liver deep to the rib cage, and obtain a soft tissue lock to assess superior-to-inferior mobility of the liver.

Notes

- The clinician can also sit or stand on the right side of the table, facing the patient to assess the inferior-to-superior mobility of the liver using the same steps.
- To assess the superior border of the liver, the patient can lie on the left side.

CLINICAL PEARL

- Restrictions in the mobility of the liver and overlying rib cage can cause right shoulder pain, right flank or thoracolumbar pain, or limited right shoulder flexion.
- Assess the mobility of the liver and rib cage while the patient is breathing. If necessary, cue the patient to take deep breaths into the clinician's hand during palpation to promote proper rib expansion.
- When palpating the upper abdominal region, the liver will move down to meet your fingertips when the patient inhales if the liver is enlarged.

Gallbladder

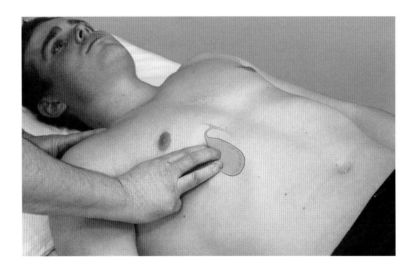

Positions

- Patient: supine, with a pillow under the knees
- Clinician: sitting or standing on the right side of the patient, facing the head of the table

Instructions

- Identify the midclavicular line on the right side.
- Palpate the right eighth and ninth costal cartilages, which are at the level of the fundus of the gallbladder.
- Sink two or three fingers in and assess the mobility of the gallbladder in all directions (right hand pictured). You should feel a small, dense structure under your fingers.

Note

Keep in mind that the gallbladder is only about 1 inch (2 to 3 centimeters) wide and approximately 2.75 to 4 inches (7 to 10 centimeters) long.

CLINICAL PEARL

Restrictions in the mobility of the gall bladder and overlying rib cage can present with upper right quadrant pain, right-side restrictions in the costovertebral joints of T7 to T9, difficulty with deep breathing, as well as many digestion problems, which may include pale stools and severe epigastric or midchest pain after meals.

Hepatopancreatic Sphincter (Sphincter of Oddi)

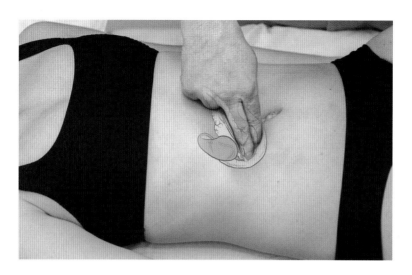

Positions
- Patient: supine, with the knees bent
- Clinician: sitting or standing on the right side, facing the head of the table

Instructions
- Identify the midclavicular line and the umbilicus.
- With two fingers, palpate about 1 inch (2 to 3 centimeters) above and slightly to the right of the umbilicus.
- Like the ileocecal valve, this is a true sphincter and usually has a denser and firmer texture compared to the surrounding structures.
- Assess the mobility of the sphincter of Oddi by moving your fingers in a clockwise and counterclockwise direction.

Note
The sphincter of Oddi is slightly inferior and deep to the gallbladder.

Zone IV: Pelvic Viscera

Urinary Bladder

Positions

- Patient: supine, with the knees bent
- Clinician: standing on either side, facing the head of the table

Instructions

- Palpate the pubic tubercle (see chapter 10) with the index finger and thumb.
- Move the fingers slightly superior to the pubic tubercle.
- Firmly, but gently, begin to sink the thumb and index fingers posteriorly.
- Depending on the fullness of the bladder, it may be located deeper.

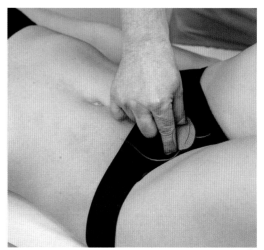

VIDEO 9.6 (FEMALE) ▶
VIDEO 9.7 (MALE) ▶

Note

Palpation of the bladder is contraindicated in the following conditions:

- Pregnancy
- Use of intrauterine device (IUD)
- Presence of tumors
- Presence of infection or stones

CLINICAL PEARL

- Restrictions in urinary bladder mobility can lead to dysfunction at T11 to L2 and at the sacroiliac and sacrococcygeal joints.
- Lower trunk rotation, unilateral heel slides, and single-leg hip external and internal rotation can all be used during visceral mobilization with movement.

Uterus

Positions

- Patient: supine, with the knees bent
- Clinician: standing on either side, facing the head of the table

Instructions

- Palpate the pubic tubercle with the index finger and thumb.
- Using the index finger and thumb, gently palpate the inferior aspect of the uterus, which is directly above the pubic tubercle. The superior end of the uterus is approximately 3 inches (7.6 centimeters) superior to the pubic tubercle.

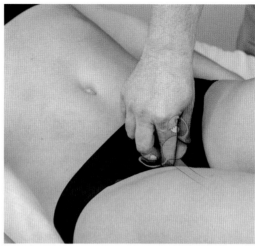

VIDEO 9.6 ▶

- Assess the lateral borders on each side of the body of the uterus, which is approximately 1.75 to 2.5 inches (4.5 to 6 centimeters) wide. You should feel a firm structure under your fingers.

Notes

- Palpation of the uterus is contraindicated in the following conditions:
  - Pregnancy (uterine or ectopic)
  - Use of intrauterine device (IUD)
  - Presence of tumors
  - Undergoing radiation treatment
- Usually, the uterus is in an anteverted and anteflexed position, but sometimes it rotates posteriorly (retroverted). This may lead to female infertility issues or difficulty conceiving.

CLINICAL PEARL

- Indications for palpation and subsequent mobilization of the uterus include low back pain, pelvic pain, dysmenorrhea, adhesions following trauma or surgery, and infertility.
- Have the patient bend the lumbar spine forward and backward and posteriorly tilt the pelvis to assess whether the uterus is restricting the mobility of the surrounding tissues.

Prostate

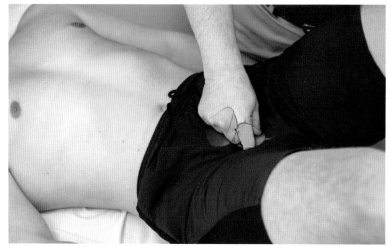

VIDEO 9.7 ▶

Positions
- Patient: supine, with the knees bent
- Clinician: standing on either side, facing the head of the table

Instructions
- Palpate the pubic tubercle with the thumb and index finger.
- Move the fingers to the inferior aspect of the pubic tubercle.
- Apply gentle, but firm, posterior pressure. The prostate is approximately 1 inch (2.5 centimeters) deep to the inferior border of the pubis.

Note
Palpation of the prostate is contraindicated in the following conditions:
- Acute prostatitis
- Signs of prostate cancer (if indicated, make a referral)

Case Study

History

A 37-year-old patient who is 6 weeks postpartum (vaginal delivery, 1 stitch required) presents to your office. The patient reports severe, intense cramping when she needs to have a bowel movement, and needs to void immediately. She reports having low back pain after delivery and sometimes has difficulty moving if she has been sitting in an unsupported position (e.g., nursing her baby) for a while. She reports having had abdominal and back labor (a small number of women report experiencing severe discomfort in the lower back that is most intense during contractions and often painful between contractions). The patient reports having bladder incontinence with her first pregnancy (2 years prior), which resolved postpartum (8 stitches required after that delivery). She reports feeling mild incontinence starting at the beginning of this pregnancy, but it was resolved with prenatal yoga. The patient denies numbness or tingling in either lower extremity. She reports having a stress fracture in her mid to low back 18 years ago caused by rowing. The patient lives with her family in an apartment with elevator access and works as a financial analyst. She was a marathoner and is looking to first get back to basic strengthening workouts and then half-marathon distance.

Examination

Past medical history	Unremarkable
Medication	Motrin
Observation	Bilateral subtalar joint pronation in weight-bearing Bilateral genu valgum Posterior left rotated innominate Decreased lumbar lordosis
Active range of motion	Trunk flexion: full, extension decreased 25%, right side-bending within normal limits, left side-bending decreased 1 inch (2.5 centimeters) from right with feeling tightness on her right, bilateral trunk rotation decreased 25% with stiffness
Passive range of motion	NA
Manual muscle testing	5/5 for all lower extremity motions except right hip flexion 4+/5, left hip flexion 4−/5, bilateral hip abductors 3+/5, bilateral hip external rotators 4/5, bilateral ankle plantar-flexion 4+/5

Special tests	McGill flexor test: 10 inches (25 centimeters)
	Positive left FABER test
	Negative distraction test
	Negative compression test
	Negative sacral thrust test
	Negative active straight-leg raise test
	Negative thigh thrust test
	Negative Gaenslen's test
Other	Normal neurological screen
	Mobility testing of lumbar spine and sacroiliac joint demonstrated hypomobility with spring testing with symptom referral up to the thoracic spine

- Based on the subjective and objective information together, what are the two most likely diagnoses? Give your rational for eliminating the third diagnosis.
- What structures should you palpate on this patient based on your differential diagnoses?
- Given all the information presented, what would you expect to find on palpation of those structures?

Case Solution and Discussion

Potential Diagnoses Based on History
- Sacroiliac joint dysfunction
- Postpartum musculoskeletal pain
- Nonspecific mechanical low back pain

Potential Diagnoses Based on History and Examination
- Postpartum musculoskeletal pain with pelvic floor dysfunction
- Nonspecific low back pain

Sacroiliac joint dysfunction: This diagnosis can be eliminated because of the lack of positive special tests based on a 2005 study by Laslett and colleagues.[15] In addition, the lack of a positive active straight-leg raise test makes sacroiliac joint instability much less likely. The findings of a posteriorly rotated left innominate and a positive left FABER test are inconsistent for sacroiliac joint dysfunction based on the current evidence.

Structures to Be Palpated
- Psoas
- Iliacus
- Adductors
- Sacrum
- Coccyx
- General visceral mobility
- Uterus
- Bladder

Palpation Findings

- Tenderness to palpation to bilateral psoas and iliacus (left > right)
- Restrictions with tenderness to palpation to uterus and bladder

Clinical Reasoning

- Nonspecific mechanical low back pain: This diagnosis is possible because of the patient's history of back labor, lack of mobility with spring testing, limited trunk mobility, and weakness in the bilateral lower extremities. However, tenderness to palpation of the uterus and bladder and the patient's report of severe, intense cramping when she needs to have a bowel movement, and the need to void immediately are inconsistent with this diagnosis.

- Postpartum musculoskeletal pain with pelvic floor dysfunction: The patient's history of two vaginal births and the reports of the pain beginning after giving birth make this a likely diagnosis. The tenderness to palpation of the psoas, iliacus, uterus, and bladder; limited trunk mobility; and the patient's report of severe, intense cramping when she needs to have a bowel movement and the need to void immediately are consistent with and indicative of postpartum musculoskeletal pain. It is possible that the trauma of pregnancy and childbirth caused scar tissue that was limiting visceral mobility and expansion (especially of the rectum, hence the need for immediate voidance). Limitations in visceral mobility can cause low back and regional discomfort. While this is not a typical pathoanatomical diagnosis, it should be distinguished from nonspecific mechanical low back pain because the treatment interventions will be different.

Case Study Questions

1. What information do the palpation findings give the clinician? How can this information be incorporated in the clinical decision-making process?
2. Think about how the subjective and objective examination findings lead to the differential diagnosis. What might you do differently?
3. What important patient education is critical in a case like this?

1. List the parts of the duodenum.
2. List the parts of the large intestine.
3. List the nerves of the sacral plexus and the muscles they innervate.
4. List the muscles that form the levator ani group.
5. Which major arteries give blood supply to the pelvis?
6. List the ligaments of the pelvis and their function.

chapter **10**

Hip and Groin Region

CHAPTER OBJECTIVES

After completing this chapter, the reader will be able to do the following:

- Identify the key bony anatomical structures of the hip and groin.
- Identify and describe the soft tissue anatomy of the hip and groin, including muscles, ligaments, nerves, arteries, and veins.
- Identify the borders of the femoral triangle and the structures located within it.
- Identify each compartment of the thigh and the muscles contained within.
- Identify on bony or skeletal models the origins and insertions of the muscles of the hip and groin to aid in understanding osteokinematic action and surface palpation.
- Palpate structures of the hip and groin.
- Integrate surface palpation findings to aid in the differential diagnosis of a patient with hip pain.

The hip and groin are responsible for producing coordinated movement in conjunction with the lumbopelvic region.[1] This coordinated movement provides controlled mobility during a variety of functional tasks. The hip joint is a ball and socket joint, very similar to the glenohumeral joint in the upper extremity. The hip permits movement in all planes and is subject to large compressive forces during activities such as walking, running, and jumping. For adequate stability to be maintained during everyday activities. a balance must exist between the passive and active structures surrounding the hip joint.[1,2]

Functions of the Hip Joint

An important function of the hip joint is proper distribution of forces down the entire kinetic chain and absorbing and dissipating forces that come up the kinetic chain during weight-bearing activities.[1] Like the glenohumeral joint in the upper extremity, the hip joint functions as a ball and socket joint to permit motion in all three cardinal planes. This allows for a wide range of functional mobility similar to that of the glenohumeral joint. However, there is more mobility in the shoulder than in the hip, while the hip has greater inherent stability than the shoulder.[1] This freedom of motion allows us to place the lower extremity, specifically the foot, in any position necessary during daily activities.

Bony Anatomy

The pelvis is shaped like a ring and is formed by the articulation of the two innominates and the sacrum. Each innominate is formed by the articulation of three bones: the ilium, the ischium, and the pubis (figure 10.1). The largest of these three bones is the ilium, which articulates with the sacrum bilaterally to form the sacroiliac joints (SIJ).[2] It is a broad bone that has several bony landmarks:

- Anterior superior iliac spine (ASIS)
- Anterior inferior iliac spine (AIIS)
- Posterior superior iliac spine (PSIS)
- Posterior inferior iliac spine (PIIS)

These landmarks are usually superficial (ASIS, PSIS) and easily palpable during the clinical examination. Also on the ilium are the anterior, posterior, and inferior gluteal lines. While not directly palpable, these landmarks serve as attachments for the gluteal muscles.[2]

Posterior and inferior to the ilium is the ischium. This bone has several important landmarks:

- Ischial tuberosity
- Ischial spine
- Greater and lesser sciatic notches

Anterior and inferior to the ilium is the pubic bone. Approximately 5 to 7 inches (13 to 18 centimeters) below the umbilicus is the symphysis pubis.[2] This joint is classified as an amphiarthrotic joint, with small amounts of movement present during activities.[1,3,4] On either side of the symphysis pubis are the superior and inferior pubic rami, which unite to form the pubic tubercle.[2]

The femur is the largest and strongest bone of the body. The large femoral head articulates with the acetabulum, forming the hip joint. The acetabulum is formed by the articulation of the ilium, the ischium, and the pubis. On the medial aspect of the femoral head is a small depression (fovea) through which blood vessels pass to bring blood supply to the femoral head and hip joint.[2]

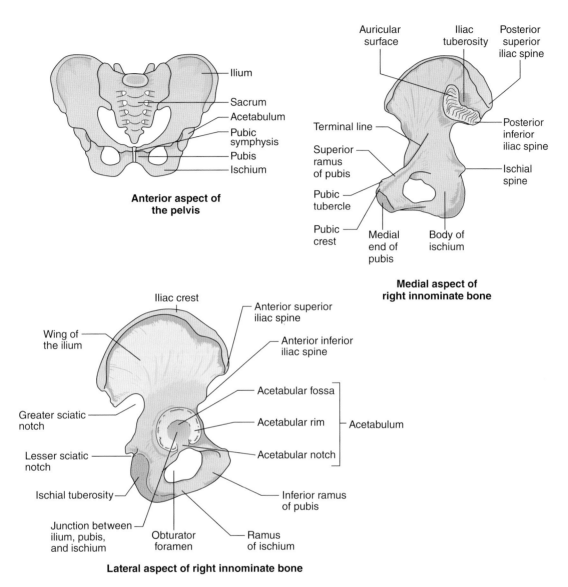

FIGURE 10.1 Bones of the pelvis.

The proximal femur includes the femoral head, the femoral neck, and the greater and lesser trochanters (figure 10.2). Between the trochanters are the intertrochanteric line anteriorly and the intertrochanteric crest posteriorly. The midshaft of the femur is where the linea aspera is found, and it serves as an attachment for several anterior and medial thigh muscles.[2]

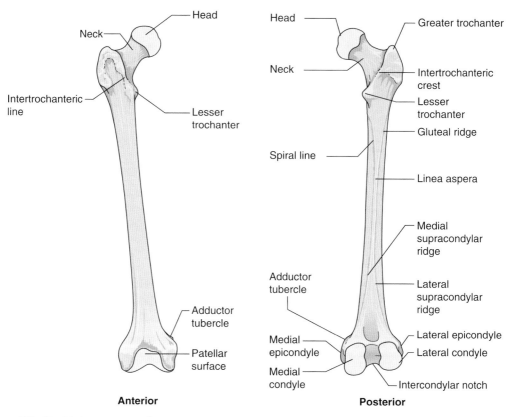

FIGURE 10.2 Aspects of the right femur.

Soft Tissue Anatomy

There are several muscles on the posterior aspect of the ilium (figure 10.3, posterior).[2]

- The gluteus maximus, which performs both hip extension and external rotation, is the largest and most superficial of these muscles.

- Proximal to the gluteus maximus is the origin of the gluteus medius, which is responsible for performing hip abduction and internal rotation.[2]

- Deep in the gluteal region are the gluteus minimus, the piriformis, the superior and inferior gemelli, the obturator internus, and the quadratus femoris.

  - The gluteus minimus is responsible for performing hip abduction and internal rotation.

  - The piriformis, gemelli muscles, and obturator internus are responsible for performing hip external rotation.

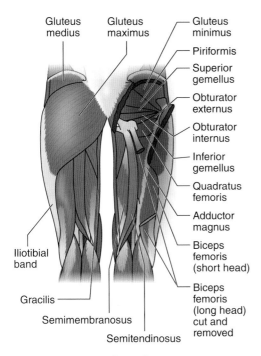

Posterior

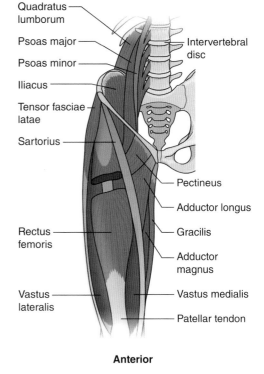

Anterior

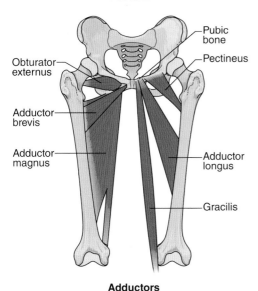

Adductors

FIGURE 10.3 Muscles of the hip.

Because these muscles can also perform other osteokinematic actions based on hip position, we highly recommend that readers review the kinesiology of the hip before proceeding to the palpation section of this chapter.[1]

The various muscles that surround the thigh can be divided into three compartments.[2]

- The anterior compartment of the thigh contains the sartorius, the tensor fasciae latae, the rectus femoris, the vastus medialis, the vastus lateralis, and the vastus intermedius (figure 10.3, anterior). Most of these muscles perform hip flexion and knee extension.

- The medial compartment of the thigh contains the adductor longus, brevis, and magnus; the gracilis; the pectineus; and the obturator externus (figure 10.3, adductors). These muscles are primarily responsible for hip adduction.

- The posterior compartment of the thigh is composed of the semitendinosus, the semimembranosus, and the biceps femoris (figure 10.3, posterior). These muscles perform hip extension and knee flexion.

In addition to the muscles surrounding the hip and groin, several ligaments provide passive stability to the region. The hip joint has three intrinsic ligaments: the iliofemoral, the ischiofemoral, and the pubofemoral. These ligaments start from the ilium, ischium, or pubis, and all insert on the femur. Collectively, these ligaments get tight during hip extension (figure 10.4).[1]

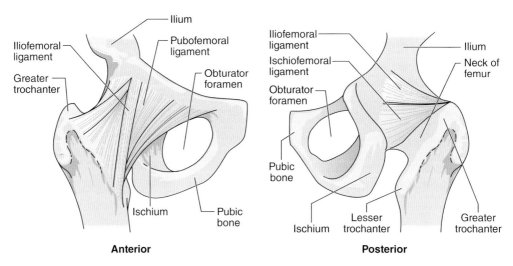

Anterior   **Posterior**

FIGURE 10.4   Ligaments of the hip.

Neurovascular Anatomy

On the anterior, medial thigh is the femoral triangle (figure 10.5).[2]

- The lateral border of the femoral triangle is the sartorius muscle.
- The medial border is the adductor longus muscle.
- The base is the inguinal ligament.
- The floor of the femoral triangle is made up of the pectineus medially and the iliopsoas laterally.

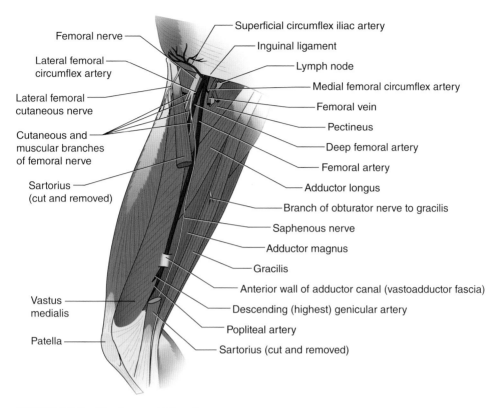

FIGURE 10.5 The femoral triangle.

Within the femoral triangle, from medial to lateral, are the femoral vein, artery, and nerve (VAN). The femoral artery is the direct continuation of the external iliac artery and is easily palpable. During palpation of the muscles that border this space, care must be taken to avoid occluding this vessel.[2] As the femoral artery travels down the anterior thigh, it gives off its largest branch, the profunda femoral artery, which is responsible for the main blood supply to the hip joint. The femoral artery then continues down the medial thigh and enters the hiatus in the adductor magnus. After exiting the hiatus, the femoral artery switches names and becomes the popliteal artery.[2]

The femoral nerve arises from the lumbar plexus (L2-L4) and travels down the anterior thigh, innervating the majority of the anterior thigh muscles, with the exception of the tensor fasciae latae (figure 10.6). Located medially in the thigh is the obturator nerve, which also arises from the lumbar plexus (L2-L4) and travels down the medial aspect of the thigh, innervating all the musculature of the medial thigh. The largest nerve aris-

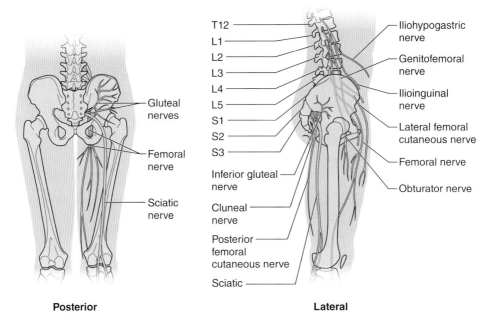

T12
L1
L2
L3
L4
L5
S1
S2
S3

Iliohypogastric nerve
Genitofemoral nerve
Ilioinguinal nerve
Lateral femoral cutaneous nerve
Femoral nerve
Obturator nerve

Gluteal nerves
Femoral nerve
Sciatic nerve

Inferior gluteal nerve
Cluneal nerve
Posterior femoral cutaneous nerve
Sciatic

Posterior   **Lateral**

FIGURE 10.6 Nerves of the hip and thigh.

ing from the sacrococcygeal plexus is the sciatic nerve (L4-S3), which runs down the posterior thigh, innervating the hamstring muscles. This nerve divides distally in the thigh into the tibial and common fibular nerves.[2]

Structural Inspection

- The clinician should start by observing the patient walking into the examining room. The ambulation pattern used by the patient can often be the first indication of a hip pathology. Particular attention should be paid to the amount of hip extension (terminal stance) the patient has bilaterally.
- Once in the examination room, the clinician can appropriately ask the patient to disrobe so both hip joints are visible as much as possible.
- The clinician should next observe for abrasions, unusual skin lesions, trophic changes, swelling, and so on.
- The clinician should next assess the levels of the ASIS and PSIS to ensure symmetry is present in standing and sitting.
- The clinician should observe from the posterior aspect to assess the overall shape and lower borders of the buttocks and to identify the gluteal folds. Asymmetry should be noted and assessed further during the remainder of the examination.

Iliac Crest

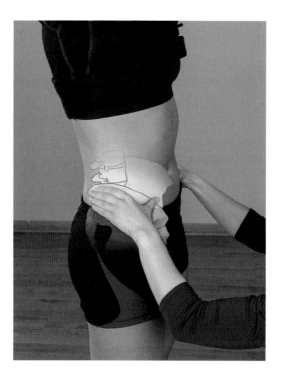

Positions
- Patient: standing, with feet shoulder-width apart
- Clinician: kneeling or seated on a low stool in front of patient

Instructions
- Visualize the umbilicus.
- At the level of the umbilicus, place both hands around the patient's waist with the thumbs pointed anteriorly.
- Slide your hands inferiorly until a prominent bony ridge is felt.

Notes
- This palpation can also be performed with the patient lying supine, sitting, or prone on a table.
- The iliac crest is usually at the level of the L4 to L5 interspace.[5,6]

Anterior Superior Iliac Spine

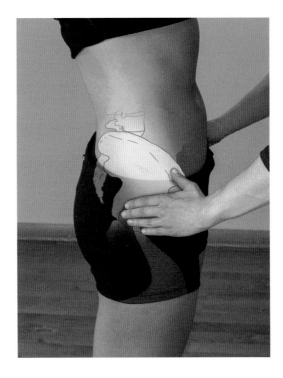

Positions
- Patient: standing, with feet shoulder-width apart
- Clinician: kneeling or seated on a low stool in front of the patient

Instructions
- Palpate the iliac crest with both hands.
- Slide your first digit inferiorly (and medially or laterally as needed) until a pointed bony prominence is felt.

Posterior Superior Iliac Spine

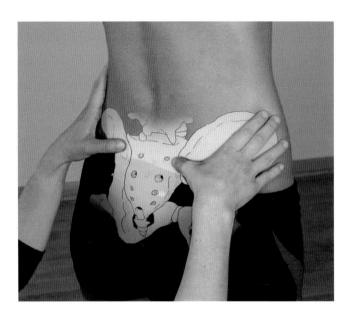

Positions

- Patient: standing, with feet shoulder-width apart
- Clinician: kneeling or seated on a low stool behind the patient

Instructions

- Palpate the posterior aspect of the iliac crests with both hands.
- Slide your first digit inferiorly and medially until a bony prominence is felt.

Note

The PSIS is at the level of S2.

Anterior Inferior Iliac Spine

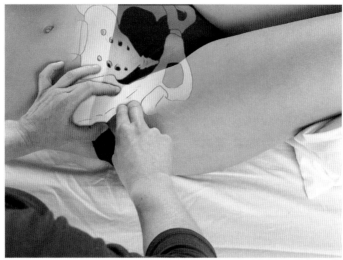

VIDEO 10.1 ▶

Positions

- Patient: supine, with hips and knees slightly flexed
- Clinician: standing, facing the patient, on the side being palpated

Instructions

- Palpate the ASIS.
- Move one or two fingers about 1 inch (2.5 centimeters) inferiorly (right hand pictured).
- Apply a firm, posteriorly directed force until a small bony prominence is felt. The anterior inferior iliac spine is not as distinct as the ASIS.

Pubic Tubercle

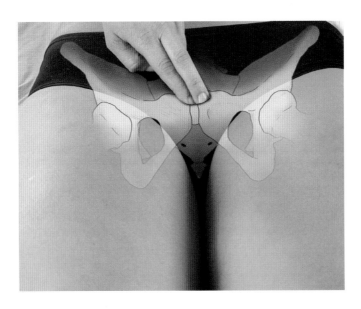

Positions
- Patient: supine, with hips and knees slightly flexed
- Clinician: standing, facing the patient, on the side being palpated

Instructions
- Visualize and palpate the umbilicus.
- Using the ulnar border of your hand, stay in midline and move inferiorly about 5 to 7 inches (13 to 18 centimeters) until you reach a bony prominence.
- Using the pads of digits 2 and 3, apply gentle but firm posterior pressure to the bony prominence.

Note
Because of its location, this palpation is very personal and may be uncomfortable for the patient. You should inform the patient about what you are doing and why it is necessary before beginning this palpation.

Pubic Ramus

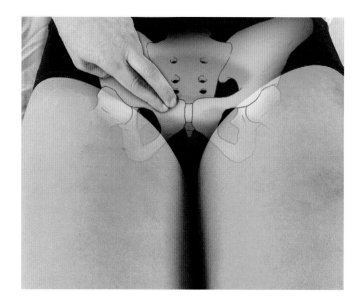

Positions
- Patient: supine, with hips and knees slightly flexed
- Clinician: standing, facing the patient, on the side being palpated

Instructions
- Palpate the pubic tubercle using two fingers.
- Follow the bony ridge laterally about one fingerwidth until a bony prominence is felt.

Note
Because of its location, this palpation is very personal and may be uncomfortable for the patient. You should inform the patient about what you are doing and why it is necessary before beginning this palpation.

Greater Trochanter

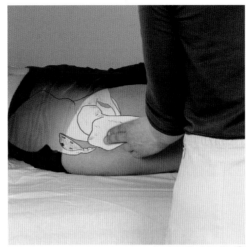

VIDEO 10.2 ▶

Positions

- Patient: supine
- Clinician: standing or sitting, facing the patient, on the side being palpated

Instructions

- Palpate the lateral aspect of the iliac crest.
- Move your second and third fingers inferiorly until a large, round, bony prominence is felt.
- To confirm palpation, have the patient internally and externally rotate the hip. You should feel the greater trochanter move under your fingers.

CLINICAL PEARL

Immediately posterior to the greater trochanter is the trochanteric bursa. Patients with greater trochanteric pain syndrome (GTPS) will have exquisite tenderness upon palpation.[7]

Ischial Tuberosity

Method 1

Positions

- Patient: side-lying, the hips and knees flexed to about 90°, with the side being palpated on top
- Clinician: standing posteriorly to the patient and slightly inferior to the patient's hips

Instructions

- Palpate the greater trochanter using two fingers.
- Slide your fingers posteriorly and inferiorly until a very large bony prominence is felt.

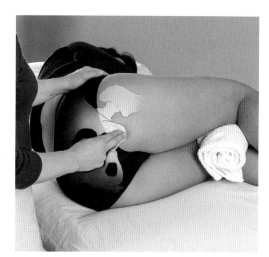

Method 2

Positions

- Patient: prone
- Clinician: standing to the side being palpated

Instructions

- Palpate the greater trochanter.
- Slide your fingers posteriorly and inferiorly until a very large bony prominence is felt.

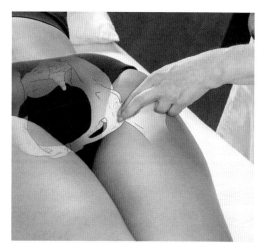

Muscles of the Hip and Thigh Regions

Muscle	Origin	Insertion	Innervation	Blood supply	Action
Tensor fasciae latae	Anterior superior iliac spine (ASIS) and anterior, lateral aspects of the external iliac crest	Iliotibial band (ITB), which inserts on Gerdy's tubercle (lateral condyle of the tibia)	Superior gluteal nerve (L4-L5)	Superior gluteal artery, lateral circumflex femoral artery	Hip flexion, abduction, and internal rotation
Sartorius	ASIS	Superior, medial aspect of the tibia (pes anserine)	Femoral nerve (L2-L4)	Femoral artery	Hip flexion, abduction, and external rotation
Rectus femoris	Anterior inferior iliac spine	Tibial tuberosity via patellar tendon	Femoral nerve (L2-L4)	Lateral circumflex femoral artery and deep femoral artery	Hip flexion and knee extension
Obturator externus	Obturator foramen and membrane	Trochanteric fossa of the femur	Obturator nerve (L2-L4)	Medial circumflex femoral artery and obturator artery	Hip external rotation, stabilization of the head of the femur in the acetabulum
Adductor longus	Body of pubis	Middle third of linea aspera of the femur	Obturator nerve (L2-L4)	Medial circumflex femoral artery and obturator artery	Hip adduction, flexion, or extension
Adductor brevis	Inferior pubic ramus	Pectineal line and proximal linea aspera of the femur	Obturator nerve (L2-L4)	Medial circumflex femoral artery and obturator artery	Hip adduction
Adductor magnus	Inferior pubic ramus and ischial tuberosity	Gluteal tuberosity, linea aspera, supracondylar line, and adductor tubercle	Obturator nerve (adductor part) (L2-L4) and sciatic nerve (hamstring part) (L4-S3)	Deep femoral artery, popliteal artery, and obturator artery	Hip adduction and extension
Pectineus	Pecten pubis	Pectineal line of femur	Femoral or obturator nerve (L2-L4)	Medial circumflex femoral artery and obturator artery	Hip adduction and flexion
Gracilis	Inferior pubic ramus	Superior, medial aspect of tibia (pes anserine)	Obturator nerve (L2-L4)	Deep femoral artery and medial circumflex femoral artery	Hip adduction and flexion and knee flexion
Gluteus maximus	Sacrum, sacrotuberous ligament, and posterior gluteal line of the ilium	ITB and gluteal tuberosity of the femur	Inferior gluteal nerve (L5-S1)	Superior and inferior gluteal arteries	Hip extension and external rotation

> continued

MUSCLES OF THE HIP AND THIGH REGIONS   > *continued*

Muscle	Origin	Insertion	Innervation	Blood supply	Action
Gluteus medius	Posterior aspect of the ilium between the anterior and posterior gluteal lines	Lateral aspect of the greater trochanter	Superior gluteal nerve (L4-S1)	Deep branch of the superior gluteal artery	Hip abduction and internal rotation
Gluteus minimus	Posterior aspect of the ilium between the anterior and inferior gluteal lines	Anterior aspect of the greater trochanter	Superior gluteal nerve (L4-S1)	Deep branch of the superior gluteal artery	Hip abduction and internal rotation
Piriformis	Anterior aspect of the sacrum	Superior aspect of the greater trochanter	Ventral rami (S1-S2)	Superior and inferior gluteal arteries and internal pudendal artery	Hip external rotation, abduction when hip is flexed
Superior gemellus	Ischial spine	Medial aspect of the greater trochanter	Nerve to obturator internus (L5-S1)	Inferior gluteal artery	Hip external rotation
Obturator internus	Obturator foramen and membrane	Medial aspect of the greater trochanter	Nerve to obturator internus (L5-S1)	Internal pudendal artery, superior gluteal artery	Hip external rotation
Inferior gemellus	Ischial tuberosity	Medial aspect of greater trochanter	Nerve to inferior gemellus (L5-S1)	Inferior gluteal artery	Hip external rotation
Quadratus femoris	Ischial tuberosity	Quadrate tubercle of the femur (medial trochanter)	Nerve to the inferior gemellus (L5-S1)	Medial circumflex femoral artery	Hip external rotation
Semiten-dinosus	Ischial tuberosity	Superior, medial aspect of the tibia (pes anserine)	Tibial division of the sciatic nerve (L4-S2)	Deep artery of the thigh, branch of the popliteal artery	Hip extension, knee flexion, and tibial internal rotation
Semimem-branosus	Ischial tuberosity	Posterior, medial condyle of tibia	Tibial division of sciatic nerve (L4-S2)	Deep artery of the thigh, branch of the popliteal artery	Hip extension, knee flexion, and tibial internal rotation
Biceps femoris	*Long head:* ischial tuberosity *Short head:* lateral lip of linea aspera, lateral supracondylar line of femur	Fibular head	*Long head:* tibial division of sciatic nerve (L4-S2) *Short head:* common fibular division of the sciatic nerve (L4-S2)	Deep artery of the thigh, branch of the popliteal artery	Hip extension *(long head only)*, knee flexion, and tibial external rotation

Zone I: Femoral Triangle

Inguinal Ligament

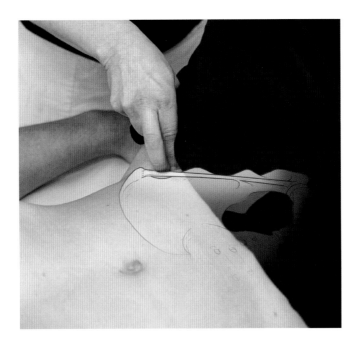

Positions
- Patient: supine with the heel of the lower extremity resting on the opposite thigh or leg in a position of slight flexion, abduction, and external rotation (FABER position)
- Clinician: standing facing the patient, on the side being palpated and with the patient's thigh resting on the clinician's thigh

Instructions
- Palpate the ASIS.
- Palpate the pubic tubercle.
- Move two fingers from the ASIS to the pubic tubercle, palpating the length of the inguinal ligament. You should feel a flat, band-like structure under your fingers.

Note
Remember that the inguinal ligament is the lower border of the external abdominal oblique muscle.

CLINICAL PEARL
During palpation, a bulge or bump may indicate an inguinal hernia. If you palpate abnormalities, refer the patient to a physician.

Femoral Artery

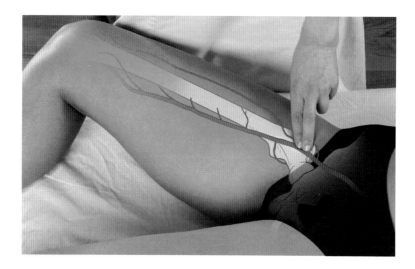

Positions

- Patient: supine, with the hip in a position of slight flexion, abduction, and external rotation (FABER position)
- Clinician: standing, facing the patient, on the side being palpated and the patient's thigh resting on the clinician's thigh or the table

Instructions

- Palpate the ASIS.
- Palpate the pubic tubercle.
- Place the pads of your second and third digits about halfway between these two structures and apply light pressure below the inguinal ligament.
- You should feel the femoral pulse under your fingers.

Note

The femoral vein and nerve are normally not palpable in the femoral triangle.

CLINICAL PEARL

Normally, the femoral pulse is very strong and easily palpated. If there is occlusion of the common iliac or external iliac arteries, the pulse may be diminished.

Sartorius

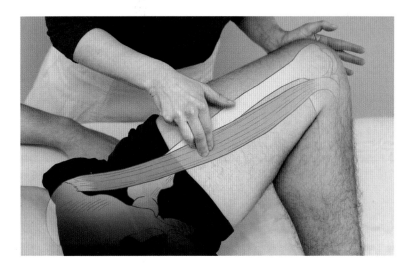

Positions

- Patient: supine, with the hip in the FABER position
- Clinician: standing, facing the patient, on the side being palpated and the patient's thigh resting on the table

Instructions

- Palpate the ASIS.
- Move your fingers just inferiorly and medially to palpate the origin of the sartorius (not shown) and continue into the medial aspect of the thigh.
- To confirm palpation, have the patient perform resisted hip flexion, abduction, and external rotation (left hand pictured). You should feel a long, slender muscle contract under your fingers (right hand pictured).

CLINICAL PEARL

In some patients there may be exquisite tenderness in the vicinity of the ASIS when the sartorius contracts. It is possible that these patients have an avulsion fracture of the ASIS. These injuries are called apophyseal injuries and are more common in adolescents than in other age groups.[8,9]

Adductor Longus

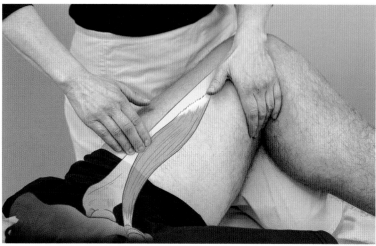

VIDEO 10.3 ▶

Positions

- Patient: supine, with the hip in the FABER position
- Clinician: standing, facing the patient, on the side being palpated and the patient's thigh resting on the clinician's thigh

Instructions

- Using two or three fingers, palpate the inferior pubic ramus.
- Move your fingers inferiorly to palpate the adductor longus.
- Follow the fibers of the adductor longus to its insertion on the linea aspera.
- To confirm palpation, have the patient perform resisted hip adduction (left hand pictured). You should feel a firm muscle contraction under your fingers (right hand pictured).

Notes

- The adductor brevis is located deep under the adductor longus and pectineus muscles. However, the depth of the adductor brevis makes it virtually impossible to isolate.
- After palpating the adductor longus, the clinician should move the fingers medially to assess for the inguinal lymph nodes. These are normally not palpable, and enlargement of these nodes could be a sign of infection or pathology and should be brought to the attention of a physician.

Zone II: Greater Trochanter

Trochanteric Bursa

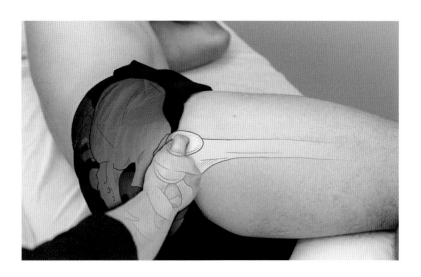

Positions
- Patient: side-lying with the affected lower extremity on top and both knees bent with a pillow between them
- Clinician: standing, facing the patient, on the side being palpated

Instructions
- Palpate the greater trochanter using two fingers.
- Palpate the soft tissues around the greater trochanter for tenderness.
- The bursa itself is not palpable, but tenderness to palpation can indicate trochanteric bursitis, now more often referred to as GTPS.[7]

Gluteus Medius

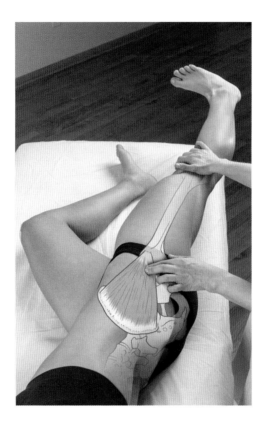

Positions

- Patient: side-lying, with the side being palpated on top, bottom leg bent approximately 90°, and the top leg straight
- Clinician: standing posterior to the patient

Instructions

- Using two fingers, palpate the posterior–lateral aspect of the iliac crest.
- Move your fingers just inferior to the iliac crest.
- To confirm palpation, have the patient perform resisted hip abduction (right hand pictured). You should feel the superior aspect of the gluteus medius contract under your fingers (left hand pictured).

CLINICAL PEARL

The gluteus medius is responsible for controlling the pelvis during the stance phase of gait. The right gluteus medius contracts to prevent the left pelvis from dropping during the right stance phase. If the left pelvis drops, the gait is called a right Trendelenburg gait.[1]

Zone III: Sciatic Nerve

Sciatic Nerve

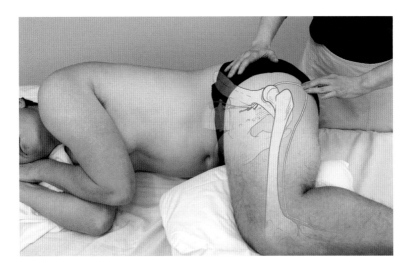

Positions
- Patient: side-lying, with the side being palpated on top and the hips flexed with a pillow between the legs
- Clinician: standing or sitting, facing the patient, on the side being palpated

Instructions
- Palpate the greater trochanter.
- Palpate the ischial tuberosity.
- Using two or three fingers, palpate the sciatic nerve halfway between the greater trochanter and ischial tuberosity by pressing firmly into the tissue (left hand pictured).

Notes
- With the hip in extension, the gluteus maximus covers the sciatic nerve, making it impossible to palpate with accuracy.
- When palpating the ischial tuberosity, remember there is a bursa overlying it.

CLINICAL PEARL
A herniated disc, muscle spasm in the piriformis muscle, or trauma to the nerve itself (e.g., a fall or poorly placed injection) may cause inflammation of the sciatic nerve. Tenderness to the bursa overlying the ischial tuberosity can be indicative of ischial bursitis. However, this is an uncommon diagnosis.

Zone IV: Hip and Pelvic Muscles

Anterior Quadrant: Flexors

Note: The sartorius was covered in the femoral triangle zone.

Tensor Fasciae Latae

Positions

- Patient: supine
- Clinician: standing, facing the patient, on the side being palpated

Instructions

- Palpate the ASIS using one or two fingers.
- Move your fingers just inferiorly and laterally.
- To confirm palpation, have the patient perform resisted hip abduction (right hand pictured). You should feel the tendon contract under your fingers (left hand pictured).

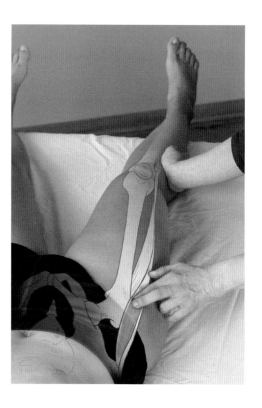

Notes

- The tensor fasciae latae inserts on the iliotibial band (ITB), which inserts on the lateral condyle of the tibia (Gerdy's tubercle).
- In some instances, fibers of the ITB insert on the lateral aspect of the patella.[2]

Rectus Femoris

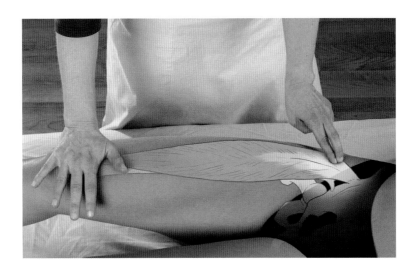

Positions

- Patient: supine
- Clinician: standing, facing the patient, on the side being palpated

Instructions

- Palpate the ASIS.
- Move one or two fingers inferiorly about 1 inch (2.5 centimeters) onto the AIIS.
- To confirm palpation, have the patient perform resisted hip flexion (right hand pictured). You should feel the tendon contract under your fingers.

CLINICAL PEARL

In some patients, there may be exquisite tenderness in the vicinity of the AIIS when the rectus femoris contracts. It is possible that these patients have an avulsion fracture of the AIIS. These injuries are called apophyseal injuries and are more common in adolescents.[8-10]

Medial Quadrant: Adductors

Note: The adductor longus was covered in the femoral triangle zone.

Adductor Magnus

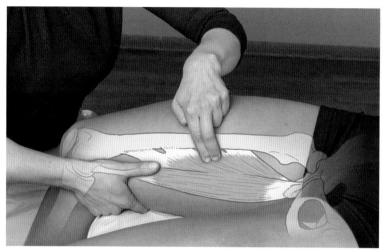

VIDEO 10.4 ▶

Positions

- Patient: supine at the end of the table, with the knees hanging off the table
- Clinician: sitting, facing the patient, on the side being palpated

Instructions

- Using two or three fingers, palpate the inferior pubic ramus.
- Move inferiorly to palpate the adductor longus.
- Move your fingers inferiorly and posteriorly to palpate the adductor magnus.
- Follow the fibers of the adductor magnus to its insertion on the adductor tubercle.
- To confirm palpation, have the patient perform resisted hip adduction and extension (right hand pictured). You should feel a large contraction under your fingers (left hand pictured).

Note

While the adductor magnus performs adduction, the majority of its fibers run posterior to the axis of rotation of the hip, and therefore it also performs hip extension. Isolation of this muscle requires minor adjustments in position and direction of applied resistance.

Pectineus

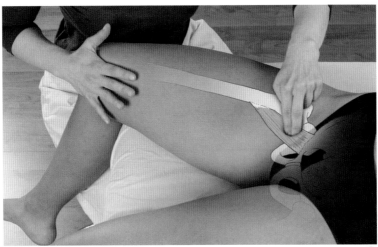

VIDEO 10.4 ▶

Positions

- Patient: supine at the end of the table, with the knees hanging off the table
- Clinician: sitting, facing the patient, on the side being palpated

Instructions

- Using two or three fingers, palpate the inferior pubic ramus.
- Move your fingers inferiorly and palpate the adductor longus.
- Move your fingers anteriorly and laterally to palpate the pectineus.
- To confirm palpation, have the patient perform resisted hip flexion and adduction (right hand pictured). You should feel a small contraction under your fingers (left hand pictured).

Gracilis

Positions

- Patient: supine at the end of the table, with the knees hanging off the table
- Clinician: sitting, facing the patient, on the side being palpated

Instructions

- Using two or three fingers, palpate the inferior pubic ramus.
- Move inferiorly to palpate the adductor longus.
- Move your fingers inferiorly and posterior–medially to palpate the gracilis. You may use three or four fingers to palpate along the belly of the muscle.
- Follow the fibers of the gracilis to the insertion on the superior, medial tibia.
- To confirm palpation, have the patient perform resisted knee flexion (right hand pictured). You should feel a small, subtle contraction under your fingers (left hand pictured).

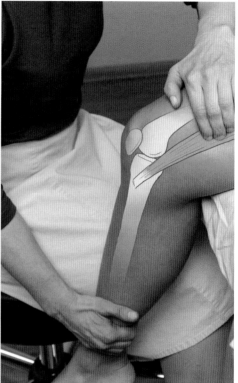

VIDEO 10.4 ▶

Note

Because the gracilis is the only adductor to cross the knee, it can be isolated from the other adductors by having the patient perform knee flexion.

CLINICAL PEARL

These muscles are commonly involved in individuals who engage in sports such as soccer, hockey, and running and have the propensity for developing tendinopathy (groin strains).[9,10] These muscles are also commonly involved in patients with low back pain or SIJ dysfunction (or both) and may contain trigger points and tender areas.

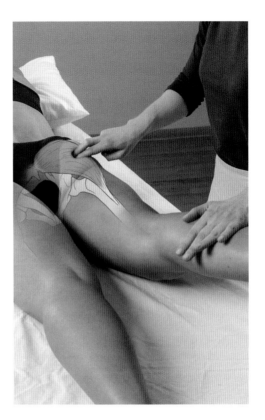
Posterior Quadrant: Extensors

Gluteus Maximus

Positions

- Patient: prone
- Clinician: standing, facing the patient, on the side being palpated

Instructions

- Palpate the posterior aspect of the gluteal region using two or three fingers.
- To confirm palpation, have the patient perform resisted hip extension (left hand pictured). You should feel a large contraction under your fingers (right hand pictured).
- To better isolate the gluteus maximus from the hamstrings, you may choose to flex the knee during this palpation.

CLINICAL PEARL

It is common to find trigger points and tender areas throughout this muscle in patients with low back pain or SIJ dysfunction. Because of its large surface area, you may need to palpate multiple areas of this muscle.

Piriformis

The piriformis is located in the center of a triangle that runs from the sacroiliac joint, greater trochanter, and ischial tuberosity. This muscle is palpated in chapter 9 as part of the pelvic region. It also functions with the global hip muscles and is therefore included here as well.

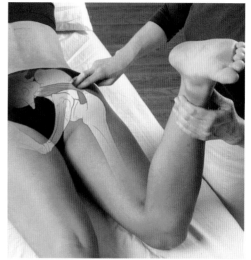

VIDEO 10.5 ◉

Positions

- Patient: prone
- Clinician: standing, facing the patient, on the side being palpated

Instructions

- Palpate the greater trochanter.
- Move your fingers posteriorly to the middle of the gluteal region.
- Using two or three fingers, palpate deep, through the gluteus maximus.
- Flex the knee to 90°.
- To confirm palpation, have the patient perform resisted hip external rotation (left hand pictured). You should feel a subtle contraction under your fingers (right hand pictured).

Note

During contraction of this muscle, it is important to tell the patient to increase the force gradually. If a large external rotational force is produced all at once, the gluteus maximus will contract, obstructing palpation of the piriformis.

CLINICAL PEARL

Because of the way its fibers run, the piriformis has multiple actions based on hip position. When the hip is in extension, it is an external rotator. At approximately 70° of hip flexion, it becomes a hip abductor. At greater than 90° of hip flexion, it is an internal rotator.[1]

Hamstrings

The origin tendon is discussed in this chapter, and individual muscles are discussed in chapter 11 because they take their insertions at the knee on the proximal tibia and fibula.

- Semitendinosus
- Semimembranosus
- Biceps femoris

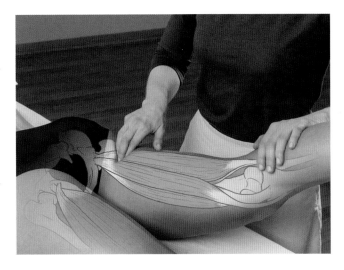

Positions

- Patient: prone
- Clinician: standing, facing the patient, on the side being palpated

Instructions

- Using three fingers, palpate the ischial tuberosity.
- Move your fingers immediately inferior to the ischial tuberosity.
- To confirm palpation, have the patient perform resisted hip extension (left hand pictured). You should feel a broad tendon contract under your fingers (right hand pictured).

CLINICAL PEARLS

Hamstring strains are a common injury, usually in people involved in sports. Often they are located proximally or in the middle of the muscle belly. These injuries can be quite debilitating and often take a while to heal. This is especially true of those located closer to the origin because of the relatively poor blood supply to the tendons.[11,12]

In some patients, there may be exquisite tenderness in the vicinity of the ischial tuberosity when the hamstrings contract. It is possible that these patients have an avulsion fracture of the ischial tuberosity. These injuries are called apophyseal injuries and are more common in adolescents than in other age groups.[8,9,11,13]

Case Study

History

A 45-year-old male presents to your clinic complaining of right hip pain. The pain began the previous month when he was playing soccer after he was leg tackled by an opponent. The patient has noticed an increase in pain over the last 2 weeks, mostly in his groin. He reports stiffness early in the morning and after being in one position for an extended period of time. He used ice to help with the pain, which did decrease it for a brief period, and reports feeling less pain after a long hot shower. The patient is single and lives in a third-floor walk-up apartment. He is the vice president of a bank, which requires sitting for many hours of the day. He plays in a soccer league on the weekends.

- Based on the subjective information only, what are the three most likely diagnoses?

Examination

Past medical history	Unremarkable
Medication	Aleve
Observation	Decreased right stance time during gait External rotation of the right lower extremity
Active range of motion	Right hip flexion = 0° to 98°, abduction = 0° to 40°, internal rotation = 0° to 15°, external rotation = 0° to 45°
Passive range of motion	Same as for active, with pain at end range of flexion and internal rotation
Manual muscle testing	Within normal limits, except right hip flexion = 4–/5 (secondary to pain), internal rotation = 3+/5 (secondary to pain)
Special tests	Positive FABER test Positive scour test Negative sacral thrust test Negative sacroiliac distraction test Negative sacroiliac compression test Negative Gaenslen's test Negative active straight-leg raise test
Other	Capsular pattern of right hip Decreased pain with long axis distraction of the right lower extremity

- Based on the subjective and objective information together, what are the two most likely diagnoses? Give your rationale for eliminating the third diagnosis.

- What structures should you palpate on this patient based on your differential diagnoses?
- Given all the information presented, what would you expect to find upon palpation of those structures?

Case Solution and Discussion

Potential Diagnoses Based on History
- Labral tear
- Onset of post-traumatic osteoarthritis
- Rectus femoris strain

Potential Diagnoses Based on History and Examination
- Onset of post-traumatic osteoarthritis
- Rectus femoris strain

Labral tear: The capsular pattern limitation of hip range of motion, along with the lack of report of clicking in the hip, allows this diagnosis to be eliminated.

Structures to Be Palpated
- Rectus femoris
- Adductor muscles (all)
- ASIS
- Psoas

Palpation Findings
- Tenderness to palpation of the rectus femoris, psoas, and all adductor muscles

Clinical Reasoning
- Onset of post-traumatic osteoarthritis: The subjective reports of stiffness in the morning and after prolonged sitting, alleviation of symptoms with heat, a positive scour test, and capsular pattern to hip motion limitations all indicate early onset of hip osteoarthritis. Sometimes arthritis is asymptomatic and remains undetected until a traumatic event occurs, with the inflammation from the event exacerbating and catalyzing the arthritic condition.
- Rectus femoris strain: The mechanism of injury, weakness and tenderness to palpation of the hip musculature, and positive FABER test are all consistent with a rectus femoris strain. However, the positive scour test and capsular pattern to the limitations of the range of motion of the hip are not consistent with this diagnosis and allow it to be ruled out.

Case Study Questions

1. What information do the palpation findings of the case give the clinician? How can this information be incorporated in the clinical decision-making process?

2. Think about how the examination findings (subjective and objective) lead to the differential diagnosis. What might you do differently?

3. Think about the long-term outcome for this patient. Is surgical intervention necessary?

CHAPTER REVIEW QUESTIONS

1. List the four spines that are found on the ilium.
2. Name the borders of the femoral triangle.
3. What structures are found in the femoral triangle?
4. List all the muscles that insert on the greater trochanter.
5. At what vertebral level can the iliac crest usually be palpated?
6. Name the branches that the abdominal aorta descends into.

chapter 11

Knee and Thigh

After completing this chapter, the reader will be able to do the following:

- Identify the key bony anatomical structures of the knee and thigh.
- Identify and describe the soft tissue anatomy of the knee and thigh, including muscles, ligaments, nerves, arteries, and veins.
- Identify the borders of the popliteal fossa and the structures located within it.
- Identify on bony or skeletal models the origins and insertions of the muscles of the knee and thigh to aid in understanding osteokinematic action and surface palpation.
- Palpate structures of the knee and thigh.
- Integrate surface palpation findings to aid in the differential diagnosis of a patient with knee pain.

The knee joint is an extremely important link in the lower kinetic chain. This joint is between the two longest bones in the body (femur and tibia), thus producing large compressive and shear forces across the joint during functional activities.[1] The knee joint is classified as a condyloid joint, which permits motion in two planes (sagittal and transverse), with the majority of motion occurring in the sagittal plane. Normal motion at this joint is necessary for tasks such as walking, running, and stair negotiation. The joint is stabilized by several ligaments that provide passive stability and muscles that provide active stability.[1]

Functions of the Knee Joint

The main function of the knee joint is flexion and extension. These osteokinematic motions provide the movement necessary for people to negotiate stairs and sit comfortably and to walk, run, and squat. The knee joint is subjected to large stresses during these activities and may, at times, become a source of pain and disability for many patients.[2] Swelling, stiffness, or weakness in or around the knee joint can have detrimental effects on the motion available, thus making activities of daily living challenging.

Bony Anatomy

Distally, the femur fans out in much the same way as the humerus, giving rise to the medial and lateral epicondyles (figure 11.1). On the medial epicondyle is a bony landmark called the adductor tubercle. Distal to the epicondyles are the articulating surfaces of the femur: the medial and lateral condyles. The condyles are convex and articulate with the proximal tibial plateaus, which are concave, to form the tibiofemoral joint. Between the medial and lateral condyles on the posterior aspect is the intercondylar notch, which is the space where the anterior cruciate ligament (ACL) and posterior cruciate ligament (PCL) are found.[3]

On the distal anterior aspect of the femur is the trochlear groove (figure 11.1). This depression is where the patella articulates, forming the patellofemoral joint

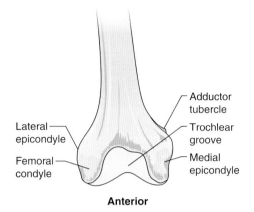

Anterior

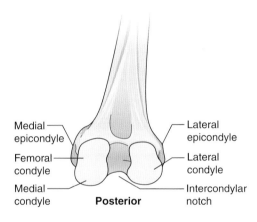

Posterior

FIGURE 11.1 Distal portion of the femur.

(PFJ). Although this joint does not provide gross motion to the knee, it is extremely important for proper knee mechanics. The patella is not a stationary bone, but rather the largest sesamoid bone in the body, and it functions to increase the mechanical advantage of the quadriceps.[1,3] The patella has three facets: a lateral facet, a medial facet, and an odd facet (figure 11.2). The odd facet is most medial and only articulates with the femur in extreme positions of knee flexion. During knee motion, the patella moves, changing its position in relation to the femur, which affects the patellofemoral contact interface. The patella moves inferiorly during knee flexion and superiorly during knee extension. In addition, the patella has the ability to tilt and rotate.[1,3]

The tibia is a long bone that helps form both the tibiofemoral and the talocrural joints. In addition to the tibial plateaus, the proximal tibia has both a medial and lateral condyle. The lateral condyle of the tibia (Gerdy's tubercle) is where the iliotibial band (ITB) inserts. Inferior to the tibial condyles, on the anterior aspect of the bone, is the tibial tuberosity (figure 11.3). This is an important landmark because it is the insertion of the

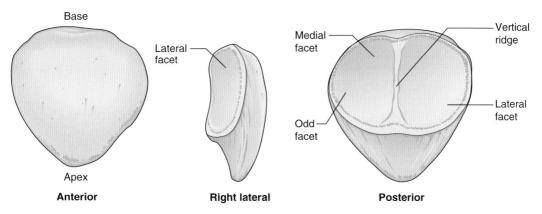

FIGURE 11.2 Aspects of the patella.

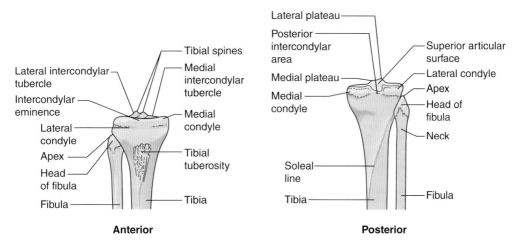

FIGURE 11.3 Proximal portion of the tibia, including tibial plateaus.

patellar tendon. On the posterior portion of the medial aspect of the tibia is the pes anserine, which is formed by three tendons: sartorius, gracilis, and semitendinosus.[1,3]

Soft Tissue Anatomy

Several muscles originate on the thigh and cross the knee joint to insert on the tibia. The large quadriceps femoris muscle is on the anterior thigh and is composed of four muscles:

- Rectus femoris
- Vastus medialis
- Vastus lateralis
- Vastus intermedius

Collectively, these muscles perform knee extension, and the rectus femoris also flexes the hip. During active quadriceps contraction, you should
be able to visualize the patella gliding superiorly (figure 11.4, anterior).[3]

On the posterior aspect of the thigh are the hamstrings. This muscle
group consists of three muscles (figure 11.4, posterior):

- Semitendinosus
- Semimembranosus
- Biceps femoris

The biceps femoris has a short head and a long head. Collectively, these
three muscles perform knee flexion, and as previously mentioned all of
them except the short head of the biceps femoris extend the hip. In addition, the hamstring muscles, with their tibial attachments, have a role
in the transverse plane motion at the knee. When the knee is flexed, the
tibia has the ability to internally and externally rotate. The medial hamstring muscles (semitendinosus and semimembranosus) internally rotate
the tibia, while the lateral hamstring muscle (biceps femoris) externally
rotates the tibia.[3]

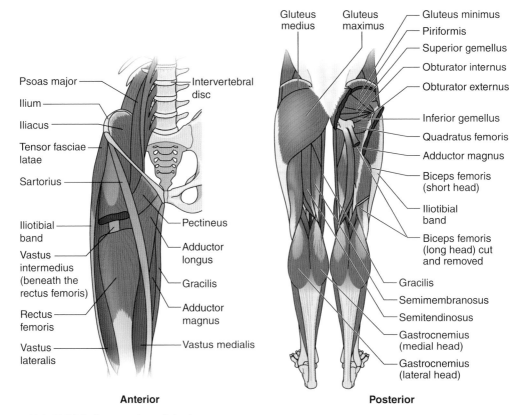

Anterior

Psoas major
Ilium
Iliacus
Tensor fasciae latae
Sartorius
Iliotibial band
Vastus intermedius (beneath the rectus femoris)
Rectus femoris
Vastus lateralis
Intervertebral disc
Pectineus
Adductor longus
Gracilis
Adductor magnus
Vastus medialis

Posterior

Gluteus medius
Gluteus maximus
Gluteus minimus
Piriformis
Superior gemellus
Obturator internus
Obturator externus
Inferior gemellus
Quadratus femoris
Adductor magnus
Biceps femoris (short head)
Iliotibial band
Biceps femoris (long head) cut and removed
Gracilis
Semimembranosus
Semitendinosus
Gastrocnemius (medial head)
Gastrocnemius (lateral head)

FIGURE 11.4 Muscles of the knee.

On the superior medial aspect of the tibia is the pes anserine.

- The sartorius, gracilis, and semitendinosus all insert here. The sartorius is the most anterior, and the semitendinosus is the most posterior.
- Deep to these three tendons is the pes anserine bursa.[3]

Apart from the bony and muscle stability around the knee joint, four major ligaments increase stability of the joint.

- Two of these ligaments, the anterior and posterior cruciate ligaments, provide anterior and posterior stability to the knee, respectively. These ligaments are intra-articular and therefore cannot be palpated.[1,3]
- The medial collateral ligament (MCL) and lateral collateral ligament (LCL) are located on the medial and lateral aspect of the joint, respectively (figure 11.5). These ligaments are extra-articular and can be palpated as part of the clinical examination. They provide medial and lateral stability to the knee joint during dynamic movements.[1,3]

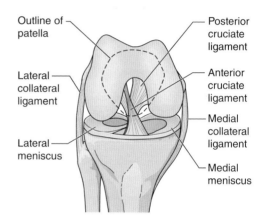

FIGURE 11.5 Ligaments of the tibiofemoral joint.

Between the femoral condyles and tibial plateaus are the menisci. The primary function of the menisci is to reduce the compressive forces between the femoral condyles and tibial plateaus.

- The medial meniscus is C-shaped, and both the MCL and semimembranosus muscle attach to it.
- The lateral meniscus is circular, and the popliteus muscle attaches to it.
- Most of the area of the menisci is avascular, mostly devoid of blood supply, and aneural, mostly devoid of nerve innervation. An exception is the outer portions (lateral one-third) of the menisci, which receive blood supply and therefore have the ability to heal on their own, especially in younger people.[1,3,4]

The popliteus muscle is extremely important for proper knee biomechanics. Because of the differences in the length of the medial and lateral femoral condyles, the tibia externally rotates during the last 10° of knee extension in order to achieve terminal (full) knee extension; this is called the *screw-home mechanism*. The popliteus is responsible for unlocking the screw-home mechanism, allowing knee flexion to occur.[1,3]

Neurovascular Anatomy

The popliteal fossa is a triangular-shaped depression on the posterior aspect of the knee. The superior borders are formed by the hamstring tendons (semitendinosus and semimembranosus medially, biceps femoris laterally), while the inferior medial and lateral borders are formed by the heads of the gastrocnemius. Deep in the popliteal fossa are the popliteal artery and vein and the tibial nerve. The popliteus muscle runs deep to these vessels. The popliteal artery is the direct continuation of the femoral artery after it exits the hiatus in the adductor magnus muscle. This artery can be palpated in the center of the popliteal fossa.[3] It travels through the hiatus of the soleus muscle before dividing into the anterior and posterior tibial arteries (figure 11.6).

Several nerves travel along the anterior and posterior aspects of the thigh (figure 11.7).[3]

- The anterior femoral cutaneous nerve travels down the anterior aspect of the thigh providing sensation to this region.

- The lateral femoral cutaneous nerve travels down the lateral aspect of the thigh providing sensation to this region.

- The saphenous nerve, which is the largest cutaneous branch of the femoral nerve, innervates the skin inferior to the patella as well as the anterior and medial aspects of the lower leg.

- The posterior femoral cutaneous nerve travels down the posterior aspect of the thigh providing sensation to this region.

Structural Inspection

- The clinician should begin by assessing the patient walking into the room, paying particular attention to the motion occurring at the knee. This should include terminal knee extension at heel strike (initial contact) and knee flexion during the swing phase of gait.

- The clinician should then assess the static position of both knees, observing for genu varum, valgum, or recurvatum.

- The clinician may now ask the patient to perform a squat while in the standing position, which will provide valuable information on the entire lower kinetic chain. Observe for asymmetrical weight-bearing, lack of closed chain dorsiflexion, and nonverbal signs that suggest increased pain.

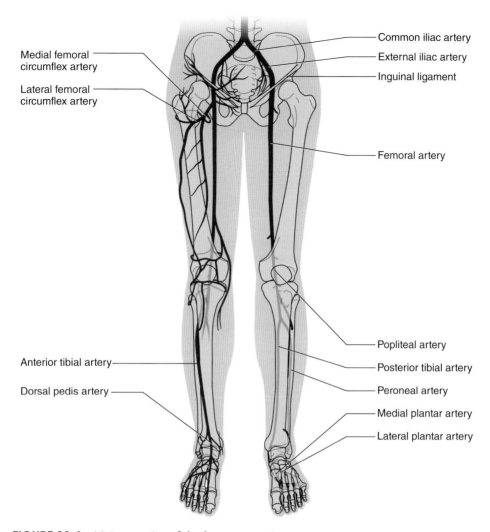

FIGURE 11.6 Major arteries of the lower extremity.

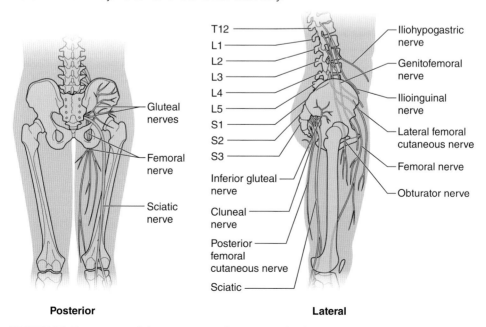

Posterior

Lateral

FIGURE 11.7 Nerves of the anterior and posterior thigh.

363

- The clinician should next assess for scars or discoloration (ecchymosis), which can be indicative of recent trauma or surgery.
- Swelling can be assessed next using the stroke test by having the patient lie supine on the examining table.[5] In the presence of a total knee replacement, where the capsule has been mostly removed, circumferential measurements can be taken as an alternative method. This can also be used to measure swelling in other pathologies.
- The clinician should also assess the muscle girth of both quadriceps, looking for signs of atrophy.

Patella

Positions

- Patient: sitting at the edge of the table, with the knees bent to 90°
- Clinician: sitting, facing the patient, on the side being palpated

Instructions

- Palpate along the anterior aspect of the distal thigh using two fingers.
- A broad bony edge (superior pole of the patella) will be felt first (right hand pictured).
- Continue to move your fingers inferiorly, palpating the body of the patella.
- The inferior pole is a narrow bony edge (left hand pictured).
- With the knee in flexion, attempt to palpate the medial

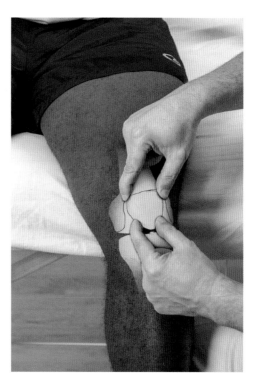

and lateral undersurface of the patella as well as the trochlear groove just above the patella in midline. Alternatively, the clinician can place the knee in terminal knee extension, with the patient in the supine position, and assess the medial and lateral aspects of the undersurface of the patella by gently pressing down on the medial or lateral side (tilting the patella) and subsequently palpating the side that is raised.

CLINICAL PEARL

When palpating the patella, it is important to assess for tenderness, swelling, or both around the entire patella.[5,6] In addition to palpating the bony landmarks, you should also assess patellar mobility by moving the patella in all directions, with the knee extended and the quadriceps relaxed, assessing for pain, hypomobility, or both.[6]

Medial Femoral Condyle

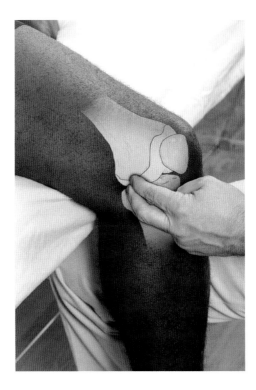

Positions

- Patient: sitting at the edge of the table, with knees bent to 90°
- Clinician: sitting, facing the patient, on the side being palpated

Instructions

- Palpate the superior pole of the patella.
- Move two fingers medially until a large bony prominence is felt on the distal, medial aspect of the femur.
- Follow the medial femoral condyle distally down to the articulation with the tibia, which provides a complete assessment of the medial femoral condyle.

Lateral Femoral Condyle

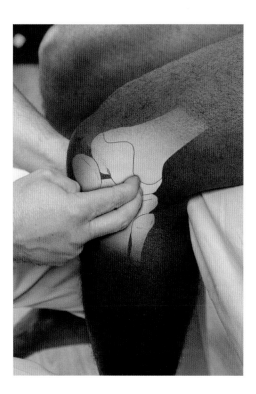

Positions
- Patient: sitting at the edge of the table, with knees bent to 90°
- Clinician: sitting, facing the patient, on the side being palpated

Instructions
- Palpate the superior pole of the patella.
- Move two fingers laterally until a large bony prominence is felt on the distal, lateral aspect of the femur.
- Follow the lateral femoral condyle distally down to the articulation with the tibia, which provides a complete assessment of the lateral femoral condyle.

Note
Because most of the lateral femoral condyle is covered by the patella, it is extremely important to flex the knee at least 90° to expose as much of it as possible.

Medial Tibial Condyle

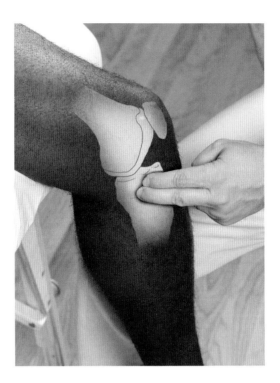

Positions

- Patient: sitting at the edge of the table, with knees bent to 90°
- Clinician: sitting, facing the patient, on the side being palpated

Instructions

- Palpate the medial femoral condyle.
- Move two fingers slightly inferiorly to palpate the joint space between the femur and tibia.
- Continue to move inferiorly until a large bony prominence is felt on the proximal, medial aspect of the tibia.

Lateral Tibial Condyle

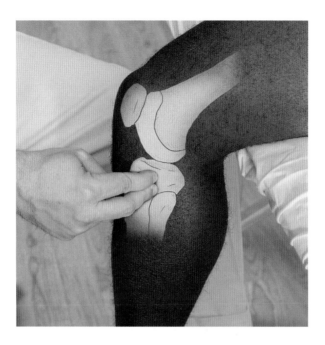

Positions
- Patient: sitting at the edge of the table, with knees bent to 90°
- Clinician: sitting, facing the patient, on the side being palpated

Instructions
- Palpate the lateral femoral condyle.
- Move two fingers slightly inferiorly to palpate the joint space between the femur and tibia.
- Continue to move inferiorly until a large bony prominence is felt on the proximal, lateral aspect of the tibia.

Tibial Tuberosity

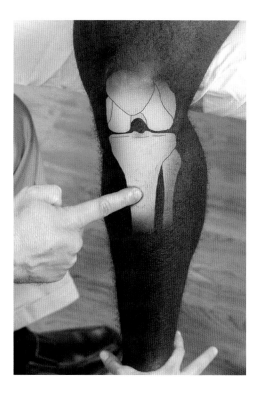

Positions

- Patient: sitting at the edge of the table, with knees bent to 90°
- Clinician: sitting, facing the patient, on the side being palpated

Instructions

- Using your second digit, palpate the inferior pole of the patella.
- Move your finger inferiorly, approximately 1 inch (2.5 centimeters).
- A sharp bony prominence will be felt.

CLINICAL PEARL

The quadriceps femoris, via the patellar tendon, inserts on the tibial tuberosity. Tenderness in this area along the patellar tendon may be a sign of patellar tendinopathy.[7,8] On the other hand, pain at the tibial tuberosity and associated enlargement and inflammation can be indicative of Osgood-Schlatter disease.[9]

Adductor Tubercle

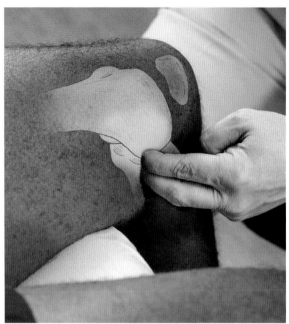

VIDEO 11.1 ▶

Positions

- Patient: sitting at the edge of the table, with knees bent to 90°
- Clinician: sitting, facing the patient, on the side being palpated

Instructions

- Palpate the medial femoral condyle.
- Move two fingers superiorly and posteriorly approximately 1 inch (2.5 centimeters) onto the medial epicondyle.
- A small bony protuberance should be felt on the superior, posterior aspect of the medial epicondyle.

CLINICAL PEARL

The adductor magnus inserts on the adductor tubercle of the femur. Tenderness in this region is common in patients with patellofemoral pain syndrome.[10]

Muscles of the Knee and Thigh Regions

Muscle	Origin	Insertion	Innervation	Blood supply	Action
Rectus femoris	Anterior inferior iliac spine	Tibial tuberosity via patellar tendon	Femoral nerve (L2-L4)	Lateral circumflex femoral artery and deep femoral artery	Knee extension and hip flexion
Vastus lateralis	Greater trochanter and lateral lip of the linea aspera	Tibial tuberosity via patellar tendon	Femoral nerve (L2-L4)	Lateral circumflex femoral artery and profunda femoral artery	Knee extension
Vastus medialis	Intertrochanteric line and the medial lip of linea aspera	Tibial tuberosity via patellar tendon	Femoral nerve (L2-L4)	Femoral and profunda femoral arteries	Knee extension
Vastus intermedius	Anterior and lateral surfaces of the body of the femur	Tibial tuberosity via patellar tendon	Femoral nerve (L2-L4)	Lateral circumflex femoral artery and profunda femoral artery	Knee extension
Sartorius	Anterior superior iliac spine	Superior medial aspect of the tibia (pes anserine)	Femoral nerve (L2-L4)	Femoral artery	Hip flexion, abduction, and external rotation; knee flexion
Gracilis	Inferior pubic ramus	Superior medial aspect of the tibia (pes anserine)	Obturator nerve (L2-L4)	Deep femoral artery and medial circumflex femoral artery	Hip adduction and flexion; knee flexion
Semitendinosus	Ischial tuberosity	Superior medial aspect of the tibia (pes anserine)	Tibial divisions of the sciatic nerve (L4-S2)	Deep artery of the thigh and branch of the popliteal artery	Hip extension, knee flexion, and tibial internal rotation
Semimembranosus	Ischial tuberosity	Posterior medial condyle of the tibia	Tibial division of the sciatic nerve (L4-S2)	Deep artery of the thigh and branch of popliteal artery	Hip extension, knee flexion, and tibial internal rotation
Biceps femoris	*Long head:* ischial tuberosity *Short head:* lateral lip of the linea aspera and the supracondylar line of the femur	Fibular head	*Long head:* tibial division of sciatic nerve (L4-S2) *Short head:* common fibular division of sciatic nerve (L4-S2)	Deep artery of the thigh and branch of the popliteal artery	Hip extension *(long head only)*, knee flexion, and tibial external rotation

Muscle	Origin	Insertion	Innervation	Blood supply	Action
Tensor fasciae latae	Anterior superior iliac spine and anterior, lateral aspects of the external iliac crest	Iliotibial band, which inserts into Gerdy's tubercle (lateral tibial condyle)	Superior gluteal nerve (L4-L5)	Superior gluteal artery and lateral circumflex femoral artery	Hip flexion, internal rotation, and abduction
Gastrocnemius	*Medial head:* medial femoral condyle *Lateral head:* lateral femoral condyle	Posterior aspect of the calcaneus via the Achilles tendon	Tibial nerve (L4-S1)	Popliteal and posterior tibial arteries	Knee flexion and ankle plantarflexion
Popliteus	Lateral meniscus and lateral femoral condyle	Posterior surface of the tibia superior to the soleal line	Tibial nerve (L4-L5)	Inferior medial and lateral genicular arteries	Knee flexion (unlocks the knee)

Zone I: Anterior Aspect

Quadriceps Femoris

The quadriceps femoris muscle group traveling from the proximal aspect of the femur to the tibial tuberosity begins to collectively narrow as it approaches the patella to insert along the anterior and medial aspects of the patella as the quadriceps tendon. This tendon attaches to the superior aspect of the patella before continuing down to insert on the tibial tuberosity via the patellar tendon. Therefore, the patella has a balance of soft tissue forces above it (quadriceps tendon) and below it (patellar tendon). During palpation, the clinician should be able to isolate and identify both the vastus medialis and vastus lateralis during knee extension because these muscles become most visible with an isometric contraction.

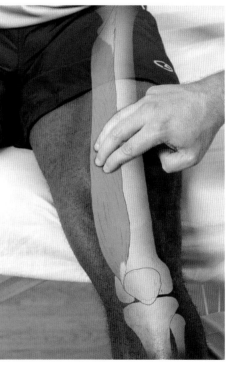

Vastus Medialis

Positions

- Patient: sitting at the edge of the table, with knees bent to 90°
- Clinician: sitting, facing the patient, on the side being palpated

Instructions

- Palpate the medial aspect of the thigh.
- With the pads of three or four fingers, follow the fibers of the vastus medialis all the way down the medial aspect of the thigh.
- To confirm palpation, have the patient perform resisted knee extension. You should feel a large contraction under your fingers.

Notes

- Collectively, the rectus femoris, vastus medialis, vastus lateralis, and vastus intermedius form the quadriceps femoris.
- The vastus intermedius is too deep to palpate.

CLINICAL PEARL

The quadriceps can be inhibited by autogenic inhibition when joint effusion is present after trauma, musculoskeletal pathology, or surgery. This can lead to poor knee control during activity or the inability to sustain knee extension or both.[5,6]

Rectus Femoris

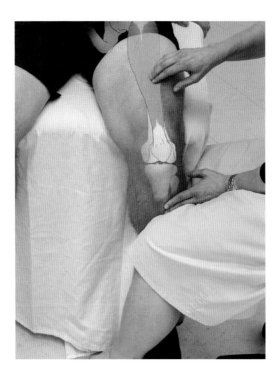

Positions

- Patient: sitting at the edge of the table, with knees bent to 90°
- Clinician: sitting, facing the patient, on the side being palpated

Instructions

- Palpate the anterior inferior iliac spine (AIIS).
- With the pads of three or four fingers, follow the fibers of the rectus femoris all the way down the anterior, middle aspect of the thigh.
- To confirm palpation, have the patient perform resisted knee extension against your leg. You should feel the muscle contract under your fingers.

Note

You can also palpate the origin tendon of the rectus femoris on the AIIS by having the patient flex the hip and palpating just below the AIIS.

Vastus Lateralis

Positions

- Patient: sitting at the edge of the table, with knees bent to 90°
- Clinician: sitting, facing the patient, on the side being palpated

Instructions

- Palpate the greater trochanter, the origin of the vastus lateralis.
- With the pads of three or four fingers, follow the fibers of the vastus lateralis all the way down the lateral aspect of the thigh.
- To confirm palpation, have the patient perform resisted knee extension against your leg.

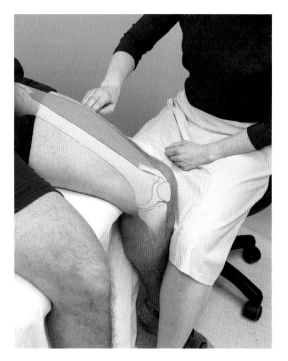

Bursae Around the Knee

Clinicians should be familiar with the important bursae that are located around the circumference of the knee. With bursitis being a fairly common clinical condition, the clinician should be able to palpate for the prepatellar bursa, superficial infrapatellar bursa, deep infrapatellar bursa, and the pes anserine bursa.

Positions

- Patient: sitting at the edge of the table, with the knees flexed to 90°
- Clinician: sitting, facing the patient, on the side being palpated

Instructions

- Palpate the anterior aspect of the patella (a). The prepatellar bursa sits superficial to the anterior aspect of the knee cap.

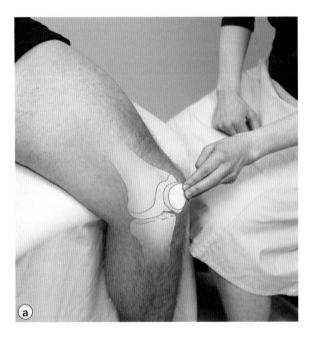

(a)

> continued

- Slide two fingers inferiorly until palpating the patellar tendon *(b)*. The superficial infrapatellar bursa lies just superficial to the tendon. The deep infrapatellar bursa is extremely difficult, if not impossible, to palpate because it is found posterior to the patellar tendon.

- Palpate the tibial tubercle and slide two fingers posterior and medial to reach the insertion of the sartorius, gracilis, and semitendinosus on the pes anserine *(c)*. The pes anserine bursa is located superficial to the tendons.

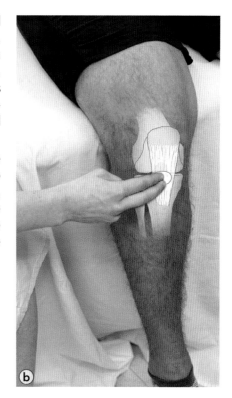

Note

Normally, the bursae around the knee are difficult to palpate. However, when they become inflamed from excessive kneeling and rubbing (friction), the bursae may fill with fluid, making it easier to palpate and assess.

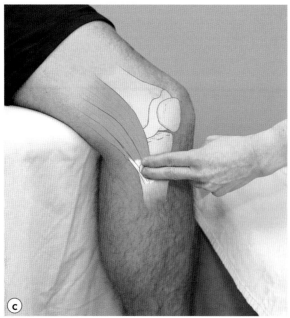

Zone II: Medial Aspect

Pes Anserine Tendons

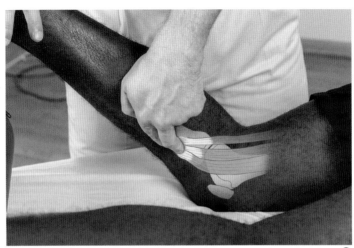

VIDEO 11.2 ▶

Positions
- Patient: prone, with legs resting on a pillow or bolster
- Clinician: standing, facing the patient, on the side being palpated

Instructions
- Place your fingers in the popliteal fossa.
- Move two fingers just medially until you feel a firm tendon.
- To confirm palpation, have the patient perform resisted knee flexion (right hand pictured); the tendon of the semitendinosus will become visible and palpable under your fingers.
- The gracilis tendon is just anterior to the semitendinosus tendon.
- The sartorius tendon is the most anterior and just anterior to the gracilis.

Notes
- Most often, the sartorius is not obvious during this palpation. However, you should be able to palpate for the tendon as it inserts near the pes anserine.
- This palpation can also be performed with the patient sitting with the knees flexed to 90° and the clinician sitting on the side being palpated. Resisted knee flexion will make the tendons visible.

Medial Collateral Ligament

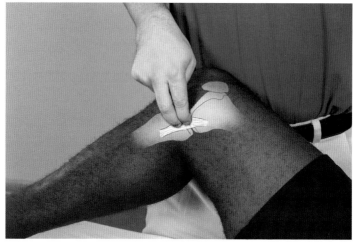

VIDEO 11.3 ▶

Positions
- Patient: supine, with the knee flexed between 70° and 90°
- Clinician: standing, facing the patient, on the side being palpated

Instructions
- Palpate the medial femoral condyle.
- Palpate the medial tibial condyle.
- Using the pads of digits 2 and 3, palpate from the medial femoral condyle to the medial tibial condyle.
- The MCL runs between these two bony landmarks as it crosses the medial joint line. You may feel a taut band-like structure under your fingers.

Note
Once you have oriented yourself and found the midsubstance of the MCL, you may want to decrease knee flexion to approximately 30° to better palpate proximal and distal portions of the MCL. At this angle, there is more tension on the MCL, making it more easily identifiable.[11]

CLINICAL PEARL
This ligament is commonly injured when the knee is subjected to a valgus force. During palpation you should assess for tenderness and gapping of the medial joint line while you apply a valgus force to the knee.[11]

Medial Meniscus

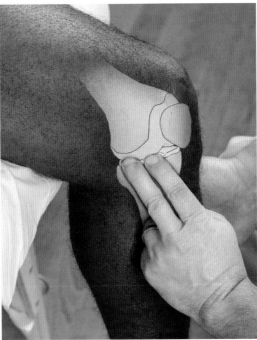

VIDEO 11.4 ▶

Positions

- Patient: sitting at the edge of the table, with knees flexed to 90°
- Clinician: sitting, facing the patient, on the side being palpated

Instructions

- Palpate the medial femoral condyle.
- Palpate the medial tibial condyle.
- Using two fingers, palpate the joint space between the medial femoral condyle and medial tibial condyle.
- Move your fingers along the joint space from anterior to posterior, assessing the entire outer edge of the medial meniscus.

CLINICAL PEARL

During palpation you should be assessing for joint line tenderness, which may be indicative of a medial meniscal tear.[12]

Zone III: Lateral Aspect

Lateral Collateral Ligament

Positions

- Patient: supine, with the lower extremity in the FABER position (hip flexion, abduction, external rotation, and knee in 90° of flexion)
- Clinician: standing, facing the patient, on the side being palpated

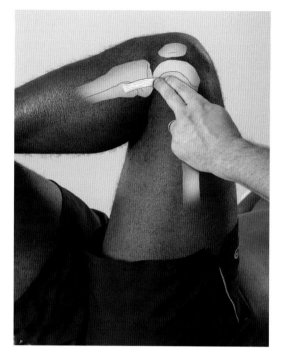

Instructions

- Palpate the lateral femoral condyle with digits 2 and 3.
- Move your fingers inferiorly to palpate the fibular head.
- Palpate from the lateral femoral condyle to the fibular head.
- The LCL runs between these two bony landmarks as it crosses over the lateral joint line.
- You should feel a taut structure similar to a guitar string.

Note

Once you have oriented yourself and found the midsubstance of the LCL, you may want to decrease knee flexion to approximately 30° to better palpate proximal and distal portions of the LCL. At this angle, there is more tension on the LCL, making it more easily identifiable.[13]

CLINICAL PEARL

This ligament is commonly injured when the knee is subjected to a varus force. During palpation, you should assess for tenderness and gapping of the lateral joint line while you apply a varus force to the knee.[13]

Lateral Meniscus

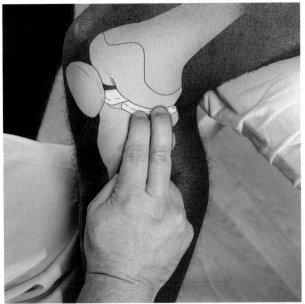

VIDEO 11.5 ▶

Positions

- Patient: sitting at the edge of the table, with the knees flexed to 90°
- Clinician: sitting, facing the patient, on the side being palpated

Instructions

- Palpate the lateral femoral condyle.
- Palpate the lateral tibial condyle.
- Using two fingers, palpate the joint space between the lateral femoral condyle and lateral tibial condyle.
- Move your fingers along the joint space from anterior to posterior, assessing the entire outer edge of the lateral meniscus.

CLINICAL PEARL

During palpation, you should be assessing for joint line tenderness, which may be indicative of a lateral meniscal tear.[12]

Tensor Fasciae Latae and Iliotibial Band

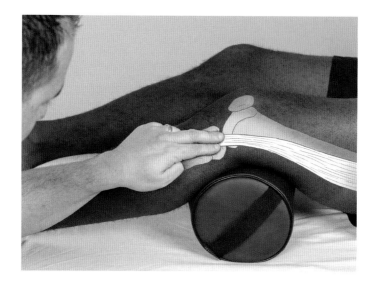

Positions

- Patient: supine, with a pillow or bolster under the knees
- Clinician: standing, facing the patient, on the side being palpated

Instructions

- Palpate the anterior superior iliac spine (ASIS) and the lateral iliac crest.
- Using the pads of two fingers, move just inferior and lateral to the ASIS.
- To confirm palpation of the tensor fasciae latae at its origin, have the patient perform resisted hip abduction.
- Move your fingers distally and continue to palpate the ITB along the lateral aspect of the thigh to its distal insertion on the lateral tibial condyle.

CLINICAL PEARL

Often the ITB can become tight and snap over the lateral tibial condyle. This can cause inflammation and pain, especially during activities involving repetitive knee flexion and extension such as running or biking. In some individuals, the ITB has fibers attaching to the lateral patellar retinaculum, which may become tight and pull the patella laterally because of the additional tension.[14]

Common Peroneal, or Fibular, Nerve

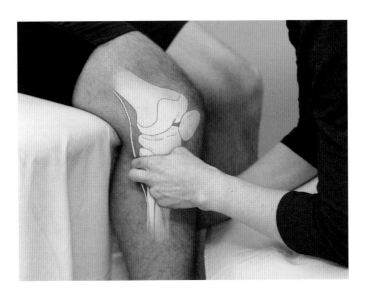

Positions

- Patient: sitting at the edge of the table, with the knee flexed to 90°
- Clinician: sitting beside the patient, on the side being palpated

Instructions

- Palpate the tendon of the biceps femoris.
- Palpate the fibular head (see chapter 12).
- Slide one or two fingers posterior to the fibular head to palpate the common fibular nerve.
- To confirm palpation, gently roll the nerve between the fibular head and your finger.

Zone IV: Posterior Aspect

Semimembranosus

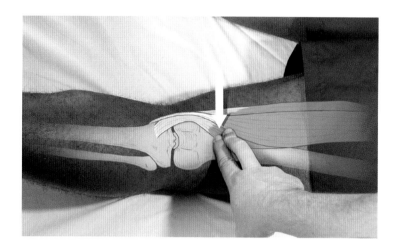

Positions
- Patient: prone, with legs resting on a pillow or bolster
- Clinician: standing, facing the patient, on the side being palpated

Instructions
- Palpate the semitendinosus tendon using two fingers.
- Add firm pressure on either side of the tendon and feel for a broader, softer structure deep to the semitendinosus.
- To confirm palpation, have the patient perform resisted knee flexion. You should feel, but not clearly see, a large bulge under the fingers.

Biceps Femoris

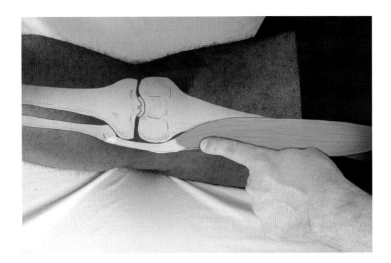

Positions
- Patient: prone, with legs resting on a pillow or bolster
- Clinician: standing, facing the patient, on the side being palpated

Instructions
- Place your fingers in the popliteal fossa.
- Move one finger laterally until you feel a firm tendon.
- To confirm palpation, have the patient perform resisted knee flexion. You should feel a firm tendon contraction.

Gastrocnemius

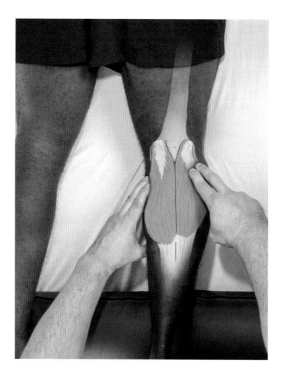

Positions

- Patient: prone, with legs resting on a pillow or bolster
- Clinician: standing, facing the patient, on the side being palpated

Instructions

- Palpate along the posterior aspect of the lower leg using two fingers.
- To confirm palpation, have the patient plantarflex the ankle.
- You can isolate the medial (left hand pictured) and lateral (right hand pictured) heads of the gastrocnemius by moving your fingers superiorly toward the knee where the heads of the gastrocnemius take their origin on the medial femoral condyle and the lateral femoral condyle, respectively.

Notes

- To palpate the soleus, passively flex the knee and move your fingers to the lateral and medial aspect of the gastrocnemius and carefully position your fingers under the gastrocnemius.
- To confirm palpation, have the patient perform ankle plantarflexion with the knee in a flexed position.

Popliteus

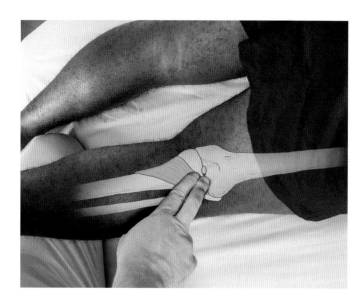

Positions

- Patient: prone, with the lower leg resting on the clinician's thigh or a bolster
- Clinician: standing on the side being palpated, slightly distal to the patient's knee (with knee up on the table, supporting the patient's lower leg)

Instructions

- Palpate the midline of the proximal gastrocnemius muscle belly.
- Slide two fingers proximally into the popliteal fossa.
- Apply firm pressure in a posterior-to-anterior direction, slowly increasing your force.
- To confirm palpation, resist knee flexion and medial tibial rotation.

Notes

- Many people have difficulty performing medial tibial rotation. In these instances, given that you are too central for the hamstring tendons and, if using enough force, too deep for the gastrocnemius, you can assume that the contraction you feel under your fingers with resisted knee flexion is that of the popliteus.
- The popliteal artery lies superficial to the popliteus muscle. After palpating the popliteus, keep the knee in flexion to slacken the fascia and posterior soft tissue and attempt to palpate the popliteal pulse.

Case Study

History

A 14-year-old female presents to your office complaining of left knee pain for 1 month. She states that the pain is localized to the front of her knee, is intermittent, and occurs with using stairs, prolonged sitting with the knee bent, and running while playing soccer. She does not recall a traumatic incident. She lives in a duplex apartment with her family, with eight stairs into the building and the entrance to her apartment on the entry level. She plays soccer, and the team practices four times a week for 2 hours, with games on the weekends.

- Based on the subjective information only, what are the three most likely diagnoses?

Examination

Past medical history	Unremarkable
Medication	Advil
Observation	Subtalar joint pronation in weight-bearing
	Genu recurvatum
Active range of motion	Within normal limits, pain at end-range flexion
Passive range of motion	Same as for active
Manual muscle testing	Within normal limits, except left quadriceps 4–/5, hip abductors 3+/5, and hip external rotators 4/5
Special tests	Positive left step-down test (pain and loss of eccentric control)
	Positive left Clarke's sign
	Positive left patellar grind test
Other	Decreased left stance time

- Based on the subjective and objective information together, what are the two most likely diagnoses? Give your rationale for eliminating the third diagnosis.
- What structures should you palpate on this patient based on your differential diagnoses?
- Given all the information presented, what would you expect to find on palpation of those structures?

Case Solution and Discussion

Potential Diagnoses Based on History
- Infrapatellar fat pad irritation
- Patellar tendonitis
- Patellofemoral pain syndrome

Potential Diagnoses Based on History and Examination

- Patellar tendonitis
- Patellofemoral pain syndrome
- Infrapatellar fat pad irritation: The location of pain and the pain occurring with prolonged sitting, in conjunction with the positive special tests, make this diagnosis unlikely. However, it cannot be completely ruled out at this point of the exam.

Structures to Be Palpated

- Patellar tendon
- Tibial tuberosity
- Adductor tubercle
- Infrapatellar fat pad*

*Note: This diagnosis relies heavily on the palpatory exam and cannot be completely ruled out until that has been completed. Therefore, the infrapatellar fat pad remains one of the structures to be palpated to affirm elimination of the possibility of this diagnosis.

Palpation Findings

- Tenderness to palpation of the left patellar tendon (proximally)
- No tenderness to palpation of the tibial tuberosity and distal patellar tendon
- Tenderness to palpation of the left adductor tubercle
- No tenderness to palpation of the left infrapatellar fat pad

Clinical Reasoning

- Patellar tendonitis: The patient's report of the location and occurrence of pain in her knee; the gait deviations; the positive special tests; and the weakness of her left quadriceps, hip abductors, and external rotators—as well as the structures that are tender to palpation—can be consistent with patellar tendonitis. While there is a strong possibility that this is the diagnosis, the reason it is not our primary diagnosis is the lack of tenderness to palpation throughout the entire patellar tendon. However, be aware that patellar tendonitis can occur in conjunction with patellofemoral pain syndrome.
- Patellofemoral pain syndrome: The patient's report of the location and occurrence of pain in her knee; gait deviations; positive special tests; and weakness of her left quadriceps, left abductors, and external rotators—along with the structures that are tender to palpation—all indicate patellofemoral pain syndrome. In addition, her posture (left subtalar joint pronation and genu recurvatum) and activity level put her at risk for patellofemoral pain syndrome.

Case Study Questions

1. What information do the palpation findings of the case give the clinician? How can this information be incorporated in the clinical decision-making process?

2. Think about how the examination findings (subjective and objective) lead to the differential diagnosis. What might you do differently?

3. Discuss the role of patient education when treating and managing a female teenager.

CHAPTER REVIEW QUESTIONS

1. List the four major ligaments of the knee.

2. Name the borders of the popliteal fossa and the contents located within it.

3. Name the muscles in the anterior compartment of the thigh and their innervation.

4. Name the muscles of the medial compartment of the thigh and their innervation.

5. Describe the blood supply to the thigh.

6. Name the common origin for the hamstring muscles.

Lower Leg, Ankle, and Foot

After completing this chapter, the reader will be able to do the following:

- Identify the key bony anatomical structures of the lower leg, ankle, and foot.
- Identify and describe the soft tissue anatomy of the lower leg, ankle, and foot, including muscles, ligaments, nerves, arteries, and veins.
- Identify the compartments of the flexor retinaculum.
- Identify on bony or skeletal models the origins and insertions of the muscles of the lower leg, ankle, and foot to aid in understanding osteokinematic action and surface palpation.
- Palpate structures of the lower leg, ankle, and foot.
- Integrate surface palpation findings to aid in the differential diagnosis of a patient with lower leg, ankle, or foot pain.

The lower leg, ankle, and foot function as a complex system of numerous bones, muscles, and joints. The foot is the segment of the kinetic chain that comes in contact with the ground during ambulation and is therefore the first link responsible for transferring the forces from the ground up through the kinetic chain.[1] Proper distribution and absorption of these forces are essential in helping prevent knee, hip, and back pain. This requires coordinated interaction of ligaments, muscles, and other soft tissues throughout the lower extremity.

Functions of the Foot and Ankle Joints

The foot and ankle—a dynamic collection of bones, joints, and soft tissues—are responsible for promoting mobility and stability throughout the gait cycle. Unlike other joints in the body, the ankle and foot are distinctive in that they do not move in the traditional cardinal planes of movement. In the ankle and foot, all motion takes place around an oblique axis, which enables the ankle and foot to have motions of pronation and supination. In open chain, supination consists of plantarflexion, inversion, and adduction. Conversely, pronation consists of dorsiflexion, eversion, and abduction.[1]

The gait cycle is quite complex, and a thorough discussion of this is beyond the scope of this book. However, briefly, the gait cycle is divided into a swing phase and a stance phase. The stance phase occurs when the foot is in contact with the ground and is subdivided into heel strike, foot flat, midstance, heel-off, and toe-off. The swing phase occurs when the foot is not in contact with the ground and is subdivided into early, mid, and late swing. For a complete discussion on gait mechanics, readers should refer to a kinesiology text.[1,2]

- From heel strike through midstance, the main function of the foot is to adapt to the ground and to transfer forces from the ground up to the ankle. This mobility is accomplished best by the efficient, coordinated interaction of multiple bones and joints. The mobility is achieved by pronation of multiple joints, essentially unlocking the ankle and foot, making them pliable in preparation for weight acceptance.

- From heel-off through toe-off, the role of the foot and ankle changes as it becomes necessary for the foot and ankle to become a rigid lever to propel the body forward. This is accomplished by supination of the multiple joints of the ankle and foot, locking the foot and creating the rigid lever required for push-off.

Bony Anatomy

The tibia and fibula (figure 12.1) both flare out to form the medial and lateral malleoli, respectively. Between the tibia and fibula is the interosseous membrane, which is responsible for increasing stability and transmitting forces between the bones.

- The distal tibia–fibula (tib–fib) articulation is considered a syndesmotic joint, with very little motion and strong ligamentous support.

- This is in contrast to the proximal tib–fib articulation, which functions as a synovial joint and has a role in ankle mobility. At the proximal tib–fib joint, the fibula moves posterior and anterior on the tibia, during dorsiflexion and plantarflexion

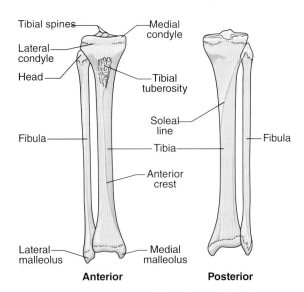

FIGURE 12.1 Aspects of the tibia and fibula.

of the ankle respectively. In addition, slight superior motion of the fibula occurs with dorsiflexion of the ankle joint.[1, 2]

Distal to the tibia and fibula are the tarsal bones. Seven tarsal bones form the ankle: the calcaneus, talus, navicular, cuneiforms (medial, intermediate, and lateral), and the cuboid (figure 12.2). The concave distal tibia and fibula articulate with the talus, forming the talocrural joint. This is a synovial joint, with the majority of its motion being dorsiflexion and plantarflexion. However, some pronation and supination occur because of the obliquity of the axis. Passive stability of the joint is provided by a collection of ligaments on both the medial and lateral aspects of the joint.[3] These ligaments are discussed later in the chapter.

Distal to the talocrural joint is the subtalar joint. The joint is formed by the calcaneus and the talus. This joint also has an oblique axis, which is angled more vertically than the axis of the talocrural joint. Several ligaments also stabilize this joint, none of which are directly palpable and therefore are not discussed in further detail.[3]

Distal to the subtalar joint is the midtarsal joint. This joint is further subdivided into the calcaneocuboid and talonavicular joints.

- The function of the calcaneocuboid joint is to increase stability of the midfoot during weight-bearing activities.
- The talonavicular joint, on the other hand, is highly mobile and allows the most amount of pronation and supination.

At the midtarsal joint, specifically the talonavicular joint, true triplanar motion is present. Closed chain supination is a combination of calcaneal inversion, talar abduction and dorsiflexion, and tibial external rotation, while closed chain pronation is a combination of calcaneal eversion, talar adduction and plantarflexion, and tibial internal rotation. This triplanar motion allows the foot to adapt to changes of terrain during ambulation.[1, 2]

The anatomy of the foot (see figure 12.2) is quite complex because of the many bones, joints, and ligaments that not only provide stability to the foot but also permit motion in multiple planes.

- Distal to the tarsal bones are the five metatarsal bones, which serve as attachments for many of the lower leg muscles.
- Distal to the metatarsals are the phalanges, which can be divided into the proximal, middle, and distal phalanges on all digits except the great toe (first digit), which has no middle phalanx.
  - These small bones help form the tarsometatarsal (TMT) joints, metatarsophalangeal (MTP) joints, proximal interphalangeal (PIP) joints, and distal interphalangeal (DIP) joints of the foot.

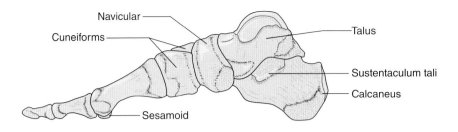

Medial

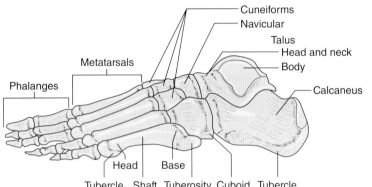

Lateral

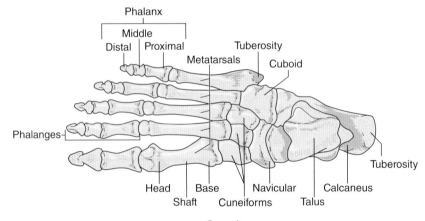

Superior

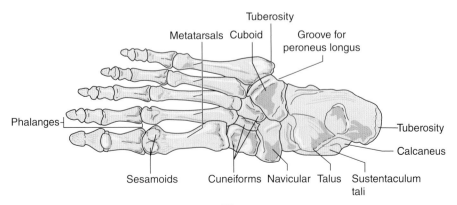

Plantar

FIGURE 12.2   Bones of the foot and ankle.

— The first MTP joint is the most important for balance and is particularly important for foot function because it permits a large amount of motion in the sagittal plane, which is necessary for proper push-off.[1,2]

Soft Tissue Anatomy

The muscles of the lower leg are divided into several compartments. The anterior compartment of the lower leg contains four important muscles: tibialis anterior, extensor digitorum longus, extensor hallucis longus, and fibularis (or peroneus) tertius (figure 12.3). Collectively, these muscles dorsiflex the ankle and extend the toes.

A tough band of fascia, called the anterior intermuscular septum, separates the anterior and lateral compartments of the lower leg. On the lateral aspect of the fibula is the lateral compartment of the lower leg. This compartment contains two muscles: the fibularis longus and fibularis brevis (also known as the peroneus longus and brevis). These muscles together perform eversion of the ankle (figure 12.3).[3]

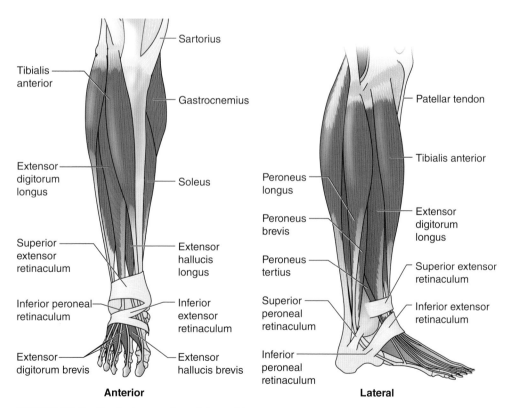

FIGURE 12.3 Extrinsic muscles of the ankle.

On the posterior aspect of the lower leg is the posterior compartment. This is the biggest of the compartments and is therefore divided into superficial and deep layers by the transverse intermuscular septum.

- The superficial posterior compartment contains three muscles that collectively perform ankle plantarflexion: the gastrocnemius, soleus, and plantaris (figure 12.4). These muscles all have a common insertion into the Achilles tendon, a thick band of connective tissue that distally attaches to the posterior aspect of the calcaneus.[3]
- In the deep posterior compartment of the lower leg are the tibialis posterior, flexor digitorum longus, and flexor hallucis longus.
  - These muscles collectively plantarflex the ankle, and the flexor digitorum longus and flexor hallucis longus perform toe flexion.
  - The tibialis posterior is also a primary invertor.
  - The tendons of these muscles in the deep posterior compartment all travel posterior to the medial malleolus and under the flexor retinaculum. From anterior to posterior, the structures are as follows: tibialis posterior; flexor digitorum longus; posterior tibial artery, vein, and nerve; and the flexor hallucis longus (figure 12.4).[3]

The sole of the foot is similar to the palm of the hand in that many muscles are located in a relatively small area. The sole of the foot has 19 intrinsic muscles. Directly under the skin is the plantar aponeurosis (fascia), which is a thick band of connective tissue that serves two functions. First, it protects vital structures that lie deep to it, and second, it is responsible for helping support the medial longitudinal arch.[3]

The muscles in the sole of the foot are divided into four layers (figure 12.5).

- Layer 1 is the most superficial and consists of the abductor hallucis, abductor digiti minimi, and flexor digitorum brevis.
- Layer 2 consists of the lumbricales and quadratus plantae as well as the tendons of the tibialis posterior, flexor digitorum longus, and flexor hallucis longus.
- Layer 3 consists of the adductor hallucis, flexor hallucis brevis, and flexor digiti minimi.
- Layer 4 is the deepest layer and consists of the plantar and dorsal interossei.

All of these muscles are innervated by either the medial or lateral plantar nerve. Collectively, these muscles are responsible for toe movement, but more importantly, they support the arch and provide stability during weight-bearing activities.[3]

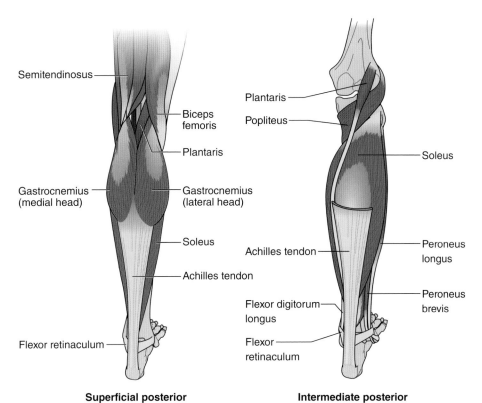

Superficial posterior

Intermediate posterior

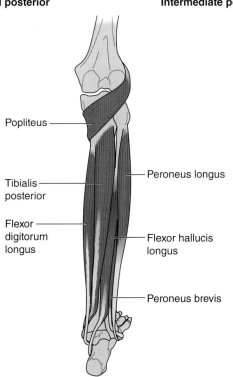

Deep posterior

FIGURE 12.4 Posterior leg muscles.

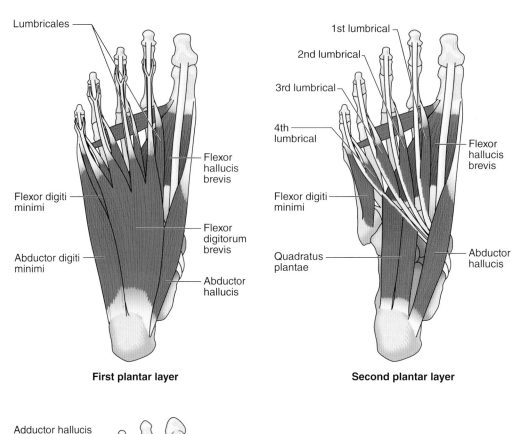

Lumbricales

Flexor hallucis brevis

Flexor digiti minimi

Flexor digitorum brevis

Abductor digiti minimi

Abductor hallucis

First plantar layer

1st lumbrical

2nd lumbrical

3rd lumbrical

4th lumbrical

Flexor hallucis brevis

Flexor digiti minimi

Quadratus plantae

Abductor hallucis

Second plantar layer

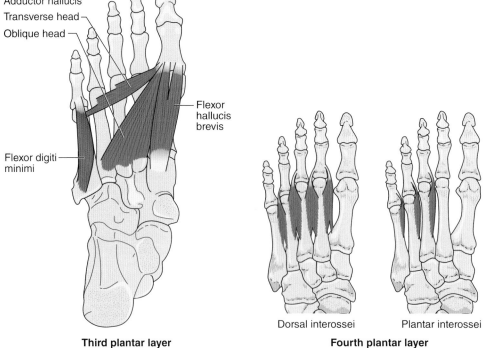

Adductor hallucis
Transverse head
Oblique head

Flexor hallucis brevis

Flexor digiti minimi

Third plantar layer

Dorsal interossei

Plantar interossei

Fourth plantar layer

FIGURE 12.5 Intrinsic plantar muscles.

Several ligaments surround the talocrural joint and provide passive stability to the ankle. These ligaments are divided into a lateral complex and a medial complex (figure 12.6). The lateral collateral ligament (lateral complex) spans the entire lateral aspect of the talocrural joint. It is composed of three separate ligaments:

- Anterior talofibular ligament (ATFL)
- Calcaneofibular ligament (CFL)
- Posterior talofibular ligament (PTFL)

Together, these ligaments protect against excessive inversion forces. The ATFL is one of the most commonly injured ligaments in the body during an inversion ankle sprain.[3]

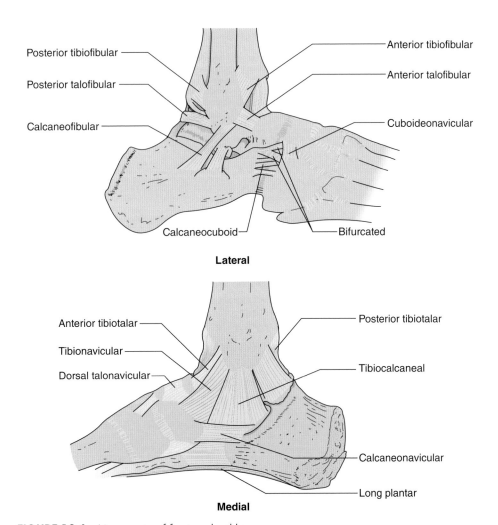

Lateral

Medial

FIGURE 12.6 Ligaments of foot and ankle.

On the medial side of the talocrural joint is the medial collateral ligament (medial complex), also referred to as the deltoid ligament. It is composed of four ligaments:

- Anterior tibiotalar ligament
- Posterior tibiotalar ligament
- Tibiocalcaneal ligament
- Tibionavicular ligament

Together these ligaments originate from the medial malleolus and protect against excessive eversion forces. Unlike the lateral collateral ligaments, the medial ankle ligaments are strong enough that they are less likely to rupture than the medial malleolus is to fracture.[3] These ligaments are more difficult to palpate.

Numerous other ligaments located throughout the foot and ankle provide passive stability. Because they are extremely difficult, if not impossible, to palpate in isolation, we will not discuss them further.

Neurovascular Anatomy

The popliteal artery divides into the anterior tibial artery and the posterior tibial artery (figure 12.7). The anterior tibial artery is responsible for the blood supply to the anterior compartment of the lower leg, while the posterior tibial artery supplies blood to the posterior compartment of the lower leg.[3]

The anterior tibial artery becomes the dorsalis pedis artery just distal to the malleoli. This artery continues into the dorsum of the foot, running between the first and second metatarsals, where it can be palpated lateral to the tendon of the extensor hallucis longus.[3] The blood supply to the

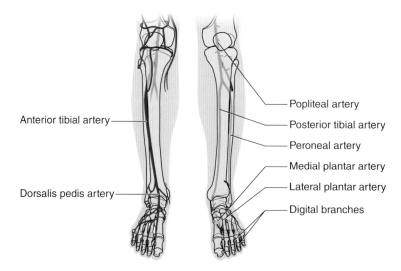

FIGURE 12.7 Arteries of the lower leg, ankle, and foot.

lateral compartment is provided by the peroneal artery, a branch of the posterior tibial artery.[3]

The posterior tibial artery travels down the posterior compartment of the lower leg and can be palpated posterior to the medial malleolus. At the origin of the soleus, the posterior tibial artery gives off its largest branch, the peroneal (fibular) artery, which is responsible for bringing blood supply to the lateral compartment of the lower leg. Distal to the medial malleolus, the posterior tibial artery divides into the medial and lateral plantar arteries, which bring blood supply to the sole of the foot.[3]

The sciatic nerve runs down the posterior thigh and divides into the common fibular and tibial nerves (figure 12.8).[3]

- The common fibular nerve then divides at the fibular head: the deep fibular nerve innervates the muscles of the anterior compartment, and the superficial fibular nerve innervates the muscles of the lateral compartment.

- The tibial nerve travels down the posterior compartment of the lower leg and innervates all the superficial and deep muscles of that compartment. This nerve divides distal to the medial malleolus into the medial and lateral plantar nerves, which innervate the muscles of the sole of the foot.

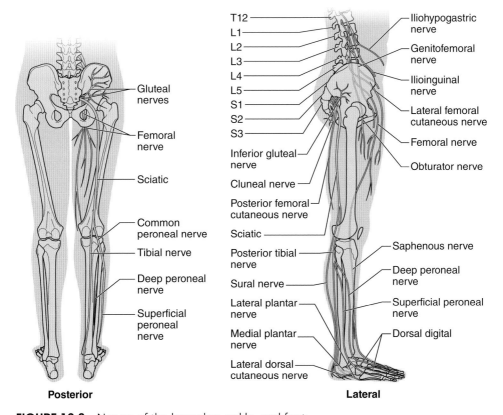

FIGURE 12.8 Nerves of the lower leg, ankle, and foot.

Structural Inspection

- The clinician should watch the patient get up from the chair in the waiting room and ambulate to the examination room. Particular attention should be given to the presence of heel strike, or lack of it, and signs of asymmetrical weight-bearing or limping.

- Once the patient is in the examination room and sitting safely in a chair or on a table, the clinician can assess the external surface of the shoe, observing for the typical wear pattern that indicates forces move from lateral to medial during the gait cycle. Areas of increased wear and tear on the bottom of the shoe may represent abnormal foot postures and loading patterns.

- After the shoes have been inspected, the clinician can observe for callus formation on the bottom of the foot, which can be indicative of increased weight-bearing forces through that area of the plantar aspect of the foot or along the medial aspect of the first metatarsophalangeal joint or both.

- While the patient is sitting, with the shoes and socks removed, the clinician should look to see if the ankle is resting in a natural position of slight plantarflexion and inversion.

- The clinician next assess the general shape and arch of the foot in a non-weight-bearing position. Observing the medial longitudinal arch, assess whether the arch is too high (pes cavus) or too low (pes planus).

- A quick screen for asymmetries of the foot and ankle should be assessed in the non-weight-bearing position. Observe and document skin breakdown, ecchymosis, swelling, or trophic changes to the skin that might indicate the presence of certain pathologies.

- The clinician should instruct the patient to stand and distribute the weight equally between both lower extremities. If unequal distribution is observed, the clinician should follow up with questions to determine the cause of the abnormal loading.

- While the patient is standing, the clinician should assess the shape of the medial longitudinal arch and compare the weight-bearing with the non-weight-bearing findings. Usually, in the weight-bearing position, the medial longitudinal arch will drop somewhat because of the weight of the body. If this is not the case, the patient may have a high arch that remains in a position of supination. On the other hand, if while in a weight-bearing position, the patient's medial longitudinal arch collapses, excessive pronation exists. Readers are referred to other texts for a full discussion of this concept.[1,2]

Fibular Head

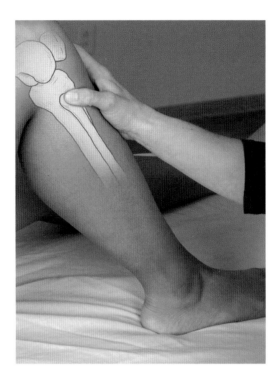

Positions
- Patient: supine, with the knee flexed to 90°
- Clinician: standing, facing the patient, on the side being palpated

Instructions
- Palpate the lateral tibial condyle.
- Move one finger posteriorly until you feel a small bony prominence.
- To confirm palpation, have the patient dorsiflex and plantarflex the ankle. You should feel the fibular head move under your fingers.

Lateral Malleolus (Key Reference Structure)

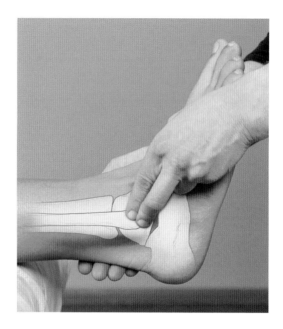

Positions
- Patient: long sitting, with the ankle slightly off the table
- Clinician: sitting or standing at the end of the table, facing the patient, on the side being palpated

Instructions
- Using two fingers, palpate the last 2 inches (5 centimeters) of the lateral aspect of the fibula.
- At the distal-most aspect of the fibula, you will feel a bony prominence.

CLINICAL PEARL
During palpation of the distal fibula and lateral malleolus, you should assess for bone tenderness, which may be an indication of fibular fracture.[4]

Sinus Tarsi Area

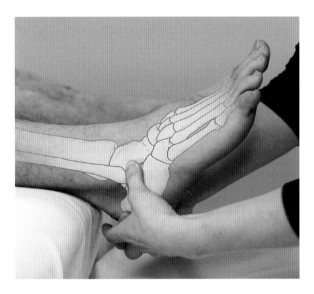

Positions
- Patient: long sitting, with the ankle slightly off the table
- Clinician: sitting or standing at the end of the table, facing the patient, on the side being palpated

Instructions
- Palpate the lateral malleolus.
- With one hand, stabilize the calcaneus (right hand pictured).
- Using the other hand, place the thumb along the soft tissue depression just anterior to the lateral malleolus.

Notes
- Located within the sinus tarsi is the extensor digitorum brevis. At times, there may also be a fat pad superficial to the extensor digitorum brevis.
- The clinician should be able to palpate the superior dorsal aspect of the calcaneus here as it articulates with the cuboid.

CLINICAL PEARL

The sinus tarsi, a concave depression located just anterior to the lateral malleolus, is often affected following an inversion ankle sprain. This is where the clinician often observes swelling and palpates the tenderness associated with a sprain of the anterior talofibular ligament. Deep tenderness within the sinus tarsi may be indicative of pathology of the subtalar joint.

Medial Malleolus (Key Reference Structure)

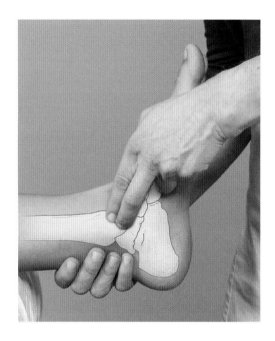

Positions
- Patient: long sitting, with the ankle slightly off the table
- Clinician: sitting or standing at the end of the table, facing the patient, on the side being palpated

Instructions
- Using two fingers, palpate the last 2 inches (5 centimeters) of the medial aspect of the tibia.
- At the distal-most aspect of the tibia, you will feel a bony prominence.

CLINICAL PEARL
During palpation of the distal tibia and medial malleolus, you should assess for bone tenderness because this may be an indication of a tibial fracture.[4]

Sustentaculum Tali

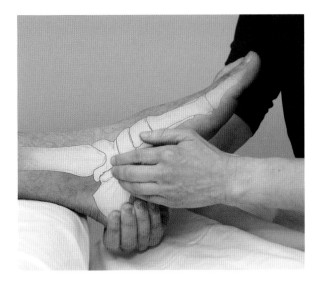

Positions
- Patient: long sitting, with the ankle slightly off the table
- Clinician: sitting or standing at the end of the table, facing the patient, on the side being palpated

Instructions
- Palpate the medial malleolus.
- Move two fingers in an inferior direction about a fingerwidth from the distal end of the medial malleolus until you feel the next bony landmark, the sustentaculum tali.

CLINICAL PEARL
This landmark, while small, has clinical significance. The sustentaculum tali, a shelflike area of the calcaneus, supports the talus and serves as an attachment for the spring ligament (plantar calcaneonavicular ligament), which, if torn or degenerated, can contribute to pes planus.[5]

Calcaneus (Key Reference Structure)

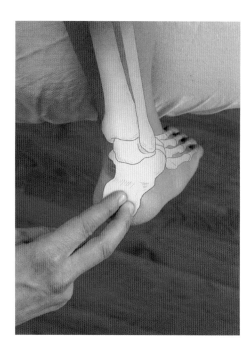

Positions
- Patient: prone, with the ankle slightly off the table
- Clinician: sitting or standing at the end of the table, facing the patient's foot, on the side being palpated

Instructions
- Palpate the middle of the heel (posterior aspect of the calcaneus).
- Move two fingers around the entire medial, lateral, posterior, and inferior aspects of the bone.

CLINICAL PEARL

The medial tubercle of the calcaneus is where the plantar fascia originates. This may be tender in people with plantar fasciitis.

Peroneal Tubercle

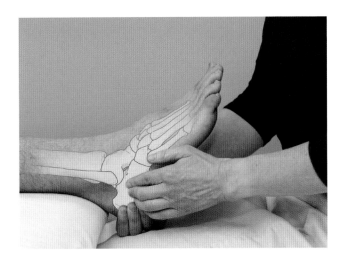

Positions

- Patient: prone, with the ankle slightly off the table
- Clinician: sitting or standing at the end of the table, facing the patient, on the side being palpated

Instructions

- Palpate the lateral malleolus.
- Palpate the lateral aspect of the calcaneus using two fingers.
- The peroneal tubercle can be palpated along the lateral aspect of the calcaneus (left hand pictured).
- It is a small bony landmark, approximately 0.25 inches (0.6 centimeter) long.

CLINICAL PEARL

This is an important anatomical landmark on the calcaneus because it separates the tendons of the fibularis longus and brevis as they pass around the calcaneus to their insertion points. The fibularis longus is inferior to the peroneal tubercle, and the fibularis brevis is superior to the peroneal tubercle.

Talar Heads

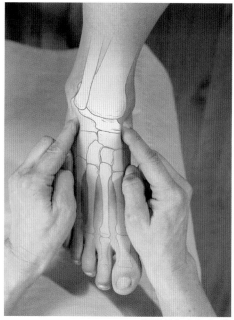

VIDEO 12.1 ▶

Positions
- Patient: long sitting, with the ankle slightly off the table
- Clinician: sitting or standing at the end of the table, facing the patient, on the side being palpated

Instructions
- Palpate the medial and lateral malleoli.
- Using the pad of digit 2 of both hands, move your fingers anteriorly into the talocrural joint space.
- Passively move the ankle into inversion to palpate and make the lateral talar head more prominent.
- Passively move the ankle into eversion to palpate and make the medial talar head more prominent.

Note
After the clinician palpates the heads of the talus, a portion of the talar dome can be palpated by placing the ankle into plantarflexion and inversion and palpating a small portion of the dome on the lateral aspect just distal to the lateral malleolus.

Distal Tibiofibular Joint

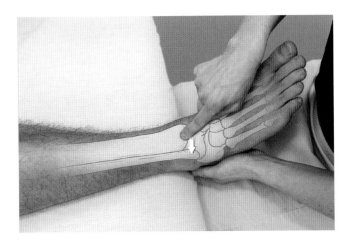

Positions
- Patient: long sitting, with the ankle slightly off the table
- Clinician: sitting or standing at the end of the table, facing the patient, on the side being palpated

Instructions
- Palpate the talus within the talocrural joint.
- Move one finger just superior to approximate the distal tibiofibular articulation.
- The anterior tibiofibular ligament is superficial to the joint, so direct palpation is not possible. However, palpating the space between the distal tibia and fibula (see the arrow) provides valuable information.

CLINICAL PEARL
An increase in space between the distal tibia and fibula can be indicative of a syndesmotic ankle sprain (high ankle sprain), in which the mechanism of injury and patient presentation is different from the typical lateral ankle sprain.

Navicular

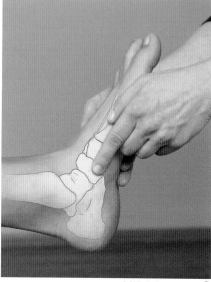

VIDEO 12.2 ▶

Positions

- Patient: long sitting, with the ankle slightly off the table
- Clinician: sitting or standing at the end of the table, facing the patient, on the side being palpated

Instructions

- Palpate the medial malleolus.
- Move one finger 0.5 inch (1.3 centimeters) inferiorly and approximately 0.5 to 1 inch (1.3 to 2.5 centimeters) anteriorly until you feel a large bony tubercle (navicular tubercle).
- Slide your finger anteriorly to palpate the dorsal aspect of the navicular.

Cuneiforms

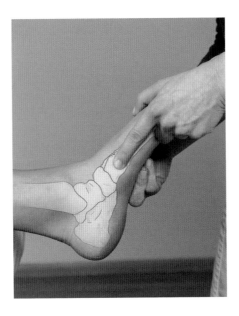

Positions

- Patient: long sitting, with the ankle slightly off the table
- Clinician: sitting or standing at the end of the table, facing the patient, on the side being palpated

Instructions

- Palpate the dorsal aspect of the navicular.
- Move one finger just distal to the navicular to palpate the medial cuneiform.
- Move your finger in a lateral direction to palpate the intermediate cuneiform.
- Continue to move your finger laterally to palpate the lateral cuneiform.

Note

The navicular articulates with all three cuneiform bones.

Cuboid

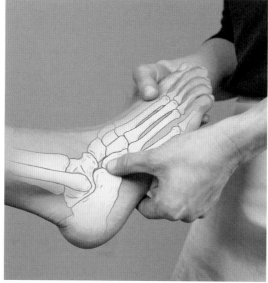

VIDEO 12.3 ▶

Positions

- Patient: long sitting, with the ankle slightly off the table
- Clinician: sitting or standing at the end of the table, facing the patient, on the side being palpated

Instructions

- Palpate the lateral malleolus.
- Move your thumb inferiorly approximately 1 inch (2.5 centimeters).
- You will feel a large bony prominence (left hand pictured).
- You should palpate the cuboid on both the dorsal and plantar surfaces of the foot.

Note

Once the cuboid has been palpated, the clinician uses a pincer grasp to palpate the dorsal and plantar aspect of the cuboid. This will permit the clinician to move the cuboid (mobilize) dorsally and plantarly.

Tuberosity of the Fifth Metatarsal

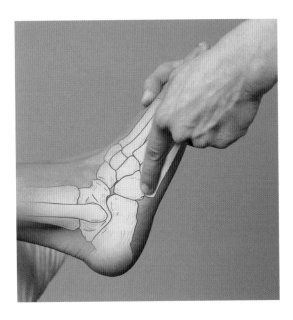

Positions

- Patient: long sitting, with the ankle slightly off the table
- Clinician: sitting or standing at the end of the table, facing the patient, on the side being palpated

Instructions

- Palpate the lateral malleolus.
- Move one finger inferiorly to the lateral border of the foot.
- Move anteriorly approximately 1 to 1.5 inches (2.5 to 4 centimeters) until you feel a bony prominence.

CLINICAL PEARL

Lateral foot pain and tenderness to the tuberosity of the fifth metatarsal may be indicative of an avulsion fracture. This usually occurs because of an inversion mechanism of injury to the foot and ankle and may accompany a lateral ankle sprain.[6]

First Ray and Sesamoids

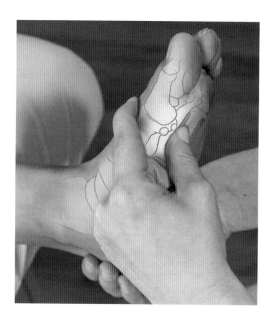

The first ray consists of the cuneiform and first metatarsal. The sesamoids are located at the base of the first MTP joint and function to protect the tendon of the flexor hallucis longus during weight-bearing activities.[1,3]

Positions

- Patient: long sitting, with the ankle slightly off the table
- Clinician: sitting or standing at the end of the table, facing the patient, on the side being palpated

Instructions

- Palpate the medial cuneiform.
- Using a pincer grasp, move distally along the dorsal and plantar surfaces of the foot until you feel a long, smooth bone (this is the first metatarsal).
- Continue distally until you feel two small bony nodules on the plantar surface of the first metatarsal, close to the MTP joint (these are the sesamoids).

CLINICAL PEARL

The first MTP joint is a common location for the development of gout, an inflammatory condition that appears to affect men more than women and people over 50 years of age. Redness, tenderness to the touch, and swelling are common body structure and function impairments seen clinically.[7] In addition, the first ray and MTP joint are susceptible to hallux valgus, a deformity consistent with lateral deviation of the first toe, in which a large painful bunion often forms on the medial aspect of the first MTP joint.[8]

Metatarsals 1 to 5

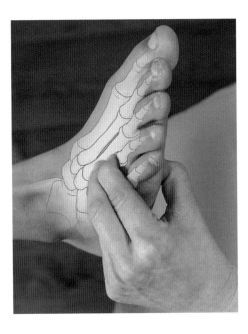

Positions
- Patient: long sitting, with the ankle slightly off the table
- Clinician: sitting or standing at the end of the table, facing the patient, on the side being palpated

Instructions
- Palpate the first metatarsal using a pincer grasp.
- Move laterally until you feel the next long smooth bone (this is the second metatarsal).
- Continue until you have palpated all five metatarsals on both the dorsal and plantar surfaces of the foot.
- While on the plantar aspect of the foot, the clinician, using the thumb, should also palpate the metatarsal heads located distally at the end of each metatarsal.

Note
Make sure that you assess the entire shaft of each metatarsal.

CLINICAL PEARL
Inflammation of the nerves that run between the metatarsals is often a cause of forefoot pain. It is most common between the third and fourth metatarsals (Morton's neuroma). The patient will present with significant tenderness to palpation of the involved joint space and with pain when all five metatarsals are compressed.[9]

Proximal Phalanges 1 to 5

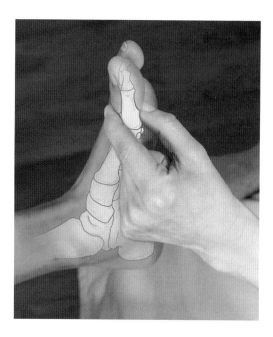

Positions

- Patient: long sitting, with the ankle slightly off the table
- Clinician: sitting or standing at the end of the table, facing the patient, on the side being palpated

Instructions

- Palpate the metatarsals, and subsequently move two fingers distally to the point where they articulate with their respective proximal phalanges.
- With two fingers (pincer grasp) encircling the bone, palpate along the shaft of the bone to the distal end.

Middle Phalanges 2 to 5

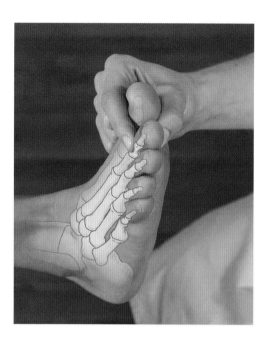

Positions

- Patient: long sitting, with the ankle slightly off the table
- Clinician: sitting or standing at the end of the table, facing the patient, on the side being palpated

Instructions

- Palpate the proximal phalanges.
- Move two fingers (pincer grasp) distally to the point where the proximal phalanges articulate with their respective middle phalanges.
- With your two fingers encircling the bone, palpate along the shaft of the bone to the distal end.

Distal Phalanges 1 to 5

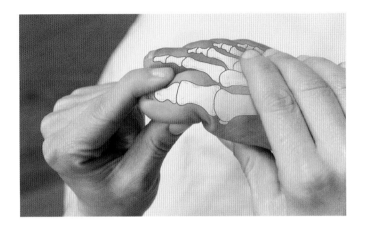

Positions
- Patient: long sitting, with the ankle slightly off the table
- Clinician: sitting or standing at the end of the table, facing the patient, on the side being palpated

Instructions
- Palpate the middle phalanges (proximal for the first digit).
- Move two fingers (pincer grasp) distally to the point where the middle phalanges articulate with their respective distal phalanges.
- With two fingers encircling the bone (left hand pictured), palpate along the shaft of the bone to the distal end.

Muscles of the Lower Leg and Sole of the Foot

Soft Tissues

Muscle	Origin	Insertion	Innervation	Blood supply	Action
LOWER LEG					
Tibialis anterior	Lateral condyle and superior half of the lateral tibia and interosseous membrane	First metatarsal and the medial and inferior aspect of the medial cuneiform	Deep fibular nerve (L4-L5)	Anterior tibial artery	Ankle dorsiflexion and inversion
Extensor digitorum longus	Lateral condyle of the tibia, superior three-fourths of the anterior surface of the fibula, and the interosseous membrane	Middle and distal phalanges of digits 2 to 5	Deep fibular nerve (L5-S1)	Anterior tibial artery	Extension of digits 2 to 5 and ankle dorsiflexion
Extensor hallucis longus	Middle part of the anterior aspect of the fibula and the interosseous membrane	Dorsal aspect of the base of the distal phalanx of the first digit	Deep fibular nerve (L5-S1)	Anterior tibial artery	Extension of the great toe and ankle dorsiflexion
Fibularis tertius	Inferior aspect of the anterior surface of the fibula and the interosseous membrane	Base of the fifth metatarsal (dorsal aspect)	Deep fibular nerve (L5-S1)	Anterior tibial artery	Dorsiflexion and eversion of the ankle
Fibularis longus	Head and superior two-thirds of the lateral aspect of the fibula	First metatarsal (plantar aspect) and lateral aspect of the medial cuneiform	Superficial fibular nerve (L5-S2)	Anterior tibial and fibular arteries	Eversion and plantarflexion of the ankle
Fibularis brevis	Inferior two-thirds of the lateral aspect of the fibula	Tuberosity of the fifth metatarsal (dorsal aspect)	Superficial fibular nerve (L5-S2)	Anterior tibial and fibular arteries	Eversion and plantarflexion of the ankle
Gastrocnemius	*Lateral head:* lateral condyle of the femur; *Medial head:* popliteal surface of the femur, superior to the medial condyle	Posterior surface of the calcaneus via the Achilles (calcaneal) tendon	Tibial nerve (S1-S2)	Popliteal and posterior tibial arteries	Plantarflexion of the ankle and flexion of the knee
Soleus	Posterior aspect of the fibular head, superior fourth of the posterior surface of the fibula, soleal line, and medial tibial border	Posterior surface of the calcaneus via the Achilles (calcaneal) tendon	Tibial nerve (S1-S2)	Popliteal, posterior tibial, and fibular arteries	Plantarflexion of the ankle

> *continued*

MUSCLES OF THE LOWER LEG AND SOLE OF THE FOOT > *continued*

Muscle	Origin	Insertion	Innervation	Blood supply	Action
LOWER LEG *continued*					
Plantaris	Inferior end of the lateral supracondylar line of the femur and oblique popliteal ligament	Posterior surface of the calcaneus via the Achilles (calcaneal) tendon	Tibial nerve (L5-S1	Popliteal artery	Assistance in plantarflexion of the ankle
Flexor digitorum longus	Medial aspect of the posterior tibia inferior to soleal line and fascia covering tibialis posterior	Base of the distal phalanges of digits 2 to 4 (plantar aspect)	Tibial nerve (L5-S2)	Posterior tibial artery	Flexion of digits 2 to 4, plantarflexion of the ankle, and support of the longitudinal arches of foot
Flexor hallucis longus	Inferior two-thirds of the posterior aspect of the fibula and distal part of the interosseous membrane	Base of the distal phalanx of the first digit (plantar aspect)	Tibial nerve (L5-S2)	Fibular artery	Flexion of first digit, support of medial longitudinal arches of the foot, weak plantarflexion of the ankle
Tibialis posterior	Interosseous membrane, posterior tibia inferior to the soleal line, and posterior surface of the fibula	Navicular tuberosity, cuneiforms, cuboid, and bases of metatarsals 2 to 4	Tibial nerve (L4-L5)	Fibular artery	Plantarflexion of the ankle, inversion of the foot, and support of the medial arches of the foot
SOLE OF THE FOOT					
Abductor hallucis brevis	Medial tubercle of the calcaneus, plantar aponeurosis, and flexor retinaculum	Medial aspect of the proximal phalanx of digit 1	Medial plantar nerve (S1-S2)	Medial plantar and first plantar metatarsal arteries	Abduction and flexion of digit 1
Abductor digiti minimi	Medial and lateral tubercles of the calcaneus and plantar aponeurosis	Lateral aspect of the proximal phalanx of digit 5	Lateral plantar nerve (S1-S2)	Medial and lateral plantar arteries and plantar digital arteries	Abduction and flexion of digit 5
Flexor digitorum brevis	Medial tubercle of the calcaneus and plantar aponeurosis	Both sides of the middle phalanges of digits 2 to 5 via tendons of the flexor digitorum longus	Medial plantar nerve (S1-S2	Medial and lateral plantar arteries and plantar digital arteries	Flexion of digits 2 to 5

Muscle	Origin	Insertion	Innervation	Blood supply	Action
Quadratus plantae	Plantar surface of the calcaneus	Tendons of the flexor digitorum longus (posterior lateral margins)	Lateral plantar nerves (S1-S3)	Medial and lateral plantar arteries	Assistance to the flexor digitorum longus in flexion of digits
Lumbricals	Tendons of the flexor digitorum longus	Extensor expansions of digits 2 to 5	Medial and lateral plantar nerves (S2-S3)	Lateral plantar artery and plantar metatarsal arteries	Flexion of the metatarso-phalangeal (MTP) joints, extension of the interpha-langeal (IP) joints
Flexor hallucis brevis	Plantar surfaces of the cuboid and lateral cuneiform	Medial and lateral aspect of the proximal phalanx of digit 1	Medial plantar nerve (S1-S2)	Medial plantar artery and first plantar metatarsal artery	Flexion of digit 1 (MTP joint)
Flexor digiti minimi brevis	Base of metatarsal 5	Proximal phalanx of digit 5	Lateral plantar nerve (S2-S3)	Lateral plantar artery and plantar digital artery to fifth digit	Flexion of digit 5 (MTP joint)
Adductor hallucis	Metatarsals 2 to 4 and ligament surrounding the MTP joints	Lateral aspect of the proximal phalanx of digit 1	Lateral plantar nerve (S2-S3)	Medial plantar and first plantar metatarsal arteries	Adduction of digit 1
Plantar interossei	Bases of the medial sides of metatarsals 3 to 5	Medial sides of the bases of the proximal phalanges of digits 3 to 5	Lateral plantar nerve (S2-S3)	Lateral plantar artery and plantar digital arteries	Adduction of digits 2 to 4, flexion of MTP joints, and extension of IP joints
Dorsal interossei	Adjacent sides of metatarsals 1 to 5	*First:* medial side of the proximal phalanx of digit 2 *Second to fourth:* lateral sides of digits 2 to 4	Lateral plantar nerve (S2-S3)	Arcuate artery, dorsal and plantar metatarsal arteries	Abduction of digits 2 to 4, flexion of MTP joints, and extension of IP joints

Zone I: Medial Aspect of the Ankle

Medial Collateral Ligament (Deltoid Ligament)

Positions

- Patient: long sitting, with the ankle slightly off the table
- Clinician: sitting or standing at the end of the table, facing the patient, on the side being palpated

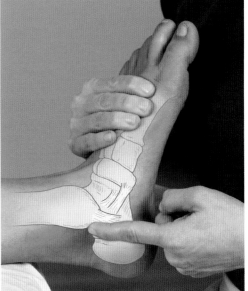

Instructions

- Palpate the proximal attachments of the anterior tibiotalar ligament, posterior tibiotalar ligament, tibionavicular ligament, and the tibiocalcaneal ligament at the medial malleolus (key reference structure).
- Move one finger inferiorly off the medial malleolus to palpate the posterior tibiotalar ligament (left hand pictured).
- Move your finger posteriorly off the medial malleolus to palpate the tibiocalcaneal ligament.
- Move your finger inferiorly and anteriorly off the medial malleolus to palpate the tibionavicular ligament.
- Move your finger anteriorly off the medial malleolus to palpate the anterior tibiotalar ligament.

Notes

- You may want to place the patient's ankle into slight passive eversion, which will place the ligaments on stretch, thereby increasing tension and making the palpation somewhat easier. The deltoid ligament is not as easy to palpate as the ligaments on the lateral side of the ankle.
- These ligaments should feel like a tight cord when assessed individually.

CLINICAL PEARL

While most ankle sprains are inversion sprains, some patients will experience an eversion ankle sprain. It is important that you know how to assess the integrity of the ligaments on the medial side of the ankle along with palpation of the medial malleolus for possible bony tenderness, a potential sign for fracture.[10]

Flexor Retinaculum

Return to the medial malleolus to reorient yourself for palpating the structures in the flexor retinaculum, a space bordered by the medial malleolus anteriorly and the Achilles tendon posteriorly.

Positions

- Patient: supine, with the ankle slightly off the table
- Clinician: sitting or standing at the end of the table, facing the patient, on the side being palpated

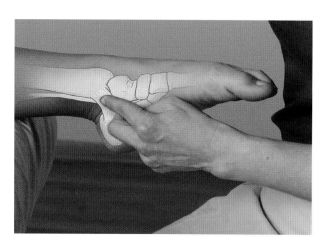

Instructions

- Palpate the medial malleolus.
- To palpate the tibialis posterior, move one finger slightly posterior to the medial malleolus.
- To confirm palpation, have the patient plantarflex and invert the ankle. You should feel the tendon contract under your finger.
- To palpate the flexor digitorum longus, continue slightly posterior to the tibialis posterior.
- To confirm palpation, have the patient perform resisted flexion of digits 2 to 5 (right hand pictured). You should feel the tendon contract under your finger (left hand pictured).

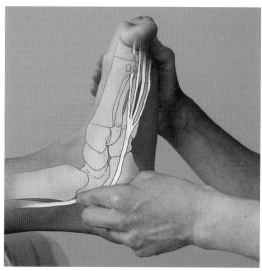

- To palpate the posterior tibial artery, continue slightly posterior to the flexor digitorum longus.
- To confirm palpation, slightly invert the ankle passively and assess for the posterior tibial pulse by applying gentle pressure using one or two fingers.

- To palpate the flexor hallucis longus, continue slightly posterior to the posterior tibial artery.
- To confirm palpation, have the patient perform resisted flexion of the first digit (right hand pictured). You may be able to feel the tendon contract under your fingers (left hand pictured). The flexor hallucis longus is extremely deep and difficult, if not impossible, to palpate.

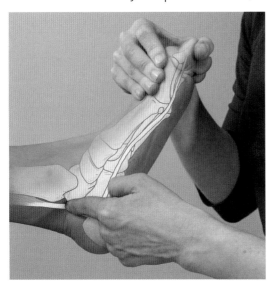
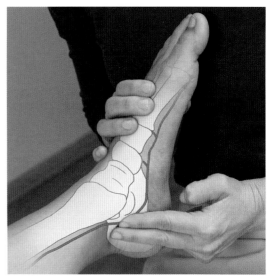

Notes

- The posterior tibial pulse is not the easiest pulse to palpate and therefore should only be assessed in a non-weight-bearing position and with the soft tissues on slack.

- While assessing the posterior tibial pulse, remember that the tibial nerve is directly posterior and lateral to the posterior tibial artery. Keep in mind that while not directly palpable, the tibial nerve travels with the posterior tibial artery and vein. Together they make up the "A Very Nervous" portion of the mnemonic for the structures in the flexor retinaculum: Tom, Dick, and A Very Nervous Harry.

- During palpation of structures around the medial malleolus, keep in mind that just anterior to the medial malleolus is the great saphenous vein, an important vein in the lower extremity that travels proximally into the medial aspect of the groin before joining other proximal veins and subsequently returning blood to the inferior vena cava. This vein often becomes varicose in older people.

CLINICAL PEARL

Tenderness to palpation posterior to the medial malleolus can be a sign of posterior tibialis tendinopathy. If this is the case, there is usually pain with resisted inversion and plantarflexion during the clinical examination.[11]

Zone II: Dorsal Aspect of the Foot Between the Malleoli

Tibialis Anterior

Positions

- Patient: long sitting, with the ankle slightly off the table
- Clinician: sitting or standing at the end of the table, facing the patient, on the side being palpated

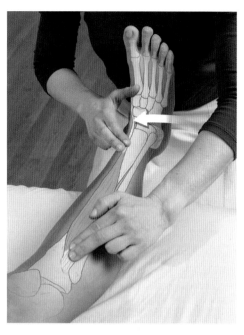

Instructions

- Using two fingers, palpate the origin of the tibialis anterior at the lateral border of the tibia (left hand pictured).
- Palpate the insertion at the medial aspect of the medial cuneiform and the first metatarsal (right hand picture).
- To confirm palpation, have the patient perform resisted ankle dorsiflexion. You should feel the muscle and tendon contract under your fingers.
- Palpate the entire muscle and tendon from origin to insertion.

Notes

- This tendon is the largest and most prominent of the anterior compartment tendons and is located most medially.
- The clinician may be able to assess the entire length of the tibialis anterior more easily if the insertion tendon is identified first and then subsequently followed proximally to the origin.
- The clinician should encourage the patient to avoid extending the toes during contraction of the tibialis anterior because the patient may compensate with the extensor digitorum longus.

CLINICAL PEARL

Weakness of the tibialis anterior caused by damage of the deep fibular nerve or compression of the L4 nerve root can cause a foot-slap gait pattern during the stance phase of gait or a foot drop during the swing phase of gait.[1,3]

Extensor Hallucis Longus

Positions

- Patient: long sitting, with the ankle slightly off the table
- Clinician: sitting or standing at the end of the table, facing the patient, on the side being palpated

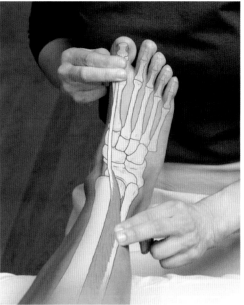

Instructions

- Using two fingers, palpate the origin of the extensor hallucis longus at the proximal, anterior aspect of the fibula (left hand pictured).
- Palpate the insertion on the distal phalanx of the first digit (right hand pictured).
- To confirm palpation, have the patient perform resisted great toe extension. You should feel the muscle and tendon contract under your fingers.
- Palpate the entire muscle and tendon from origin to insertion.

Notes

- This tendon lies immediately lateral to the tibialis anterior tendon.
- The clinician may be able to assess the entire length of the extensor hallucis longus more easily if the insertion tendon is identified first and then subsequently followed proximally to the origin.
- The clinician can encourage the patient to attempt to isolate movement to the big toe only.

Extensor Digitorum Longus

Positions

- Patient: long sitting, with the ankle slightly off the table
- Clinician: sitting or standing at the end of the table, facing the patient, on the side being palpated

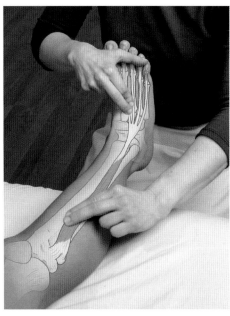

Instructions

- Using two fingers, palpate the origin of the extensor digitorum longus at the lateral border of the tibia and anterior aspect of the fibula (left hand pictured).
- Palpate the insertion at the dorsal aspect of the middle and distal phalanges of digits 2 to 5.
- To confirm palpation, have the patient perform resisted toe extension. You should feel the muscle and tendons contract under your fingers.
- Palpate the entire muscle and all tendons from origin to insertion.

Notes

- This tendon lies lateral to the extensor hallucis longus.
- The clinician may be able to assess the entire length of the extensor digitorum longus more easily if the insertion tendon is identified first and then subsequently followed proximally.
- In this case, the clinician can encourage the patient to attempt to isolate movement to the toes only, using the extensor digitorum longus.

Dorsalis Pedis Pulse

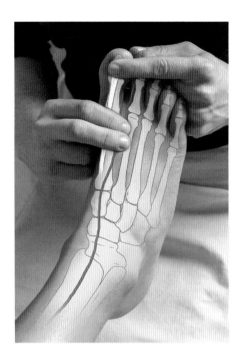

Positions
- Patient: long sitting, with the ankle slightly off the table
- Clinician: sitting or standing at the end of the table, facing the patient, on the side being palpated

Instructions
- Palpate the first and second metatarsals.
- Palpate the tendon of the extensor hallucis longus.
- Move two fingers lateral to the tendon, between metatarsals 1 and 2.
- Apply gentle pressure with the pads of your second and third digits to assess the pulse (right hand pictured).

Notes
- The dorsalis pedis artery is located between the tendons of the extensor hallucis longus and the extensor digitorum longus.
- Palpation of the dorsalis pedis pulse is much easier than assessing for the posterior tibial pulse because this structure is more superficial.
- This pulse may be absent in some people; therefore, while a comparison to the other side is always needed, it is particularly important in this case.

Zone III: Lateral Aspect of the Ankle

Lateral Collateral Ligament

Positions

- Patient: long sitting, with the ankle slightly off the table
- Clinician: sitting or standing at the end of the table, facing the patient, on the side being palpated

Instructions

- Palpate the proximal attachments of the anterior talofibular ligament, calcaneofibular ligament, and posterior talofibular ligament at the lateral malleolus (key reference structure).

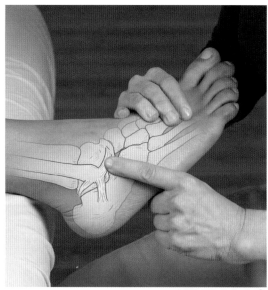

VIDEO 12.4 ►

- Move one finger anteriorly off the lateral malleolus to palpate the anterior talofibular ligament (left hand pictured).
- Move your finger inferiorly off the lateral malleolus to palpate the calcaneofibular ligament. It often inserts posterior to the peroneal tubercle.
- Move your finger posteriorly off the lateral malleolus to palpate the posterior talofibular ligament. This is the strongest of the ligaments on the lateral aspect of the ankle and predominantly functions to prevent anterior displacement of the fibula on the talus.

Notes

- The clinician may want to passively place the ankle into inversion, putting the ligaments on stretch, to make the palpation easier.
- These ligaments should feel like a tight cord when assessed individually.

CLINICAL PEARL

When managing lateral ankle sprains, clinicians often make the mistake of palpating only the anterior talofibular ligament. It is important to evaluate all the ligaments of the ankle because different grades of sprains involve other ligaments. A grade I inversion ankle sprain involves only the anterior talofibular ligament. A grade II inversion ankle sprain involves both the anterior talofibular ligament and the calcaneofibular ligament. A grade III inversion ankle sprain involves all three ligaments.[12]

Fibularis Longus and Brevis

Positions

- Patient: side-lying, with the ankle slightly off the table
- Clinician: sitting or standing, facing the patient, on the side being palpated

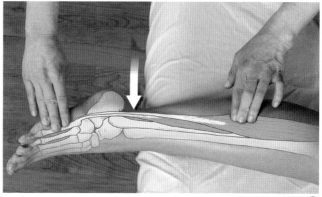

VIDEO 12.5 ▶

Instructions

- Starting from the proximal, lateral tibia, palpate the muscle bellies as a group using three fingers (left hand pictured).
- To confirm palpation, have the patient perform resisted ankle eversion (right hand pictured). You should feel a large contraction under your fingers.

Notes

- The clinician should make every effort to follow the fibularis brevis down to its insertion on the tuberosity of the fifth metatarsal. It hugs the lateral malleolus as it travels distally toward its insertion.
- The fibularis longus travels just posterior to the fibularis brevis. As these tendons pass the calcaneus, they are separated by the peroneal tubercle.

CLINICAL PEARL

These muscles are extremely important following an inversion ankle sprain. Because passive stability is now lost, it is necessary to increase the strength and dynamic control of these muscles during functional activities. It is common for these muscles and their tendons to be irritated and tender after forcefully contracting during an inversion ankle sprain. Despite this anatomical and kinesiological theoretical construct for targeting these muscles after an inversion ankle sprain, the literature supporting this theory is scarce and instead emphasizes the importance of the strength in the dorsiflexors following an inversion ankle sprain. Clinicians should consider both groups of muscles in the formal rehabilitation of people with lateral ankle sprains.[13] In addition, these tendons are covered by a tendon sheath (peroneal retinaculum) that can become inflamed (tenosynovitis) with overuse injuries. The tendons themselves can also become problematic, leading to peroneal (fibularis) tendinopathy.[14]

Extensor Digitorum Brevis

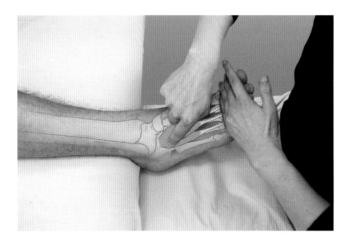

Positions

- Patient: long sitting, with the ankle slightly off the table
- Clinician: sitting or standing at the end of the table, facing the patient, on the side being palpated

Instructions

- Palpate the lateral malleolus.
- Move one or two fingers just anterior into the region of the sinus tarsi.
- To confirm palpation, have the patient perform resisted toe extension (left hand pictured). You should feel the contraction of the extensor digitorum brevis (right hand pictured).

Zone IV: Posterior Aspect of the Ankle

Gastrocnemius

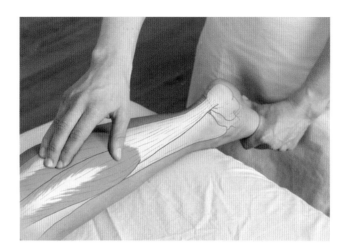

Positions
- Patient: prone, with the ankle slightly off the table
- Clinician: sitting or standing, facing the patient, on the side being palpated

Instructions
- Palpate the entire posterior region of the calf using three fingers (right hand pictured).
- To confirm palpation, have the patient perform resisted ankle plantarflexion (left hand pictured). You should feel a large contraction under your fingers.
- Palpate the muscle from origin to its insertion via the Achilles tendon on the posterior aspect of the calcaneus (key reference structure).

Note
Because the gastrocnemius is a two-joint muscle, ankle dorsiflexion may be limited when the knee is extended. Dorsiflexion range of motion needs to be assessed with the knee both flexed and extended.

Soleus

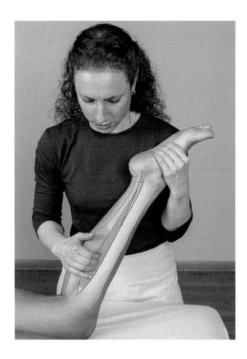

Positions
- Patient: prone, with the knee flexed to approximately 70°
- Clinician: sitting or standing, facing the patient, on the side being palpated

Instructions
- Palpate the gastrocnemius.
- Move three fingers deep to, and to the sides of, the gastrocnemius (right hand pictured).
- To confirm palpation, have the patient perform resisted ankle plantarflexion (left hand pictured). You should feel a subtle contraction under your fingers.

Notes
- You may be able to differentiate between the gastrocnemius and soleus by palpating the soleus more distally and then working your way proximally.
- The gastrocnemius and soleus have a common insertion on the Achilles tendon, the thickest and strongest tendon in the body.
- When the Achilles tendon is torn, the clinician will be able to palpate a defect in the continuity of the Achilles tendon.

Retrocalcaneal Bursa

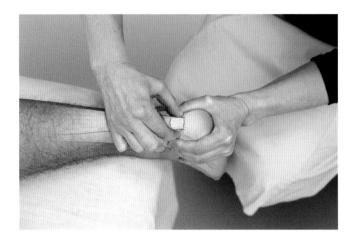

Positions
- Patient: prone, with the ankle slightly off the table
- Clinician: sitting or standing at the end of the table, facing the patient, on the side being palpated

Instructions
- Palpate the calcaneus.
- The retrocalcaneal bursa is between the anterior aspect of the Achilles tendon and the superior aspect of the calcaneus. This bursa can be palpated when the clinician pinches (pincer grasp) the soft tissues anterior to the Achilles tendon (right hand pictured).

CLINICAL PEARL

Any thickening, swelling, tenderness to palpation, or a combination of these findings may be indicative of bursitis of either the retrocalcaneal or calcaneal bursa.[15]

Calcaneal Bursa

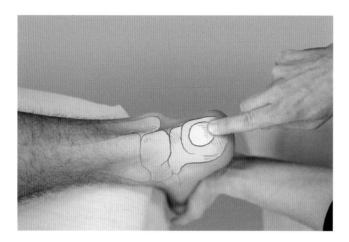

Positions
- Patient: prone, with the ankle slightly off the table
- Clinician: sitting or standing at the end of the table, facing the patient, on the side being palpated

Instructions
- Palpate the calcaneus using one finger.
- The calcaneal bursa is located between the insertion of the Achilles tendon and the skin. This bursa can be palpated when the clinician lifts the skin up posterior to the Achilles tendon (right hand pictured).

CLINICAL PEARL
Any thickening, swelling, tenderness to palpation, or a combination of these findings may be indicative of bursitis of either the retrocalcaneal or calcaneal bursa.[15]

Zone V: Plantar Aspect of the Foot

Plantar Fascia

Positions

- Patient: long sitting, with the ankle slightly off the table
- Clinician: sitting or standing at the end of the table, facing the patient, on the side being palpated

Instructions

- Passively dorsiflex the ankle and extend digits 1 to 5 (right hand pictured).
- Using two fingers, palpate the medial tubercle of the calcaneus (left hand pictured).
- Follow the plantar fascia from the medial tubercle of the calcaneus to its insertion at the metatarsal heads of digits 1 to 5.

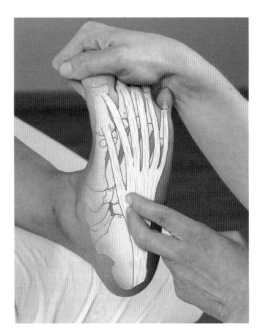

Note

The intrinsic muscles of the sole of the foot are deep to the plantar fascia. Due to thickness of the fascia, it is extremely difficult to palpate each muscle individually. However, certain muscles, such as the abductor hallucis brevis and abductor digiti minimi, can be identified. In addition, the dorsal interossei are palpable between the shafts of the metatarsals.

CLINICAL PEARL

Plantar fasciitis is a common inflammatory or degenerative condition of the plantar fascia and affects many people who spend long hours on their feet. In addition, shortness of the gastrocnemius–soleus complex, plantar fascia, or other more proximal two-joint muscles, along with intrinsic muscle weakness, a lack of dorsiflexion, and other factors may all increase the chances of developing plantar fasciitis.[16,17]

Abductor Hallucis Brevis

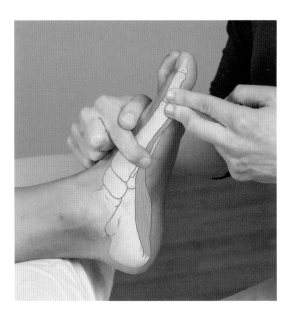

Positions

- Patient: long sitting, with the ankle slightly off the table
- Clinician: sitting or standing at the end of the table, facing the patient, on the side being palpated

Instructions

- Palpate the origin of the abductor hallucis brevis at the medial tubercle of the calcaneus.
- Palpate the insertion at the medial aspect of the proximal phalanx of digit 1.
- Follow the fibers from origin to insertion using one finger (right hand pictured).
- To confirm palpation, have the patient perform resisted abduction of digit 1 (left hand pictured).

Abductor Digiti Minimi

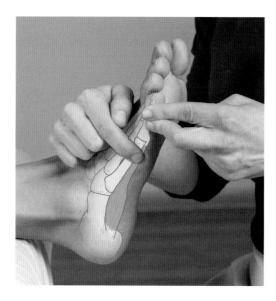

Positions

- Patient: long sitting, with the ankle slightly off the table
- Clinician: sitting or standing at the end of the table, facing the patient, on the side being palpated

Instructions

- Palpate the origin of the abductor digiti minimi at the lateral tubercle of the calcaneus.
- Palpate the insertion at the lateral aspect of the proximal phalanx of digit 5.
- Follow the fibers from origin to insertion using one finger (right hand pictured).
- To confirm palpation, have the patient perform resisted abduction of digit 5 (left hand pictured).

Dorsal Interossei

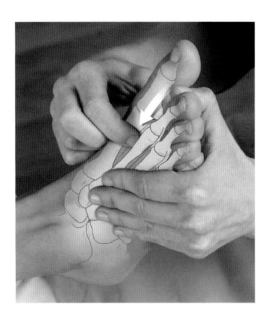

Positions

- Patient: long sitting, with the ankle slightly off the table
- Clinician: sitting or standing at the end of the table, facing the patient, on the side being palpated

Instructions

- Palpate metatarsals 1 and 2 on the dorsal aspect of the foot.
- Place the pad of one finger between the first and second metatarsals (right hand pictured).
- To confirm palpation of the first dorsal interossei, have the patient perform resisted abduction of digit 2 (left thumb pictured).
- Follow the same instructions to palpate the other dorsal interossei

Note

The midline of the foot is the second digit. Therefore, digit 2 can abduct toward the big toe (performed by the first dorsal interossei) or abduct away from the big toe (performed by the second dorsal interossei).

Case Study

History

A 17-year-old male is referred to you by his coach, having "landed wrong" after going for a rebound during a game earlier that day. The patient reports landing on another player's foot and twisting his left ankle. He felt a sharp pain on the outside of his ankle and fell to the floor. He had trouble putting weight on his foot and had to be helped off the court. The trainer at the game iced his ankle, applied an ace wrap, and gave him a pair of crutches. The patient lives in a four-story house with his family and dog. He is the starting point guard for his high school team and is being actively recruited by some Division I schools.

- Based on the subjective information only, what are the three most likely diagnoses?

Examination

Past medical history	Osgood-Schlatter disease at 14 years old
Medication	Denies taking medication, vitamins, or supplements
Observation	Diffuse swelling of the lateral aspect of the left ankle Ace wrap around his left ankle
Active range of motion	Dorsiflexion = 0° (neutral), plantarflexion = 0° to 30°, inversion = 0° to 5°, eversion = 0° to 10°
Passive range of motion	Same as for active
Manual muscle testing	Dorsiflexors 4/5, plantarflexors 2+/5 (with pain), inversion 4/5, eversion 3/5 2° to pain (all within available range)
Special tests	Positive anterior drawer test Negative external rotation stress test Negative lower leg squeeze test
Other	Patient ambulating with bilateral axillary crutches (minimal weight-bearing on left lower extremity)

- Based on the subjective and objective information together, what are the two most likely diagnoses? Give your rationale for eliminating the third diagnosis.
- What structures should you palpate on this patient based on your differential diagnoses?
- Given all the information presented, what would you expect to find on palpation of those structures?

Case Solution and Discussion

Potential Diagnoses Based on History

- Ankle fracture
- High ankle sprain (syndesmotic)
- Lateral ankle sprain

Potential Diagnoses Based on History and Examination

- High ankle sprain (syndesmotic)
- Lateral ankle sprain

Ankle fracture: The lack of ecchymosis on the lateral ankle, in addition to the ability to bear some weight on the ankle, is not suggestive of an ankle fracture. However, this cannot be completely ruled out at this point of the exam.

Structures to Be Palpated

- Medial malleolus
- Lateral malleolus
- Tuberosity of the fifth metatarsal
- Distal 2.5 inches (about 6 centimeters) of the tibia and fibula
- Anterior talofibular ligament
- Calcaneofibular ligament
- Posterior talofibular ligament

Note: The decision to refer the patient for radiographs relies heavily on the palpatory exam, and the possibility of a fracture cannot be completely ruled out until that has been completed. Therefore, the bony structures of the distal ankle that are listed remain part of the palpatory exam to enable you to make this decision.

Palpation Findings

- Significant tenderness to palpation of the left anterior talofibular ligament and calcaneofibular ligament
- Tenderness to palpation throughout the left fibularis longus and brevis

Clinical Reasoning

- High ankle sprain (syndesmotic): The patient's report of the mechanism of injury, location of pain, and difficulty bearing weight may be indicative of a syndesmotic sprain. However, the negative special tests performed for a syndesmotic sprain allow this diagnosis to be ruled out.

- Lateral ankle sprain: The patient's report of the mechanism of injury, the location of pain, and the difficulty in bearing weight can be indicative of a lateral ankle sprain. Diffuse swelling, and often ecchymosis (not present in this case), are common with lateral ankle sprains, as are tenderness to palpation of the anterior talofibular ligament and calcaneofibular ligament, along with the positive anterior drawer test. Collectively, these findings confirm this diagnosis.

Case Study Questions

1. What information do the palpation findings of the case give the clinician? How can this information be incorporated in the clinical decision-making process?
2. Think about how the examination findings (subjective and objective) lead to the differential diagnosis. What might you do differently?
3. Discuss the treatment approach for a young patient with a lateral ankle sprain.

CHAPTER REVIEW QUESTIONS

1. List the ligaments on the lateral side of the ankle.
2. List the ligaments on the medial side of the ankle.
3. List the structures found in the anterior compartment of the lower leg.
4. List the structures in the posterior compartment of the lower leg.
5. Describe the blood supply to the lower leg and foot regions.
6. Describe the function of the plantar fascia.

References

Chapter 1

1. Beaman FD, Kransdorf MJ, Andrews TR, Murphey MD, Arcara LK, Keeling JH. Superficial soft-tissue masses: Analysis, diagnosis, and differential considerations. *Radiographics*. 2007;27(2):509-523. doi:10.1148/rg.272065082

2. Yang SW, Geng ZJ, Ma K, Sun XY, Fu XB. Comparison of the histological morphology between normal skin and scar tissue. *J Huazhong Univ Sci Technolog Med Sci*. 2016;36(2):265-269. doi:10.1007/s11596-016-1578-7

3. Gerwin RD, Shannon S, Hong CZ, Hubbard D, Gevirtz R. Interrater reliability in myofascial trigger point examination. *Pain*. 1997;69(1-2):65-73.

4. Njoo KH, Van der Does E. The occurrence and inter-rater reliability of myofascial trigger points in the quadratus lumborum and gluteus medius: A prospective study in non-specific low back pain patients and controls in general practice. *Pain*. 1994;58(3):317-323.

5. Mehta P, Rand EB, Visco CJ, Wyss J. Resident accuracy of musculoskeletal palpation with ultrasound verification. *J Ultrasound Med*. 2018;37(7):1719-1724. doi:10.1002/jum.14523

6. Azer SA. The place of surface anatomy in the medical literature and undergraduate anatomy textbooks. *Anat Sci Educ*. 2013;6(6):415-432. doi:10.1002/ase.1368

7. Davis A, Wilhelm MP, Pendergrass TJ, et al. Anatomical relationship of palmar carpal bone landmarks used in locating the lunate and capitate during palpation: A cadaveric investigation. *J Hand Ther*. 2019;32(4):463-469. doi:10.1016/j.jht.2018.02.002

8. Levine D, Walker JR, Marcellin-Little DJ, Goulet R, Ru H. Detection of skin temperature differences using palpation by manual physical therapists and lay individuals. *J Man Manip Ther*. 2018;26(2):97-101. doi:10.1080/10669817.2018.1427908

9. Dvorak J, Dvorak V. Genral principles of palpation. In: Gilliar W, Greenman P, eds. *Manual Medicine Diagnostics*. 2nd ed. Thieme; 1990:71-75.

10. Dyson M, Suckling J. Stimulation of tissue repair by ultrasound: A survey of the mechanisms involved. *Physiotherapy*. 1978;64(4):105-108.

11. Hsieh CY, Hong CZ, Adams AH, et al. Interexaminer reliability of the palpation of trigger points in the trunk and lower limb muscles. *Arch Phys Med Rehabil*. 2000;81(3):258-264.

12. Beynon AM, Hebert JJ, Walker BF. The interrater reliability of static palpation of the thoracic spine for eliciting tenderness and stiffness to test for a manipulable lesion. *Chiropr Man Therap*. 2018;26:49. doi:10.1186/s12998-018-0218-7

13. Ponce BA, Archie AT, Watson SL, et al. Sternoclavicular joint palpation pain: The shoulder's Waddell sign? *J Shoulder Elbow Surg*. 2018;27(7):e203-e209. doi:10.1016/j.jse.2018.02.056

14. Beckenkamp PR, Lin CC, Macaskill P, Michaleff ZA, Maher CG, Moseley AM. Diagnostic accuracy of the Ottawa ankle and midfoot rules: A systematic review with meta-analysis. *Br J Sports Med*. 2017;51(6):504-510. doi:10.1136/bjsports-2016-096858

15. Frymann V. Palpation, its study in the workshop. *AAO Yearbook*. 1963:16-31.

16. Keating J, Matyas TA, Bach TM. The effect of training on physical therapists' ability to apply specified forces of palpation. *Phys Ther*. 1993;73(1):45-53.

17. Kothari SF, Kothari M, Zambra RF, Baad-Hansen L, Svensson P. Standardization of muscle palpation: Methodological considerations. *Clin J Pain*. 2014;30(2):174-182. doi:10.1097/AJP.0b013e31828c893d

18. Maitland G, Hengeveld E, Banks K, English K. *Maitland's Vertebral Manipulation*. 7th ed. Elsevier; 2006.

19. Moore H, Nichols C, Engles M. Tissue reponse. In: Donatelli RA, Wooden MJ, eds. *Orthopaedic Physical Therapy*. 4th ed. Elsevier; 2010.

20. Childs DR, Murthy AS. Overview of wound healing and management. *Surg Clin North Am*. 2017;97(1):189-207. doi:10.1016/j.suc.2016.08.013

21. Agur AM, Dalley AR. *Moore's Essential Clinical Anatomy*. 6th ed. Lippincott, Williams, & Wilkins; 2019.

22. Magee D. *Orthopedic Physical Assessment*. 6th ed. Elsevier; 2014.

23. Sturgill LP, Snyder-Mackler L, Manal TJ, Axe MJ. Interrater reliability of a clinical scale to assess knee joint effusion. *J Orthop Sports Phys Ther*. 2009;39(12):845-849. doi:10.2519/jospt.2009.3143

24. Johnson GS. Soft tissue mobilization. In: Donatelli RA, Wooden MJ, eds. *Orthopaedic Physical Therapy*. 4th ed. Elsevier; 2010:612-613.

25. Waugh EJ. Lateral epicondylalgia or epicondylitis: What's in a name? *J Orthop Sports Phys Ther*. 2005;35(4):200-202. doi:10.2519/jospt.2005.0104

26. Ling SK, Lui TH. Posterior tibial tendon dysfunction: An overview. *Open Orthop J*. 2017;11:714-723. doi:10.2174/1874325001711010714

27. Frank CB. Ligament structure, physiology and function. *J Musculoskelet Neuronal Interact*. 2004;4(2):199-201.

28. Schultz G, Rotatori DS, Clark W. EGF and TGF-alpha in wound healing and repair. *J Cell Biochem*. 1991;45(4):346-352. doi:10.1002/jcb.240450407

29. Birch R, Misra P, Stewart MP, et al. Nerve injuries sustained during warfare: part II: Outcomes. *J Bone Joint Surg Br*. 2012;94(4):529-535. doi:10.1302/0301-620X.94B4.28488

30. Elliott M, Coventry A. Critical care: The eight vital signs of patient monitoring. *Br J Nurs*. 2012;21(10):621-625. doi:10.12968/bjon.2012.21.10.621

Chapter 2

1. Nassif NJ, Al-Salleeh F, Al-Admawi M. The prevalence and treatment needs of symptoms and signs of temporomandibular disorders among young adult males. *J Oral Rehabil*. 2003;30(9):944-950.

2. Shaffer SM, Brismee JM, Sizer PS, Courtney CA. Temporomandibular disorders. Part 1: anatomy and examination/diagnosis. *J Man Manip Ther*. 2014;22(1):2-12. doi:10.1179/2042618613Y.0000000060

3. Shaffer SM, Brismee JM, Sizer PS, Courtney CA. Temporomandibular disorders. Part 2: conservative management. *J Man Manip Ther*. 2014;22(1):13-23. doi:10.1179/2042618613Y.0000000061

4. Agur AM, Dalley AR. *Moore's Essential Clinical Anatomy*. 6th ed. Lippincott, Williams, & Wilkins; 2019.

5. Murray GM, Bhutada M, Peck CC, Phanachet I, Sae-Lee D, Whittle T. The human lateral pterygoid muscle. *Arch Oral Biol*. 2007;52(4):377-380. doi:10.1016/j.archoralbio.2006.10.002

6. Kuroda M, Otonari-Yamamoto M, Araki K. Evaluation of lateral pterygoid muscles in painful temporomandibular joints by signal intensity on fluid-attenuated inversion recovery images. *Oral Radiol*. 2018;34(1):17-23. doi:10.1007/s11282-017-0272-1

7. Neumann DA. *Kinesiology of the Musculoskeletal System: Foundations for Rehabilitation*. 3rd ed. Elsevier; 2017.

8. Okeson JP. *Management of Temporomandibular Disorders and Occlusion*. 6th ed. Elsevier; 2005.

9. Manfredini D, Tognini F, Zampa V, Bosco M. Predictive value of clinical findings for temporomandibular joint effusion. *Oral Surg Oral Med Oral Pathol Oral Radiol Endod*. 2003;96(5):521-526. doi:10.1016/S107921040300475X

Chapter 3

1. Pegreffi F, Paladini P, Campi F, Porcellini G. Conservative management of rotator cuff tear. *Sports Med Arthrosc Rev*. 2011;19(4):348-353. doi:10.1097/JSA.0b013e3182148dc6

2. Picavet HS, Schouten JS. Musculoskeletal pain in the Netherlands: Prevalences, consequences and risk groups, the DMC(3)-study. *Pain*. 2003;102(1-2):167-178.

3. Neumann DA. *Kinesiology of the Musculoskeletal System: Foundations for Rehabilitation*. 3rd ed. Elsevier; 2017.

4. Agur AM, Dalley AR. *Moore's Essential Clinical Anatomy*. 6th ed. Lippincott, Williams, & Wilkins; 2019.

5. Thompson JC. *Netter's Concise Orthopaedic Anatomy*. 2nd ed. Elsevier; 2016.

6. Burkart AC, Debski RE. Anatomy and function of the glenohumeral ligaments in anterior shoulder instability. *Clin Orthop Relat Res*. 2002;(400):32-39. doi:10.1097/00003086-200207000-00005

7. Tillander B, Norlin R. Intraoperative measurements of the subacromial distance. *Arthroscopy*. 2002;18(4):347-352.

8. Shah AA, Butler RB, Sung SY, Wells JH, Higgins LD, Warner JJ. Clinical outcomes of suprascapular nerve decompression. *J Shoulder Elbow Surg*. 2011;20(6):975-982. doi:10.1016/j.jse.2010.10.032

9. Steinmann SP, Wood MB. Pectoralis major transfer for serratus anterior paralysis. *J Shoulder Elbow Surg*. 2003;12(6):555-560. doi:10.1016/S1058274603001745

10. Ludewig PM, Cook TM. Translations of the humerus in persons with shoulder impingement symptoms. *J Orthop Sports Phys Ther*. 2002;32(6):248-259. doi:10.2519/jospt.2002.32.6.248

11. Kibler WB, Sciascia A, Wilkes T. Scapular dyskinesis and its relation to shoulder injury. *J Am Acad Orthop Surg*. 2012;20(6):364-372. doi:10.5435/JAAOS-20-06-364

12. Mattingly GE, Mackarey PJ. Optimal methods for shoulder tendon palpation: A cadaver study. *Phys Ther*. 1996;76(2):166-173. doi:10.1093/ptj/76.2.166

13. Prentice WE. *Principles of Athletic Training: A Guide to Evidence-Based Clinical Practice*. 16th ed. McGraw-Hill; 2017.

14. Waugh EJ. Lateral epicondylalgia or epicondylitis: What's in a name? *J Orthop Sports Phys Ther*. 2005;35(4):200-202. doi:10.2519/jospt.2005.0104

Chapter 4

1. Agur AM, Dalley AR. *Moore's Essential Clinical Anatomy*. 6th ed. Lippincott, Williams, & Wilkins; 2019.

2. Neumann DA. *Kinesiology of the Musculoskeletal System: Foundations for Rehabilitation*. 3rd ed. Elsevier; 2017.

3. Collins CK, Johnson VS, Godwin EM, Pappas E. The reliability and validity of the Saliba postural classification system. *Journal of Manual & Manipulative Therapy*. 2016;24(3):174-181. doi:10.1080/10669817.2016.1138599

4. Kendall F, P., McCreary E, K., Provance P, G., Rodgers M, M., Romani W, A. *Muscles Testing and Function With Posture and Pain*. 5th ed. Lippincott, Williams, & Wilkins; 2005.

5. Bourghli A, Fabre A. Proximal end clavicle fracture from a parachute jumping injury. *Orthop Traumatol Surg Res*. 2012;98(2):238-241. doi:10.1016/j.otsr.2011.09.021

6. Thompson JC. *Netter's Concise Orthopaedic Anatomy*. 2nd ed. Elsevier; 2016.

7. Banerjee R, Waterman B, Padalecki J, Robertson W. Management of distal clavicle fractures. *J Am Acad Orthop Surg*. 2011;19(7):392-401.

8. Lindgren KA, Leino E, Hakola M, Hamberg J. Cervical spine rotation and lateral flexion combined motion in the examination of the thoracic outlet. *Arch Phys Med Rehabil*. 1990;71(5):343-344.

9. Tillander B, Norlin R. Intraoperative measurements of the subacromial distance. *Arthroscopy*. 2002;18(4):347-352.

10. Borstad JD. Measurement of pectoralis minor muscle length: Validation and clinical application. *J Orthop Sports Phys Ther*. 2008;38(4):169-174. doi:10.2519/jospt.2008.2723

11. Lewis JS, Valentine RE. The pectoralis minor length test: A study of the intra-rater reliability and diagnostic accuracy in subjects with and without shoulder symptoms. *BMC Musculoskelet Disord*. 2007;8:64. doi:10.1186/1471-2474-8-64

12. Turgut E, Duzgun I, Baltaci G. Stretching exercises for subacromial impingement syndrome: Effects of 6-week program on shoulder tightness, pain, and disability status. *J Sport Rehabil*. 2018;27(2):132-137. doi:10.1123/jsr.2016-0182

Chapter 5

1. Neumann DA. *Kinesiology of the Musculoskeletal System: Foundations for Rehabilitation*. 3rd ed. Elsevier; 2017.

2. Agur AM, Dalley AR. *Moore's Essential Clinical Anatomy*. 6th ed. Lippincott, Williams, & Wilkins; 2019.

3. Akalin E, El O, Peker O, et al. Treatment of carpal tunnel syndrome with nerve and tendon gliding exercises. *Am J Phys Med Rehabil*. 2002;81(2):108-113.

4. Regan WD, Korinek SL, Morrey BF, An KN. Biomechanical study of ligaments around the elbow joint. *Clin Orthop Relat Res*. 1991;(271):170-179.

5. Moore AR, Fleisig GS, Dugas JR. Ulnar Collateral Ligament Repair. *Orthop Clin North Am*. 2019;50(3):383-389. doi:10.1016/j.ocl.2019.03.005

6. Gonzalez-Iglesias J, Cleland JA, del Rosario Gutierrez-Vega M, Fernandez-de-las-Penas C. Multimodal management of lateral epicondylalgia in rock climbers: A prospective case series. *J Manipulative Physiol Ther*. 2011;34(9):635-642. doi:10.1016/j.jmpt.2011.09.003

7. Kraushaar BS, Nirschl RP. Tendinosis of the elbow (tennis elbow): Clinical features and findings of histological, immunohistochemical, and electron microscopy studies. *J Bone Joint Surg Am*. 1999;81(2):259-278.

8. Camp CL, Fu M, Jahandar H, et al. The lateral collateral ligament complex of the elbow: Quantitative anatomic analysis of the lateral ulnar collateral, radial collateral, and annular ligaments. *J Shoulder Elbow Surg*. 2019;28(4):665-670. doi:10.1016/j.jse.2018.09.019

Chapter 6

1. Neumann DA. *Kinesiology of the Musculoskeletal System: Foundations for Rehabilitation*. 3rd ed. Elsevier; 2017.

2. Agur AM, Dalley AR. *Moore's Essential Clinical Anatomy*. 6th ed. Lippincott, Williams, & Wilkins; 2019.

3. Kitay A, Wolfe SW. Scapholunate instability: Current concepts in diagnosis and management. *J Hand Surg Am*. 2012;37(10):2175-2196. doi:10.1016/j.jhsa.2012.07.035

4. Corella F, Del Cerro M, Ocampos M, Simon de Blas C, Larrainzar-Garijo R. Arthroscopic scapholunate ligament reconstruction, volar and dorsal reconstruction. *Hand Clin*. 2017;33(4):687-707. doi:10.1016/j.hcl.2017.07.019

5. Padua L, Coraci D, Erra C, et al. Carpal tunnel syndrome: Clinical features, diagnosis, and management. *Lancet Neurol*. 2016;15(12):1273-1284. doi:10.1016/S1474-4422(16)30231-9

6. Akalin E, El O, Peker O, et al. Treatment of carpal tunnel syndrome with nerve and tendon gliding exercises. *Am J Phys Med Rehabil*. 2002;81(2):108-113.

7. Fowler JR, Hughes TB. Scaphoid fractures. *Clin Sports Med*. 2015;34(1):37-50. doi:10.1016/j.csm.2014.09.011

8. Ring D, Schnellen A. Patient-centered care of de Quervain's disease. *J Hand Microsurg*. 2009;1(2):68-71. doi:10.1007/s12593-009-0018-3

9. Feldman G, Rozen N, Rubin G. Dupuytren's contracture: Current treatment methods. *Isr Med Assoc J*. 2017;19(10):648-650.

10. Shah A, Rettig M. Trigger finger location and association of comorbidities. *Bull Hosp Jt Dis (2013)*. 2017;75(3):198-200.

Chapter 7

1. Croft PR, Lewis M, Papageorgiou AC, et al. Risk factors for neck pain: A longitudinal study in the general population. *Pain*. 2001;93(3):317-325.

2. Bialosky JE, Bishop MD, George SZ. Regional interdependence: A musculoskeletal examination model whose time has come. *J Orthop Sports Phys Ther*. 2008;38(3):159-160. doi:10.2519/jospt.2008.0201

3. Wainner RS, Whitman JM, Cleland JA, Flynn TW. Regional interdependence: A musculoskeletal examination model whose time has come. *J Orthop Sports Phys Ther*. 2007;37(11):658-660. doi:10.2519/jospt.2007.0110

4. Agur AM, Dalley AR. *Moore's Essential Clinical Anatomy*. 6th ed. Lippincott, Williams, & Wilkins; 2019.

5. Neumann DA. *Kinesiology of the Musculoskeletal System: Foundations for Rehabilitation*. 3rd ed. Elsevier; 2017.

6. Beer A, Treleaven J, Jull G. Can a functional postural exercise improve performance in the cranio-cervical flexion test? A preliminary study. *Man Ther*. 2012;17(3):219-224. doi:10.1016/j.math.2011.12.005

7. Kelly M, Cardy N, Melvin E, Reddin C, Ward C, Wilson F. The craniocervical flexion test: An investigation of performance in young asymptomatic subjects. *Man Ther*. 2013;18(1):83-86. doi:10.1016/j.math.2012.04.008

8. Diab AA. The role of forward head correction in management of adolescent idiopathic scoliotic patients: A randomized controlled trial. *Clin Rehabil*. 2012;26(12):1123-1132. doi:10.1177/0269215512447085

9. Diab AA, Moustafa IM. The efficacy of forward head correction on nerve root function and pain in cervical spondylotic radiculopathy: A randomized trial. *Clin Rehabil*. 2012;26(4):351-361. doi:10.1177/0269215511419536

10. Ulbrich EJ, Aeberhard R, Wetli S, et al. Cervical muscle area measurements in whiplash patients: Acute, 3, and 6 months of follow-up. *J Magn Reson Imaging*. 2012;36(6):1413-1420. doi:10.1002/jmri.23769

Chapter 8

1. Delitto A, George SZ, Van Dillen L, et al. Low back pain. *J Orthop Sports Phys Ther*. 2012;42(4):A1-A57. doi:10.2519/jospt.2012.42.4.A1

2. Hoy D, Bain C, Williams G, et al. A systematic review of the global prevalence of low back pain. *Arthritis Rheum*. 2012;64(6):2028-2037. doi:10.1002/art.34347

3. Walker BF. The prevalence of low back pain: A systematic review of the literature from 1966 to 1998. *J Spinal Disord*. 2000;13(3):205-217.

4. Sueki DG, Cleland JA, Wainner RS. A regional interdependence model of musculoskeletal dysfunction: Research, mechanisms, and clinical implications. *J Man Manip Ther*. 2013;21(2):90-102. doi:10.1179/2042618612Y.0000000027

5. Bialosky JE, Bishop MD, George SZ. Regional interdependence: A musculoskeletal examination model whose time has come. *J Orthop Sports Phys Ther*. 2008;38(3):159-160. doi:10.2519/jospt.2008.0201

6. Wainner RS, Whitman JM, Cleland JA, Flynn TW. Regional interdependence: A musculoskeletal examination model whose time has come. *J Orthop Sports Phys Ther*. 2007;37(11):658-660. doi:10.2519/jospt.2007.0110

7. Neumann DA. *Kinesiology of the Musculoskeletal System: Foundations for Rehabilitation*. 3rd ed. Elsevier; 2017.

8. Goode A, Hegedus EJ, Sizer P, Brismee JM, Linberg A, Cook CE. Three-dimensional movements of the sacroiliac joint: A systematic review of the literature and assessment of clinical utility. *J Man Manip Ther*. 2008;16(1):25-38. doi:10.1179/106698108790818639

9. Vleeming A, Schuenke M. Form and force closure of the sacroiliac joints. *PM&R*. 2019;11:S24-S31. doi:10.1002/pmrj.12205

10. Vleeming A, Schuenke MD, Masi AT, Carreiro JE, Danneels L, Willard FH. The sacroiliac joint: An overview of its anatomy, function and potential clinical implications. *J Anat*. 2012;221(6):537-567. doi:10.1111/j.1469-7580.2012.01564.x

11. Agur AM, Dalley AR. *Moore's Essential Clinical Anatomy*. 6th ed. Lippincott, Williams, & Wilkins; 2019.

12. Cleland JA, Koppenhaver S, Su J. *Netter's Orthopaedic Clinical Examination: An Evidence-Based Approach*. 3rd ed. Elsevier; 2016.

13. Hides JA, Belavy DL, Cassar L, Williams M, Wilson SJ, Richardson CA. Altered response of the anterolateral abdominal muscles to simulated weight-bearing in subjects with low back pain. *Eur Spine J*. 2009;18(3):410-418. doi:10.1007/s00586-008-0827-2

14. Hides JA, Stanton WR, McMahon S, Sims K, Richardson CA. Effect of stabilization training on multifidus muscle cross-sectional area among young elite cricketers with low back pain. *J Orthop Sports Phys Ther*. 2008;38(3):101-108. doi:10.2519/jospt.2008.2658

15. Hodges PW. Is there a role for transversus abdominis in lumbo-pelvic stability? *Man Ther*. 1999;4(2):74-86. doi:10.1054/math.1999.0169

16. Hodges PW, Cholewicki J, Popovich JM, Jr., et al. Building a collaborative model of sacroiliac joint dysfunction and pelvic girdle pain to understand the diverse perspectives of experts. *PM&R*. 2019;11:S11-S23. doi:10.1002/pmrj.12199

17. Hodges PW, Richardson CA. Altered trunk muscle recruitment in people with low back pain with upper limb movement at different speeds. *Arch Phys Med Rehabil*. 1999;80(9):1005-1012.

18. Lee D. *The Pelvic Girdle: An Integration of Clinical Expertise and Research*. 4th ed. Elsevier; 2011.

19. Beynon AM, Hebert JJ, Walker BF. The interrater reliability of static palpation of the thoracic spine for eliciting tenderness and stiffness to test for a manipulable lesion. *Chiropr Man Therap*. 2018;26:49. doi:10.1186/s12998-018-0218-7

20. Chakraverty R, Pynsent P, Isaacs K. Which spinal levels are identified by palpation of the iliac crests and the posterior superior iliac spines? *J Anat*. 2007;210(2):232-236. doi:10.1111/j.1469-7580.2006.00686.x

21. Chakraverty RC, Pynsent PB, Westwood A, Chakraverty JK. Identification of the correct lumbar level using passive intersegmental motion testing. *Anaesthesia*. 2007;62(11):1121-1125. doi:10.1111/j.1365-2044.2007.05189.x

22. Kim HW, Ko YJ, Rhee WI, et al. Interexaminer reliability and accuracy of posterior superior iliac spine and iliac crest palpation for spinal level estimations. *J Manipulative Physiol Ther*. 2007;30(5):386-389. doi:10.1016/j.jmpt.2007.04.005

Chapter 9

1. O'Sullivan P, Caneiro JP, O'Keeffe M, O'Sullivan K. Unraveling the complexity of low back pain. *J Orthop Sports Phys Ther*. 2016;46(11):932-937. doi:10.2519/jospt.2016.0609

2. Gilroy AM. *Anatomy: An Essential Textbook*. 2nd ed. Thieme; 2017.

3. Hides JA, Belavy DL, Cassar L, Williams M, Wilson SJ, Richardson CA. Altered response of the anterolateral abdominal muscles to simulated weight-bearing in subjects with low back pain. *Eur Spine J.* 2009;18(3):410-418. doi:10.1007/s00586-008-0827-2

4. Hides JA, Stanton WR, McMahon S, Sims K, Richardson CA. Effect of stabilization training on multifidus muscle cross-sectional area among young elite cricketers with low back pain. *J Orthop Sports Phys Ther.* 2008;38(3):101-108. doi:10.2519/jospt.2008.2658

5. Hodges PW. Is there a role for transversus abdominis in lumbo-pelvic stability? *Man Ther.* 1999;4(2):74-86. doi:10.1054/math.1999.0169

6. Hodges PW, Cholewicki J, Popovich JM, Jr., et al. Building a collaborative model of sacroiliac joint dysfunction and pelvic girdle pain to understand the diverse perspectives of experts. *PM&R.* 2019;11:S11-S23. doi:10.1002/pmrj.12199

7. Hodges PW, Richardson CA. Altered trunk muscle recruitment in people with low back pain with upper limb movement at different speeds. *Arch Phys Med Rehabil.* 1999;80(9):1005-1012.

8. Moses KP, Banks Jr. JC, Nava PB, Petersen DK. *Atlas of Clinical Gross Anatomy.* 2nd ed. Elsevier; 2013.

9. Vleeming A, de Vries HJ, Mens JM, van Wingerden JP. Possible role of the long dorsal sacroiliac ligament in women with peripartum pelvic pain. *Acta Obstet Gynecol Scand.* 2002;81(5):430-436.

10. Vleeming A, Schuenke M. Form and force closure of the sacroiliac joints. *PM&R.* 2019;11:S24-S31. doi:10.1002/pmrj.12205

11. Vleeming A, Schuenke MD, Masi AT, Carreiro JE, Danneels L, Willard FH. The sacroiliac joint: An overview of its anatomy, function and potential clinical implications. *J Anat.* 2012;221(6):537-567. doi:10.1111/j.1469-7580.2012.01564.x

12. Barral JP. *Visceral Manipulation II.* Eastland Press; 2007.

13. Hazama D, Johnson GS. *Visceral Functional Mobilization.* Institute of Physical Art; 2018.

14. Nielsen OH, Gjorup T, Christensen FN. Gastric emptying rate and small bowel transit time in patients with irritable bowel syndrome determined with ^{99m}Tc-labeled pellets and scintigraphy. *Dig Dis Sci.* 1986;31(12):1287-1291. doi:10.1007/bf01299804

15. Laslett M, Aprill CN, McDonald B, Young SB. Diagnosis of sacroiliac joint pain: Validity of individual provocation tests and composites of tests. *Man Ther.* 2005;10(3):207-218. doi:10.1016/j.math.2005.01.003

Chapter 10

1. Neumann DA. *Kinesiology of the Musculoskeletal System: Foundations for Rehabilitation.* 3rd ed. Elsevier; 2017.

2. Agur AM, Dalley AR. *Moore's Essential Clinical Anatomy.* 6th ed. Lippincott, Williams, & Wilkins; 2019.

3. Vleeming A, Schuenke M. Form and force closure of the sacroiliac joints. *PM&R.* 2019;11:S24-S31. doi:10.1002/pmrj.12205

4. Vleeming A, Schuenke MD, Masi AT, Carreiro JE, Danneels L, Willard FH. The sacroiliac joint: An overview of its anatomy, function and potential clinical implications. *J Anat.* 2012;221(6):537-567. doi:10.1111/j.1469-7580.2012.01564.x

5. Chakraverty R, Pynsent P, Isaacs K. Which spinal levels are identified by palpation of the iliac crests and the posterior superior iliac spines? *J Anat.* 2007;210(2):232-236. doi:10.1111/j.1469-7580.2006.00686.x

6. Chakraverty RC, Pynsent PB, Westwood A, Chakraverty JK. Identification of the correct lumbar level using passive intersegmental motion testing. *Anaesthesia.* 2007;62(11):1121-1125. doi:10.1111/j.1365-2044.2007.05189.x

7. Mulligan EP, Middleton EF, Brunette M. Evaluation and management of greater trochanter pain syndrome. *Phys Ther Sport*. 2015;16(3):205-214. doi:10.1016/j.ptsp.2014.11.002

8. McKinney BI, Nelson C, Carrion W. Apophyseal avulsion fractures of the hip and pelvis. *Orthopedics*. 2009;32(1):42.

9. Prentice WE. *Principles of Athletic Training: A Guide to Evidence-Based Clinical Practice*. 16th ed. McGraw-Hill; 2017.

10. Avrahami D, Choudur HN. Adductor tendinopathy in a hockey player with persistent groin pain: A case report. *J Can Chiropr Assoc*. 2010;54(4):264-270.

11. Hickey JT, Timmins RG, Maniar N, et al. Pain-free versus pain-threshold rehabilitation following acute hamstring strain injury: A randomized controlled trial. *J Orthop Sports Phys Ther*. 2020;50(2):91-103. doi:10.2519/jospt.2020.8895

12. Ali K, Leland JM. Hamstring strains and tears in the athlete. *Clin Sports Med*. 2012;31(2):263-272. doi:10.1016/j.csm.2011.11.001

13. Macdonald B, McAleer S, Kelly S, Chakraverty R, Johnston M, Pollock N. Hamstring rehabilitation in elite track and field athletes: Applying the British Athletics Muscle Injury Classification in clinical practice. *Br J Sports Med*. 2019;53(23):1464-1473. doi:10.1136/bjsports-2017-098971

Chapter 11

1. Neumann DA. *Kinesiology of the Musculoskeletal System: Foundations for Rehabilitation*. 3rd ed. Elsevier; 2017.

2. Smith BE, Selfe J, Thacker D, et al. Incidence and prevalence of patellofemoral pain: A systematic review and meta-analysis. *PLoS One*. 2018;13(1):e0190892. doi:10.1371/journal.pone.0190892

3. Agur AM, Dalley AR. *Moore's Essential Clinical Anatomy*. 6th ed. Lippincott, Williams, & Wilkins; 2019.

4. Barber-Westin SD, Noyes FR. Clinical healing rates of meniscus repairs of tears in the central-third (red-white) zone. *Arthroscopy*. 2014;30(1):134-146. doi:10.1016/j.arthro.2013.10.003

5. Sturgill LP, Snyder-Mackler L, Manal TJ, Axe MJ. Interrater reliability of a clinical scale to assess knee joint effusion. *J Orthop Sports Phys Ther*. 2009;39(12):845-849. doi:10.2519/jospt.2009.3143

6. Magee D. *Orthopedic Physical Assessment*. 6th ed. Elsevier; 2014.

7. Malliaras P, Cook J, Purdam C, Rio E. Patellar tendinopathy: Clinical diagnosis, load management, and advice for challenging case presentations. *J Orthop Sports Phys Ther*. 2015;45(11):887-898. doi:10.2519/jospt.2015.5987

8. Pascarella A, Alam M, Pascarella F, Latte C, Di Salvatore MG, Maffulli N. Arthroscopic management of chronic patellar tendinopathy. *Am J Sports Med*. 2011;39(9):1975-1983. doi:10.1177/0363546511410413

9. Holden S, Rathleff MS. Separating the myths from facts: Time to take another look at Osgood Schlatter "disease." *Br J Sports Med*. 2019;54(14):824-825. doi:10.1136/bjsports-2019-101888

10. Frommer C, Masaracchio M. The use of patellar taping in the treatment of a patient with a medial collateral ligament sprain. *N Am J Sports Phys Ther*. 2009;4(2):60-69.

11. Laprade RF, Wijdicks CA. The management of injuries to the medial side of the knee. *J Orthop Sports Phys Ther*. 2012;42(3):221-233. doi:10.2519/jospt.2012.3624

12. Couture JF, Al-Juhani W, Forsythe ME, Lenczner E, Marien R, Burman M. Joint line fullness and meniscal pathology. *Sports Health*. 2012;4(1):47-50. doi:10.1177/1941738111422330

13. Meister BR, Michael SP, Moyer RA, Kelly JD, Schneck CD. Anatomy and kinematics of the lateral collateral ligament of the knee. *Am J Sports Med*. 2000;28(6):869-878. doi:10.1177/03635465000280061601

14. Strauss EJ, Kim S, Calcei JG, Park D. Iliotibial band syndrome: Evaluation and management. *J Am Acad Orthop Surg.* 2011;19(12):728-736.

Chapter 12

1. Neumann DA. *Kinesiology of the Musculoskeletal System: Foundations for Rehabilitation.* 3rd ed. Elsevier; 2017.

2. Loudon JK, Manske RC, Reiman MP. *Clinical Mechanics and Kinesiology.* Human Kinetics; 2013.

3. Agur AM, Dalley AR. *Moore's Essential Clinical Anatomy.* 6th ed. Lippincott, Williams, & Wilkins; 2019.

4. Stiell I, Wells G, Laupacis A, et al. Multicentre trial to introduce the Ottawa ankle rules for use of radiography in acute ankle injuries. *BMJ.* 1995;311(7005):594-597. doi:10.1136/bmj.311.7005.594

5. Kelly M, Masqoodi N, Vasconcellos D, et al. Spring ligament tear decreases static stability of the ankle joint. *Clin Biomech (Bristol, Avon).* 2019;61:79-83. doi:10.1016/j.clinbiomech.2018.11.011

6. Zwitser EW, Breederveld RS. Fractures of the fifth metatarsal; diagnosis and treatment. *Injury.* 2010;41(6):555-562. doi:10.1016/j.injury.2009.05.035

7. Hainer BL, Matheson E, Wilkes RT. Diagnosis, treatment, and prevention of gout. *Am Fam Physician.* 2014;90(12):831-836.

8. Doty JF, Harris WT. Hallux valgus deformity and treatment: A three-dimensional approach. *Foot Ankle Clin.* 2018;23(2):271-280. doi:10.1016/j.fcl.2018.01.007

9. Adams WR, 2nd. Morton's neuroma. *Clin Podiatr Med Surg.* 2010;27(4):535-545. doi:10.1016/j.cpm.2010.06.004

10. Crim J. Medial-sided ankle pain: Deltoid ligament and beyond. *Magn Reson Imaging Clin N Am.* 2017;25(1):63-77. doi:10.1016/j.mric.2016.08.003

11. Ling SK, Lui TH. Posterior tibial tendon dysfunction: An overview. *Open Orthop J.* 2017;11:714-723. doi:10.2174/1874325001711010714

12. Vuurberg G, Hoorntje A, Wink LM, et al. Diagnosis, treatment and prevention of ankle sprains: Update of an evidence-based clinical guideline. *Br J Sports Med.* 2018;52(15):956. doi:10.1136/bjsports-2017-098106

13. Hall EA, Docherty CL, Simon J, Kingma JJ, Klossner JC. Strength-training protocols to improve deficits in participants with chronic ankle instability: A randomized controlled trial. *J Athl Train.* 2015;50(1):36-44. doi:10.4085/1062-6050-49.3.71

14. Davda K, Malhotra K, O'Donnell P, Singh D, Cullen N. Peroneal tendon disorders. *EFORT Open Rev.* 2017;2(6):281-292. doi:10.1302/2058-5241.2.160047

15. Tu P. Heel pain: Diagnosis and management. *Am Fam Physician.* 2018;97(2):86-93.

16. Huffer D, Hing W, Newton R, Clair M. Strength training for plantar fasciitis and the intrinsic foot musculature: A systematic review. *Phys Ther Sport.* 2017;24:44-52. doi:10.1016/j.ptsp.2016.08.008

17. Luffy L, Grosel J, Thomas R, So E. Plantar fasciitis: A review of treatments. *JAAPA.* 2018;31(1):20-24. doi:10.1097/01.JAA.0000527695.76041.99

18. Beckenkamp PR, Lin CC, Macaskill P, Michaleff ZA, Maher CG, Moseley AM. Diagnostic accuracy of the Ottawa ankle and midfoot rules: A systematic review with meta-analysis. *Br J Sports Med.* 2017;51(6):504-510. doi:10.1136/bjsports-2016-096858

19. Toney CM, Games KE, Winkelmann ZK, Eberman LE. Using tuning-fork tests in diagnosing fractures. *J Athl Train.* 2016;51(6):498-9. doi:10.4085/1062-6050-51.7.06

20. Kaminski TW, Needle AR, Delahunt E. Prevention of lateral ankle sprains. *J Athl Train.* 2019;54(6):650-661. doi:10.4085/1062-6050-487-17

Index

Note: The italicized *f* and *t* following page numbers refer to figures and tables, respectively.

About the Authors

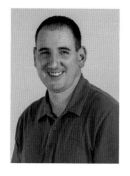

Michael Masaracchio, PT, DPT, PhD, OCS, FAAO-MPT, is an associate professor and the chairperson of the department of physical therapy at Long Island University in Brooklyn. He is also the current director of the anatomy lab at Long Island University, where he was awarded the David Newton Award for Excellence in Teaching in 2018. He is board certified in orthopedic physical therapy by the American Physical Therapy Specialization Council and served on the Specialization Academy of Content Experts for the sports physical therapy examination from 2013 to 2016. A long-time practicing physical therapist, he is currently the clinical director at Masefield and Cavallaro Physical Therapy, where he specializes in the examination and management of orthopedic and sport-related pathologies.

Dr. Masaracchio completed his manual therapy fellowship from Regis University in 2013 and is a fellow in the American Academy of Orthopedic Manual Physical Therapists. He served as the Brooklyn/Staten Island chapter director for the New York Physical Therapy Association (NYPTA) from 2014 to 2018. He also was the member-at-large and sat on the executive committee for the NYPTA in 2016. Dr. Masaracchio has published 22 articles, a textbook, and a book chapter, and he has presented at local, national, and international conferences.

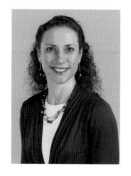

Chana Frommer, PT, DPT, OCS, SCS, RISPT, CCI, is an adjunct associate professor in the department of physical therapy at Long Island University in Brooklyn. A long-time practicing physical therapist, she is currently a senior staff physical therapist at Nola Physical Therapy + Performance where she focuses on treating people with orthopedic and sports pathologies. Dr. Frommer is board certified in orthopedics and sports by the American Physical Therapy Specialization Council. She served on the Specialization Academy of Content Experts for both the orthopedic and sports physical therapy examinations, and she was a reviewer for ABPTS Specialist Re-certification Committee. She is also certified as a clinical instructor (CCI) by the American Physical Therapy Association and serves as an instructor and mentor for physical therapy students during their clinical rotations. Dr. Frommer is a Registered International Sports Physical Therapist and has served as a Medical Captain for the New York City Marathon medical team for a number of years. She has also been the lead author on two articles related to pediatric and adolescent sports injuries, has coauthored a textbook, and has presented at a national conference.

Contributors

Dean Hazama, PT, CFMT, FFMT, FAAOMPT

Clinical Director and Instructor of Functional Manual Therapy Fellowship, IPA
Manhattan Physical Therapy

Gregory Scott Johnson, PT, FFFMT, FAAOMPT

Codirector and Cofounder, Institute of Physical Art
Vice President, Functional Manual Therapy Foundation
Director, Functional Manual Therapy Fellowship Program

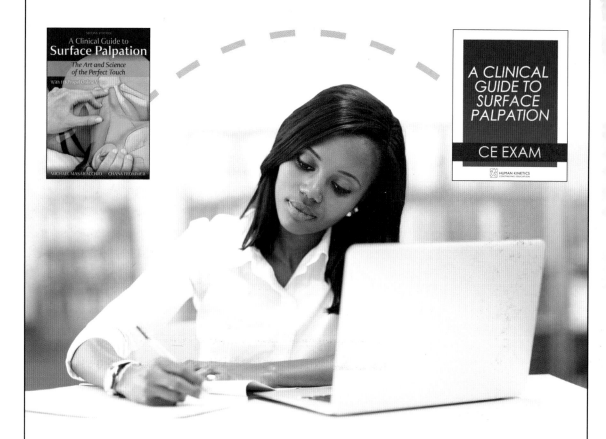
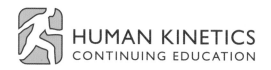